Forging
CAMINOS

Pathways to Becoming a Bilingual
Mental Health Professional

Forging
CAMINOS

Edited by

Maciel Campos ▪ Yessenia Mejia ▪ Andrés J. Consoli

AMERICAN PSYCHOLOGICAL ASSOCIATION

Published by
American Psychological Association
750 First Street, NE
Washington, DC 20002
https://www.apa.org

Order Department
https://www.apa.org/pubs/books
order@apa.org

Typeset in Charter and Interstate by Circle Graphics, Inc., Reisterstown, MD

Printer: Gasch Printing, Odenton, MD
Cover Designer: Anthony Paular Design, Newbury Park, CA

Library of Congress Cataloging-in-Publication Data

Names: Campos, Maciel editor | Mejia, Yessenia editor | Consoli, Andrés,
  1961- editor
Title: Forging caminos : pathways to becoming a bilingual mental health
  professional / [edited] by Maciel Campos, Yessenia Mejia, and Andrés J.
  Consoli.
Description: Washington, DC : American Psychological Association, [2026] |
  Includes bibliographical references and index.
Identifiers: LCCN 2025013744 (print) | LCCN 2025013745 (ebook) |
  ISBN 9781433842665 paperback | ISBN 9781433849718 pdf |
  ISBN 9781433842672 epub
Subjects: LCSH: Mental health services--Vocational guidance | Bilingualism
Classification: LCC RA790.75 .F67 2026 (print) | LCC RA790.75 (ebook)
LC record available at https://lccn.loc.gov/2025013744
LC ebook record available at https://lccn.loc.gov/2025013745

https://doi.org/10.1037/0000481-000

Printed in the United States of America

10 9 8 7 6 5 4 3 2 1

Contents

Contributors

Hector Y. Adames, PsyD, College of Professional Psychology, The Chicago School, Chicago, IL, United States

Kimberly Alba, PsyD, Sana Healing Spaces, Inc., Valhalla, NY, United States

Maira Anaya-López, MA, University of California, Santa Barbara, CA, United States

Maciel Campos, PsyD, Program Director, Child & Adolescent Outpatient Psychiatry Center, Kings County Hospital, Brooklyn, NY, United States

Cristalís Capielo Rosario, PhD, University of Arizona, Tempe, AZ, United States

Jeanett Castellanos, PhD, University of California, Irvine, CA, United States

Nayeli Y. Chavez-Dueñas, PhD, College of Professional Psychology, The Chicago School, Chicago, IL, United States

Jorge Cienfuegos Szalay, PhD, NYU Langone, New York, NY, United States

Andrés J. Consoli, PhD, Department of Counseling, Clinical & School Psychology, University of California, Santa Barbara, CA, United States

Edward A. Delgado-Romero, PhD, University of Georgia, Athens, GA, United States

Melanie M. Domenech Rodríguez, PhD, Utah State University, Logan, UT, United States

Erick Felix, PhD, Educational Outreach and Student Services, Arizona State University, Tempe, AZ, United States

Geysa Flores, PhD, Camino Psychological Services, LLC, Cumming, GA, United States

Veronica Franco, PhD, Department of Counseling, Clinical, and School Psychology, University of California, Santa Barbara, CA, United States

Jacqueline Fuentes, MEd, MSW, PhD, Children's Hospital Los Angeles and University of Southern California, Los Angeles, CA, United States

Alberta M. Gloria, PhD, University of Wisconsin–Madison, Madison, WI, United States

Karen E. Godinez Gonzalez, PhD, Department of Counseling Psychology, California State University, Fullerton, CA, United States

Jessica Gomez, PsyD, Momentous Institute, Dallas, TX, United States

Candice N. Hargons, MA, Arizona State University, Tempe, AZ, United States

Isabel López, MA, University of California, Santa Barbara, CA, United States

Yessenia Mejia, PsyD, Clinical Assistant Professor, Department of Child & Adolescent Psychiatry, Grossman School of Medicine, New York University; and Family Health Centers of NYU Langone, New York, NY United States

Evelyn A. Melendez, MA, University of California, Santa Barbara, CA, United States

Jasmine A. Mena, PhD, Bucknell University, Lewisburg, PA, United States

Charmaine Mora-Ozuna, PhD, Emory University School of Medicine, Atlanta, GA, United States

Vanesa Mora Ringle, PhD, Lehigh University, Bethlehem, PA, United States

Yvette Ramírez-Gutiérrez, MA, University of California, Santa Barbara, CA, United States

Génesis Ramos Rosado, PhD, Emory University, Atlanta, GA, United States

Raquel Sosa, MEd, Lehigh University, Bethlehem, PA, United States

Grevelin Ulerio, MA, PhD, DePaul University, Chicago, IL, United States

Yesenia Uribe, BA, University of Wisconsin–Madison, Madison, WI, United States

Eckart Werther, MSW, PhD, Clayton State University, Morrow, GA, United States

An essential resource that serves as both a guide and a map—offering clear direction, practical wisdom, and profound insight for Latinxs seeking to forge a path as a bilingual mental health professional, researcher, or educator. Drawing deeply from their own lived experiences, the contributors illuminate the journey with compassion and clarity, making the road ahead both accessible and inspiring. *Este libro es clave para la formación bilingüe en salud mental.*
—**Dr. Carlos P. Zalaquett, PhD, MA, Lic., LMHC,** Professor—Catedrático, The Pennsylvania State University, University Park, PA, United States

A timely and comprehensive resource authored by leading experts in the field! This book is essential reading for anyone working with bilingual Latine students, patients, and families. An invaluable guide for trainers, supervisors, and practitioners committed to culturally responsive care.
—**Milton A. Fuentes, PsyD,** Montclair State University, Montclair, NJ, United States

The authors offer a thoughtful developmental approach to becoming a bilingual mental health professional, from one's undergraduate experiences to those of postgraduate status. Individuals' personal language, bilingual competency, and cultural heritage are described as assets for engaging in bilingual mental health interventions. *Dichos* and other cultural resources are shared to enrich one's bilingual (mental health) practice.
—**Dr. Patricia Arredondo, EdD,** President, Arredondo Advisory Group; Faculty, Fielding Graduate University, Santa Barbara, CA, United States; and Founding President of the National Latinx Psychological Association

Finally! This much-needed guidebook is useful for bilingual Latine students pursuing careers in mental health, but also essential for the faculty, families, and institutions that support them. Chapters thoughtfully trace developmental milestones of bilingual students and early career professionals, all the while celebrating the richness of Latine language, culture, and identity. With practical advice and honest reflections, the authors (all experts in Latine psychology) affirm the experiences of those too often left out of dominant narratives.
—**Ana J. Bridges, PhD,** Distinguished Professor and Director of Clinical Training, University of Arkansas, Fayetteville, AR, United States; and Past President of the National Latinx Psychological Association

In *Forging Caminos*, Doctores Campos Mejia y Consoli offer a deeply insightful and timely guide for mental health professionals seeking to expand their practice across linguistic and cultural lines. With clarity, compassion, and hard-earned experience, they illuminate the unique challenges—and profound rewards—of working bilingually in research, training, and the clinical setting. As a friend and fellow advocate for equitable mental health care, I've witnessed their dedication to building authentic, culturally attuned therapeutic relationships. This book is more than a manual—it's a call to action for clinicians to embrace language as both a tool and a bridge to underserved communities. Whether you're just beginning your journey or are a seasoned clinician looking to grow, *Forging Caminos* is an essential companion. It will inspire you, challenge you, and remind you why this work matters.

—Alexandra Canetti, MD, Program Medical Director of the Special Need Clinic, Cochair of the Diversity and Inclusion Alliance, and Associate Professor of Psychiatry, Columbia University Irving Medical Center, New York, NY, United States

As a graduate student, I struggled to find training, education, and supervision experiences to hone my Spanish language skills as a budding bilingual clinician. This is the book I wish I had! It is a comprehensive guide for mental health professionals at all stages of training or anywhere in their career journey. The book is full of reflections, advice, and concrete steps people can take to forge their unique bilingual and/or bicultural professional identity.

—Timothy Stahl, PhD, Licensed Clinical Psychologist

Foreword: *Compromisos* and Visibility

JESSICA GOMEZ

I still remember the first word I ever learned in *español*. I was sitting on the back porch of our home in the South Side of Chicago, Illinois, with my *abuela*, and she was giving me my first "formal" lesson in *español*: REFRIGERADOR. *¡R-E-F-R-I-G-E-R-A-D-O-R!* Not *gato*, not *perro*, not even *tortilla*, but *refrigerador*. Five-year-old me did not understand that my grandmother was planting a seed that would long influence the trajectory of both my personal and professional lives. She was going to challenge me; she was going to instill in me the love for my *cultura, raíces*, and language. These lessons have continued throughout my life and opened a path for me to becoming the bilingual clinical psychologist I am today.

Growing up in Chicago, it was important to my *familia* that I learn about where I came from. In fact, to this day my parents and grandmother still remind me, *"Nunca te olvides de dónde vienes."* They were wise in nurturing my strong roots in my *cultura latina* because they knew my path in the United States would likely open my world in ways they could only imagine. Having a solid footing in my identity would help anchor me as I stepped out of my home.

This emphasis on *cultura* and language stemmed from my needed role as cultural and language broker for my family. At the bank, as a child I could barely reach the counter to hand the teller the English form for my grandfather to cash his paycheck. When I accompanied my grandparents to their medical appointments I had to communicate back and forth in both English and Spanish. Other times, I helped my parents sign up to volunteer at my school to help pay for the tuition. These experiences would allow me a unique perspective as a first-generation Mexican American woman. I had one foot in each world: coming home to the safety of my *cultura* and *idioma* and walking out into the United States.

These early experiences started to plant the seeds for a career dedicated to helping provide equitable access to mental health services. This motivation reached a critical point when I, myself, needed to seek treatment. I was 10 years old when I built up the courage to tell *mi amá* that I woke up most mornings feeling really, really sad and that at times it felt like the walls were going to close in on me. I did my best to describe what I now know was the beginning of a battle with depression and anxiety. It would take my family years to find the care I needed from a culturally and linguistically competent mental health provider.

During one of these sessions, I made a commitment, a commitment that I would do whatever it took to lower the barriers to mental health care for diverse people, including Spanish-speaking *familias* and *familias latinas*. My focus was fueled by my desire to ensure that no other child would have to sit across from a therapist and translate for their parents during therapy, explain cultural norms, or feel shame because of their culture. This commitment led me to become a bilingual psychologist, moving to *Tejas*, where there is a critical need for bilingual providers, training the next generation of psychologists and mental health providers, and now being the first person of color and Latina to lead an over 100-year-old nonprofit that specializes in mental health care.

As I began to read *Forging* Caminos*: Pathways to Becoming a Bilingual Mental Health Professional,* I had to stop and process. It was a powerful and emotional experience to read each chapter, as I saw parts of my journey shared by others. This book is what I needed as an undergraduate, graduate, and postgraduate student. As noted throughout the collection of chapters, for Latine individuals, the academic journey to obtaining a professional degree in psychology is often a lonely one. This book is an *acompañante* that offers collective wisdom and practical guidance on how to navigate various parts of the journey.

I wish I had such an insightful resource to guide me during those early years because I would have benefited from being challenged to find people to uplift me when I had self-defeating thoughts, as suggested in Chapter 2. I would have appreciated the prod to explore intersecting identities, as written about in Chapter 3, especially when I struggled to define my identity as a Latina, but not "just" a Latina. Even today, when I am at my midcareer point, this book has an uncanny ability to provide words for and context to the challenges and stressors that are ever-present for a bilingual, bicultural mental health professional and leader. Chapter 9's reference to the stress of serving clients who are traumatized and monolingual Spanish-speaking, and the high potential for burnout that accompanies this work, reflects my lived experience. Chapter 10's exploration of individualism versus collectivism put into words the tension that exists as I navigate cultures within innumerable cultures.

These insights inspired renewed reflection. I now recognize that practicing as a bilingual psychologist in *Tejas* has exposed me to sitting across from families with trauma that was raw and often included fear about what was happening in their *comunidad* and to their families. *Sus miedos* were palpable in the therapy room. It had me reflecting on the resources and courage my parents needed when they decided to immigrate to Chicago, a city with one of the largest populations of Mexican immigrants. In *Tejas*, I encountered much more diversity with waves of immigrants who have just arrived and had a limited resource safety net.

This new reality meant that I had to quickly learn how to access resources for my client families in a state with restricted supports for this population. It also meant I had to adapt to a diversity of Spanish dialects. I still remember having to fine-tune my ear to the linguistic cadence of my clients from El Salvador, Venezuela, or Puerto Rico, among many others. The risk of vicarious trauma and burnout became a reality during my internship and early licensure years. There was such a significant need for Spanish-speaking mental health providers, and the caseloads never ceased to get larger.

It was through these experiences that I learned to advocate for my needs as a bilingual provider and set healthy boundaries on how much I could take on while still offering quality care. I still remember telling my supervisor that one of my goals was to balance my caseload with English-speaking cases. They looked at me with curiosity as I shared that I needed to practice and become more comfortable offering therapy in English. I also needed to have diversity in my caseload, varying clinical presentations and the needs of the children and families with whom I was working. I wanted to ensure that my clinical skill set was comprehensive.

Chapter 12's encouragements to accept the torch and take the right next steps to strengthen our field are, in essence, a rallying cry. As I grew in experience, I felt ready to meet the clinical training demands of the next generation. I became one of the first bilingual and bicultural psychologists on the doctoral training committee for future psychologists for a community organization, whose primary population was Latinx. No *presión, ¿verdad?* I felt the moral imperative to help train the next generation. What would it have been for me to have experienced a supervisor who spoke my language, was part of my culture, and even looked like me? As we often say, representation matters. Thus began my journey as a bilingual supervisor, and this has encompassed developing standards, best practices, didactics, and the very intentional super-vision of students. It has helped bake into a system the cultural lens that is so important to quality care.

Reading this collection of wisdom in *Forging* Caminos, from the many pioneers in the field of bilingual mental health, was a validation my soul needed. As I read *consejos, dichos,* and encouragement, I was reminded that I simply am not alone. This book is a road map for anyone considering a career as a bilingual mental health provider or anyone working alongside these trailblazers.

As I write this Foreword, I want to thank the many clients with whom I have had the privilege of working. Each of them has offered the best training and lessons, rivaling those of even the most culturally sensitive of books. The *camino* to becoming a well-trained bilingual psychologist will continue to be a lifelong journey, one that started with lessons on how to pronounce and spell *R-E-F-R-I-G-E-R-A-D-O-R.* One that included finding my place in academia and persisting through graduate school as the path became lonelier. One that involved finding allies, resources, books, and experiences that nurtured my growth. This journey required humility to learn from my mistakes and from others. It involved accepting that the *camino* is one for trailblazers and is best traveled with friends and allies.

I dream of the day that bilingual psychologists will make up significantly more than the current 5% of the profession. These numbers are not much better when you look at other fields in mental health. We understand that the population growth in the United States will continue to be significant for Latines from a variety of backgrounds. The responsibility for training the next generation is significant; it is a moral imperative to increase access to competent mental health providers. Travel safe, *comxadres.* May this book be your guide as your *camino* continues to challenge, shape, and nourish you both personally and professionally.

¡Echa pa'lante!

Foreword: *¡Date Puesto!*

MELANIE M. DOMENECH RODRÍGUEZ

Bienvenides a Forjando Caminos. If you are a bilingual, Latinx professional—you too, students!—then, *tú sabes*. You know about the constant translations running in the backgrounds and foregrounds of our lives. You know about the literal translation of language and about the metaphorical translations of values, beliefs, practices that require constant checks of assumptions, motives, and strategies. Metaphorical translation is known as *biculturalism*. Bilingualism and biculturalism are specific skills that we can nurture; they represent significant assets for each of us and for the teams and communities of which we are a part.

As an academic, I have felt the bone-tired exhaustion of the constant exercise *de forjar caminos entre mundos* and the profound benefits it entails. *Forjar caminos entre mundos* is not something you can put down and take a break from, and yet, for me, the benefits have far exceeded the costs. I want to focus on the benefits. As you walk this path, my greatest hope for you is that you know your worth. Go ahead, *¡Date puesto!* Because that expression (which roughly translates to "Assume or project the respect you deserve from others") can be tied to arrogance, let me clarify that I believe *que te puedes dar puesto* and walk in the world with humility, warmth, and grace. *Te puedes dar puesto* and be collegial and collaborative. My mother likes to say, *"Quien mucho se agacha, el trasero enseña"* (albeit using slightly more colorful language). As Jacqueline Fuentes et al. so clearly communicate in Chapter 6, your bilingual and bicultural skills are not there to be exploited by supervisors or mentors but instead form part of your worth as a professional. If you know your worth, you can keep the unveiling of your rear end under your control so you can flaunt it only as you wish.

The cognitive and social benefits of bilingualism and biculturalism are noteworthy. The literature shows benefits, ranging from improved cognitive flexibility (Kim & Runco, 2022; Xia et al., 2022) and metacognitive skills (Abu Rabia, 2019) to delayed onset of dementia and other milder cognitive impairment (Taylor et al., 2022; Venugopal et al., 2024). Bilingual and bicultural folks also show benefits in social domains, specifically greater flexibility and more frequent social contact (Ikizer & Ramírez-Esparza, 2018). These social skills—ease in navigating and adapting to new social contexts and reading social cues—are critically important in psychological services work as well as is navigating teams and collaborations.

In academic environments, collaborations are essential to knowledge production. The bilingual/bicultural professional brings in varied perspectives based on lived experiences that are likely to be unique to the group. In my own experience, I find that I am often the person in a group who is asking for the unstated assumptions to be stated: What is our goal in this space? What is our plan for getting to the goal? How will each of us contribute, and how will we actively collaborate toward the goal? I think this is partly due to my experience with missteps whereby my assumptions have been incorrect because of cultural and linguistic misunderstandings. The more I engage in this exercise, the more I realize how critical it is to developing competence in multicultural settings and to practicing consistent and effective inclusion.

In academic research, the bilingual/bicultural professional can be a particular asset in the formulation of research questions, the methods or research design, and even in understanding lessons learned. In addition to the excellent points made by Vanesa Mora Ringle and Raquel Sosa (Chapter 11) regarding the ability to produce research specific to Latinx mental health and bilingualism, I would also encourage you, *querides lectores*, to consider that the cognitive and social flexibility afforded by your bilingualism, biculturalism, and broad lived experiences position you well to collaborate broadly (on any topic, in either language!) and to be more creative about the questions you pose and the methods you use (see Chapter 7).

Déjame hacerte un cuento. Years ago, I led a randomized controlled trial with Latine families in Logan, Utah, United States. Our team started data collection, following existing norms for randomized controlled trials: We set up individual appointments in a controlled setting—a university laboratory— to ensure that privacy was maintained, per ethical guidelines and research protections policies. Families interested in participating often missed appointments or called to reschedule. Some families "came up the hill" to the university and were lost. I met families in the middle of the street to direct them to the parking area and walk them to our research space. At one point, I mused how I wished that we could run our randomized controlled trial like physicians ran their practices in Puerto Rico. Patients are given a morning or afternoon appointment, and they are *atendides* in the order in which they arrive, at a very familiar location. The funny musing turned into a reality when, in collaboration with my local institutional review board (Domenech Rodríguez et al., 2017), we figured out a path for day-long data collection at a local school. The shift allowed us to assess families in a timely and efficient fashion, with flexibility. Families seemed happy to have the flexibility, and some even reported that they enjoyed being around other families who were also participating in the research. It occurred to me that "privacy" could be scary, especially for undocumented families.

In the United States, being bilingual and bicultural sometimes leads to experiences of marginalization. I would offer to you that, within limits, these experiences can help us build critical academic skills. *Te hago otro cuento.* In another research project in Oregon, United States, we were conducting focus groups with Latine parents when a member of the research team came running in to find me, asking for language support. I was a little surprised. This team member was bilingual, but given that English was their *lengua materna*, I thought perhaps their Spanish-language skills were not as advanced as I had assumed. Imagine my surprise when I also struggled to communicate! This Latina mother was not speaking Spanish; she was speaking an Indigenous language. It was a sobering moment. I reflected on how White supremacy was present in my own program of research (see Chapter 4). I reflected on the pain that mother felt at being excluded from a space that she was told had been created for her. Discrimination from within our own identity groups hurts (Hook et al., 2016; Mata-Greve & Torres, 2019). *Me pude haber resguardado en un análisis intelectual acerca de la opresión internalizada* (Gale et al., 2020), *pero en realidad me tocó asumir la responsabilidad y el bochorno de haber causado daño a una de las personas que más me interesaba atender* (do you ever notice that your deepest emotions just have to be stated in Spanish?).

We were lucky to find someone on our team who could communicate our deepest apologies and assurance that we would correct the errors that led to this mother's wasted time and exclusion. If memory serves, we paid her for her participation. For that specific project, the correction was minor: Spanish language fluency was added to the inclusion criteria. That event represented a major pivot in my personal and scholarly consideration of colonization, imperialism, and racism within Latine groups, within myself. There is emic within the emic (see Chapter 7). I have tried to honor this mother by retaining her experience front and center in my consciousness. This lesson has shaped my teaching and research. My experiences with exclusion allowed for real empathy and productive guilt to propel me to work toward justice within my academic activities.

In teaching, supervision, and mentorship, bilingualism and biculturalism are also invaluable assets. Many authors in this volume speak to the value of mentees having a bilingual mentor or supervisor. Others speak to the value of connecting to identity through working in Latine contexts, national and international. I would add to these excellent points the ability to build bridges of understanding between students and the material taught in class and in practice-oriented educational offerings. A very special example for me was the development of Heart2Heart (https://osf.io/7vjxp/), an intervention to address discrimination-based stress that I codeveloped with Shari Linares. Shari first came to me as a high school student. She had done a survey of her peers and learned that her ethnic and racially minoritized peers were having experiences with discrimination that were affecting their mental health. She wanted to do something about it. We started with a very small project (a single-case design), and together we built an intervention. Eventually, Shari enrolled at Utah State University, and we continued our work together through her entire undergraduate career.

Along the way, Shari learned about applying for awards and then for grants. She learned about how to develop an intervention, and then deliver it, and then evaluate the impact after delivery. She learned that the constructs that she deeply cared about (e.g., discrimination stress) were constructs of scholarly focus in psychology and allied fields. She learned about best practices in protecting participants and eventually obtained a part-time job in the Human Research Protections Program Office at Utah State. Our meetings were in Spanish, English, and Spanglish. There was no questioning of experiences with discrimination, only deep discussions about how to understand them and their impact on mental health and wellness. She wrote an honors thesis that was based on all her work. I would like to believe that, as Shari enters a doctoral program, she learned about research methods, specific areas of important psychological scholarship, ethics, and the many aspects of navigating psychology as a professional. Our shared bilingualism and biculturalism supported every point of our connection and collaboration.

I am also keenly aware of my unique ability to support Spanish speakers writing in English. As a mentor to undergraduate and graduate students and early career professionals, I have noticed time and again that I can "decode" English language sentences that my monolingual colleagues might simply mark as "awkward." For example, in a recent paper review I noted what appeared to be a sentence fragment. The authors were located in a Spanish-speaking country. When that same sentence was translated into Spanish it clearly provided a full idea. Rather than pointing to sentence fragment (because it was not a fragment if you consider the intended meaning), I alerted the authors to the need to say more clearly what they intended to say. I received a note from the authors saying that they figured out I spoke Spanish from the way I provided the feedback. In the context of supervision, a colleague approached me with chronic concerns about the clinical documentation completed by a student I had mentored. My colleague perceived the student as recalcitrant and was frustrated that the student was not following their feedback and recommendations. The student, on the other hand, was spending countless hours trying to be responsive to feedback and frustrated that they continued to receive critical feedback on their notes. Realizing that both people were trying their best to support the other, I asked to see the notes and immediately recognized the long and convoluted sentences that are so valued in Spanish-language writing. I was able to tell my colleague that the student was writing in Spanish style with English words. The student and I then discussed my observation about their style, and I recommended using short and simple sentences. The quality of the notes improved. More important, the relationship between the supervisor and the student improved while each developed a greater awareness of the experience of the other.

Now in my role as a journal editor, I am working to decolonize the publishing process. It turns out that is much easier said than done. Transparency is a huge part of the process. I have noticed how most of the reviewers and advisory board editorial members of this international journal are based in the United States. I also have noticed how it is very easy for me to center the United States as part of a location, and so I have made efforts to make visible the locations (e.g., Logan, Utah, United States, rather than Logan, Utah) whenever needed. I have asked authors to make visible the location of U.S. samples—have you ever noticed in articles how location is not mentioned when manuscripts are based in the United States? I have requested that authors add a notation for currency when reporting payment to participants in the United States. I have also requested that authors use the term "United Statesian" to refer to people from the United States rather than use the term "American." These are all details, but they are notable points on the journey thus far. I would have never known that "United Statesian" was a term if I had not grown up with the term *estadounidense.* I was absolutely delighted when I searched for a translation for *estadounidense* and learned that "United Statesian" is a real and valid word! My bilingualism and biculturalism are deeply implicated in my ability to see what changes need to be made, and I am hopeful that my relationships with diverse authors, reviewers, and advisory editors lead me to see more areas in need of transparency and decentering.

Bueno. Aquí entre cuento y cuento, I hope that I have highlighted the benefits of bilingualism and biculturalism in an academic context. Every day I am grateful for my *puertorriqueñidad,* for my bilingualism, and for the cognitive flexibility and the social benefits that these have afforded me. *Querides lectores,* we are better off *forjando caminos, aun cuando nos cansamos.* We bring important skills to our academic communities. Bilingualism is not just about speaking two languages; language is a portal to multiple worldviews.

This book uncovers some important information that we can put in our backpacks while we are *forjando caminos.* For example, the deep and nuanced exploration of the terms "Hispanic," "Latinx," and so on, provides exceptional degree and detail. As those of us *que forjamos caminos entre mundos* know, good bridges are flexible. The information provided in Chapter 1 helps us understand how terms came to be; this not only helps us inform others but also helps inform our own decisions. As a scholar, when I am writing a paper, I tend to favor the terms "Latinx" and "Latine." However, when I am working with students who prefer the term "Hispanic" or "Spanish," I use that. Knowing where terms come from and what they might mean to myself, and to others, helps me be intentional in my preferences as well as flexible in meeting others where they are and respecting their preferences. This extends, for example, to people's preferences for the use of traditional accents in their names and surnames and preferences in greetings. Although I personally always accent Rodríguez and insist on using my paternal and maternal surnames, I always ask students about their preferences and traditions, and I respect those. Similarly, I tend to default to a kiss on the cheek as a baseline greeting and often negotiate with mentees and colleagues for what their preference and comfort is. *El forjar caminos* requires that we connect with our fellow *caminantes* in a respectful way. Our bilingualism and biculturalism afford us the sensitivity to know what to negotiate as well as when and how. The contents of this book give us a breadth and depth of areas to consider and a joyful opportunity to feel seen and understood on this phenomenal journey toward constantly becoming our best professional selves.

If you are still reading, *gracias.* Notions of *respeto* in our communities have shaped you and I to listen attentively to our elders. As the grooves in my skin, the sparkles in my hair, and the length of my curriculum vitae morph into something consistent with elderhood, I have become keenly aware of what a privilege it is to be able to share stories and be heard, seen, and acknowledged. *Gracias de todo corazón. Espero que nuestros caminos se crucen pronto.*

REFERENCES

Abu Rabia, S. (2019). The effect of degrees of bilingualism on metacognitive linguistic skills. *The International Journal of Bilingualism, 23*(5), 1064–1086. https://doi.org/10.1177/1367006918781060

Domenech Rodríguez, M. M., Corralejo, S. M., Vouvalis, N., & Mirly, A. K. (2017). Institutional review board: Ally not adversary. *Psi Chi Journal of Psychological Research, 22*(2), 76–84. https://doi.org/10.24839/2325-7342.JN22.2.76

Gale, M. M., Pieterse, A. L., Lee, D. L., Huynh, K., Powell, S., & Kirkinis, K. (2020). A meta-analysis of the relationship between internalized racial oppression and health-related outcomes. *The Counseling Psychologist, 48*(4), 498–525. https://doi.org/10.1177/0011000020904454

Hook, J. N., Farrell, J. E., Davis, D. E., DeBlaere, C., Van Tongeren, D. R., & Utsey, S. O. (2016). Cultural humility and racial microaggressions in counseling. *Journal of Counseling Psychology, 63*(3), 269–277. https://doi.org/10.1037/cou0000114

Ikizer, E. G., & Ramírez-Esparza, N. (2018). Bilinguals' social flexibility. *Bilingualism: Language and Cognition, 21*(5), 957–969. https://doi.org/10.1017/S1366728917000414

Kim, D., & Runco, M. A. (2022). Role of cognitive flexibility in bilingualism and creativity. *Journal of Creativity, 32*(3), 100032. https://doi.org/10.1016/j.yjoc.2022.100032

Mata-Greve, F., & Torres, L. (2019). Rejection and Latina/o mental health: Intragroup marginalization and intragroup separation. *American Journal of Orthopsychiatry, 89*(6), 716–726. https://doi.org/10.1037/ort0000368

Taylor, C., Hall, S., Manivannan, S., Mundil, N., & Border, S. (2022). The neuroanatomical consequences and pathological implications of bilingualism. *Journal of Anatomy, 240*(2), 410–427. https://doi.org/10.1111/joa.13542

Venugopal, A., Paplikar, A., Varghese, F. A., Thanissery, N., Ballal, D., Hoskeri, R. M., Shekar, R., Bhaskarapillai, B., Arshad, F., Purushothaman, V. V., Anniappan, A. B., Rao, G. N., & Alladi, S. (2024). Protective effect of bilingualism on aging, MCI, and dementia: A community-based study. *Alzheimer's & Dementia, 20*(4), 2620–2631. https://doi.org/10.1002/alz.13702

Xia, T., An, Y., & Guo, J. (2022). Bilingualism and creativity: Benefits from cognitive inhibition and cognitive flexibility. *Frontiers in Psychology, 13*, 1016777. https://doi.org/10.3389/fpsyg.2022.1016777

Forging
CAMINOS

¡BIENVENIDE!

An Introduction to *Forging* Caminos

MACIEL CAMPOS, YESSENIA MEJIA, AND ANDRÉS J. CONSOLI

For decades now, the varied mental health fields that seek to understand and address the needs of Spanish speakers in the United States have required tenacious, resilient, and dedicated researchers and professionals *como tú*. We all have paved *caminos* in innovative and groundbreaking fashion for future bilingual (i.e., English–Spanish) professionals. Although bilingual mental health training, research, and therapeutic services continue to face formidable challenges, resource sharing and community building empower and promote the development of our academic and professional workforce. This book builds on these *tradiciones*, intentionally increasing access to guidance for competent bilingual mental health training, research, practice, and advocacy. It also provides advice on the recruitment, retention, graduation, and promotion of aspiring bilingual scientists and practitioners, emphasizing the nuances and unique skill sets necessary for success.

https://doi.org/10.1037/0000481-001
Forging Caminos: *Pathways to Becoming a Bilingual Mental Health Professional*,
M. Campos, Y. Mejia, and A. J. Consoli (Editors)
Copyright © 2026 by the American Psychological Association. All rights reserved.

FORGING *CAMINOS*

You can expect this book to offer much-needed parameters for effectively navigating the multiple and complex systems of higher education and the health care field, parameters that are relevant to bilingual mental health scientists, practitioners, and advocates. We take a developmental approach, one that celebrates and underscores the strengths and unique contributions made to communities and society by bilingual individuals and professionals. We embrace the intersectionality between bilingualism and the different stages of professional development and affirm *colores* in all their shades. We intentionally chose to use Spanish and English throughout this book to highlight the importance of operating in both languages and of feeling more comfortable as providers speaking, thinking, and using Spanish in a professional and educational setting.

"*Unides jamás seremos vencides*" frames the purpose of creating a consolidated resource that centers the expertise, knowledge, innovation, and resilience of professionals and researchers; our collective, lived experiences in bilingual training, research, advocacy, and professional development are shaping bilingual mental health in the United States. This book is a proactive response to the call to action in the recruitment, training, and retention of competent bilingual mental health scientists and practitioners who currently accompany, or seek to accompany, Spanish-speaking communities.

If you identify as a bilingual graduate student and early-career professional in the mental health field, *este libro es para ti*. In it, you can expect a guide that addresses each stage of your professional development and does so sequentially. As a how-to guide, this book is infused with *consejos*, *reflexiones*, relatable stories, and action plans to inform and inspire your personal and professional trajectory throughout your professional life span.

The notable group of contributing authors to this book are leaders in the field; they embody the practice of equity and justice, with a focus on creating *caminos* for future generations of bilingual clinicians, supervisors, academics, and researchers. Through their contributions, the book underscores the numerous ways in which mentorship, community, solidarity, empowerment, knowledge, competency, humility, and structural justice can facilitate the affirmation of a proficient bilingual mental health workforce. Chapter authors, your *guías* on this journey, are experts in the unique intersection of bilingualism and different stages of your professional development. They share their *consejos y sabiduría* on important milestones.

Each chapter is designed to review a specific *camino* in readers' development as bilingual mental health scientist practitioners. Although the chapters are anchored in a developmental framework that follows the process sequentially, they also serve as stand-alone chapters that readers can select according to their educational and professional needs. Two psychology experts in bilingual mental health care, academia, training, research, and leadership have ushered your arrival to these *caminos* with the wisdom they shared in the opening Forewords. The central themes of Chapter 1 are the current state of affairs and foundational matters that are relevant to bilingual mental health training, such as definitions, history, and the role of language. Chapter 2 sets the stage for your graduate school application process as a bilingual student, guiding you to maximize your bilingualism experiences for your successful acceptance to graduate programs. The unique adjustment for bilingual, racialized, and/or first-generation students is addressed in Chapter 3, whose authors provide examples of lived experiences and offer tips and encouragement. The initial stages of beginning your graduate program *camino* are complemented with Chapter 4, whose contributors anchor us all in a decolonized perspective that names anti-Blackness and anti-Indigeneity within Latinx culture and, by proxy, bilingual scientist–practitioners. This chapter questions White supremacy and *mestizaje* ideologies that often underlie approaches intended to shape bilingual mental health training and related services, and it centers the experiences of Afro and Indigenous Latinxs toward the goal of liberation.

Chapter 5 takes a closer look at bilingual students' graduate school experience as they engage in theory, research, and practice. You will find an overview of the invaluable roles of supervision and mentorship for bilingual students looking to further advance their bilingual skills in Chapter 6. Chapter 7 is designed to orient you to salient considerations of and nuances in bilingual research. The internship process is the focus of Chapter 8, which is meant to assist in maximizing your skills, experience, goals, and values as a developing bilingual professional.

As you round out your training and begin to make decisions about your postgraduation career, Chapter 9 provides guidance for choosing between *caminos* and how to go about this process in a way that honors your goals of growing as a bilingual early-career professional. Chapter 10 offers insights into a *camino* focused on clinical work, and Chapter 11 provides *una mirada* into the academic *camino*. Our developmental trajectory concludes with a discussion in Chapter 12 of anticipations for the near future, salient themes affecting bilingual populations within mental health, and a renewed invitation to engage in advocacy and leadership as a bilingual professional.

All of your *guías* have curated each of these *caminos* with the goals of supporting you on this increasingly traveled journey that is bilingual mental health training and professional development. *¡Ahora que sabes* what lies ahead; allow us to introduce ourselves!

MEET THE COEDITORS

> Always believe that the impossible is possible.
>
> —Selena Quintanilla

We come from different walks of life, and *nuestros caminos se han encontrado* in this pivotal moment. We are *unidxs* in our desire to continuously enrich the existing foundation that has been paved, to ensure competent teaching, training, research, and care. As coeditors of this book, we have dedicated ourselves to providing a comprehensive guide for those interested in becoming bilingual mental health academics, researchers, and providers and to exploring all facets of this role, including leadership and advocacy. As a team, we embody a variety of intersecting identities, many of which we share with the Latinx communities we seek to accompany and of which we are a part. We aim to center our values and put theory into practice while evoking *conocimiento* for readers for the sake of our communities who are not only in need but are deserving of *apoyo*.

Maciel Campos, PsyD (She, Her, *Ella*)

"*¿Qué? Háblame en español que aquí no se habla inglés*" was how my immigrant Dominican mother and Salvadorian father responded to my younger sister and me, both bilingual and born in Brooklyn, New York, when we spoke English at home. Despite this early exposure, I grew up during a time when Latinx and Spanish representation was fairly limited. As a *primogénita* and a member of the first generation born in the United States, the awkward "*ni de aquí ni de allá*" tightrope walk felt thrilling yet overbearing. Deciding to correct mispronunciations of my name, translating, and navigating uncharted waters were some examples of this balance. Movies like *Stand and Deliver* were my early narratives and reference points as I navigated my working-class background and academic goals through higher education. At every *paso*, I directly experienced the need for and impact of bicultural and bilingual mentorship. *Cada cual pone un grano de arroz*, and mine is to self-locate within my privileges of proximity to Whiteness, a cisgender– heterosexual female identity, and English fluency to advocate for bilingual mental health. I identify as Latina.

Yessenia Esther Mejia Perez, PsyD (She, Her, *Ella*)

It took me a long time to love all my names. Today, I hold onto them with *orgullo* as a reminder not only of *quién soy* but also of who and where I came from. I am a White heterosexual cisgender Latina first-born *hija* to immigrant parents from Colombia. Being born and raised in a multigenerational household in one of the most ethnically diverse neighborhoods in the borough of Queens, New York, was paradise. I learned Spanish in my family home; over summers in Barranquilla, Colombia; and in school as my "second language," making me a heritage speaker. I ethnically identify as Latina or *colombiana*, which encompasses my family origins. Code switching between "Colombian" and "*gringa*" identities helped me straddle two worlds and made me privy to the ways in which both were plagued by the same systemic oppression. As I found myself bridging a White- and English-dominant discipline and Latinx communities, I also confronted numerous challenges that evidenced a lack of intentional training for bilingual and bicultural students. As I finished my training, I vowed that I would help pave the way to a *nuevo amanecer* for our culture, community, and field.

Andrés J. Consoli (He/Him/*Él*)

I am an immigrant from Argentina, where I was raised monolingually in Spanish and earned a *licenciatura* in clinical psychology. Learning English as an adult was and continues to be a sizable challenge. The accent in my written and spoken English leads to the inevitable question, "Where are you from?" It has also been accompanied by many instances of discrimination, and with some people speaking louder and more slowly to me—their own version of "sheltered" English. I have sought to put my binational and bilingual identities to good use through a career characterized by international engagement and by bilingual teaching, mentoring, research, leadership, and service. I identify as a recovering prejudist; although my culture of origin fostered in me commitments of which I am proud, such as the power of the collective (e.g., *juntes somos más*), it also taught me to discriminate on the basis of matters such as phenotype. The road to recovery is a lifelong one.

The authors who have contributed chapters to this book, your *guías* on each of the *caminos* ahead, bring additional lived experiences and identities for a more comprehensive perspective. *Te invitamos* to bring your full authentic self on this journey to increase representation of views that might be missing.

DIME CON QUIÉN ANDAS, Y TE DIRÉ QUIÉN ERES

Settling on one singular term to collectively address a widely diverse population of bilingual Spanish-speakers *es todo un reto*. Although we acknowledge the ways many terms fall short of their intended goal, we have decided to use the terms "Latinx" and "Latine" interchangeably to refer to individuals living in the United States who have roots in Latin America, the latter understood here broadly and encompassing the Caribbean, México, Central America, South America, and their corresponding diasporas. Our decision to use "Latinx" and "Latine" are grounded in values of equity and justice and aims to promote inclusivity across intersecting identities.

From your personal and/or professional experience you may already understand that many terms have been used interchangeably to denote a people's connections to the Spanish language and Latin America. A history of the evolution of these terms as used in the United States is presented in Chapter 1. The term you use for yourself and for the Spanish-speaking communities you accompany is important and requires an intentional, informed approach. The selection of this term is a fluid process that might generate a changing identification with different terms over time on the basis of additional perspectives that inform your worldview. Furthermore, clients, participants, and communities are likely to have their own ways to identify themselves; dialoguing to understand their views of themselves is paramount. Most importantly, our *camino* forward recognizes that multiple identities need to be honored in this process. We acknowledge the limitations of many of these terms that intend to unite yet perpetuate the exclusion and erasure of a range of experiences, identities, and heritage. Similarly, experiences with multilingualism are varied throughout Latinx communities and transcend the Spanish–English binary. Although the scope of this book is limited to Spanish–English bilingualism as the authors' areas of expertise, *esperamos* that the tips and themes reviewed in the chapters are relevant to and helpful across multilingual Latinx communities.

EL CAMINO HACIA ADELANTE

Social responsibility, justice, equity, and intentionality serve as foundations for this book as we identify salient issues that truly competent bilingual scientists–practitioners need to keep in mind when working with Spanish-speaking populations in the United States within the context of oppressive and colonized–colonizing systems (e.g., academia, research, health care).

In this vein, the contributing authors identify concrete avenues for advocacy in recognition of these issues in all settings that are bound to thrive from the participation of Spanish-speaking communities. To achieve radical comprehensiveness, this discourse must include colorism, racism, and anti-Blackness in Latin American cultures; liberation psychology; and centering U.S. Latinx and bilingual Spanish-speaking *comunidades*, including bilingual Spanish-speaking mental health scientists and practitioners. In this capacity, we invite you to consider the relevance and importance of affirming spirituality and decolonizing curricula and practice, exploring borderlands and Latinidad, and centering Afro descendance and Indigeneity. The chapter authors share from a lens of personal experiences and wisdom aimed at validating, affirming, and inspiring the reader while celebrating the power of a bilingual identity. Too often these central and critical themes, which can amount to *vida o muerte*, are relegated to add-on topics, as if though theory and practice exist in a vacuum, free of oppression. Accordingly, we bring attention to liberation and centering Blackness and Indigeneity early in this book, in Chapter 4, to contextualize the *caminos* that lie ahead.

We also include action plans, reflective exercises, and *consejos* to assist with your *caminos*. Be it through elders, *hermanes mayores, alebrijes*, or *ángeles*, these *guías* are important characters in our *historias*, especially in the United States. We hope to accompany you, our reader, on your journey, with the intent of offering *sabiduría, apoyo, y fortaleza. Reconocemos que este camino es difícil* and often is met with a multitude of barriers related to systemic oppression, racism, and prejudice. Therefore, we seek to empower and bestow on you the generational and collective knowledge that has been acquired over time. *Te invitamos a este proceso* of learning and unlearning, reflection and growth. *¡Pa'lante, pa'trás ni pa' tomar impulso!*

Our goals as editors, authors, and contributors have led to many nuanced discussions about you, our reader, and increasing access for bilingual English–Spanish-speaking communities and professionals. In meeting this goal and forging *caminos* we acknowledge the at-times erroneous overidentification between Spanish language and Latinx culture. Over time, Spanish, the colonizer's language, has become the de facto language in a particular region. However, we all know that the two can be mutually exclusive depending on the context. Speaking Spanish does not confirm *latinidad*, and vice versa. And yet it is our experience that for many people it remains fairly difficult to extricate these two from each other. You will notice on this *camino*, as outlined in the chapters ahead, as well as in your day-to-day life, that at times the conversation may veer from bilingualism and Spanish language to *latinidad*. Why is that? Although we do not have the answers, we note an intentional effort to address bilingualism in these *caminos* while also sharing here a transparent challenge in separating language from culture. Our endeavor that lies ahead is one that actively welcomes non-Latinx bilingual English- and Spanish-speaking providers while also maintaining mindfulness of power and privilege and the underrepresentation of Latinx communities and their intersecting identities in higher education. It is our duty as mental health scientists–practitioners to pioneer efforts to increase and improve equitable mental health care and pertinent linguistic access for Latinxs. This includes buttressing training for all bilingual providers; identifying *caminos* through standards of training, care, and advocacy; and building upon existing foundations. So, *adelante—que aquí cabemos todes.*

1

HA LLEGADO EL MOMENTO

The Intentional Becoming of a Bilingual Mental Health Professional in the United States

MACIEL CAMPOS, YESSENIA MEJIA, AND ANDRÉS J. CONSOLI

We open doors so others can walk through them.

—Alexandria Ocasio-Cortez

Becoming a bilingual mental health professional in the United States requires intentionality in training, education, and experience. It is crucial to understand language, bilingualism, and the communities bilingual mental health professionals aim to accompany in the context of mental health fields and services. Accordingly, our *camino* begins with a brief look at bilingualism from a cognitive perspective and how this connects to experiences specific to mental health and psychology.[1] A review of Latinx communities and related terminology adds understanding of the peoples addressed in this *guía*. The intentionality for this beginning *camino* continues with an examination of current training standards and an exploration of ethics and competencies for

---

[1] A note to readers regarding intentional choices we made about language: First, we have italicized certain words and phrases to signal that they are written and formatted in Spanish; second, we elected not to translate into English words and phrases written in Spanish because the intended readership is one journeying the bilingual *caminos*.

https://doi.org/10.1037/0000481-002
Forging Caminos: *Pathways to Becoming a Bilingual Mental Health Professional*, M. Campos, Y. Mejia, and A. J. Consoli (Editors)

bilingual mental health training. Such information will be imperative for shaping your upcoming journey.

Language is central to people's lives and daily experiences, and facilitating thinking, processing, and encoding. It is essential to the organization of people's identity, memories, and emotions (Kokaliari et al., 2013), and its role prompts many questions about experiences related to multilingualism. Early theories of bilingualism proposed different methods of second-language acquisition, be it simultaneously or sequentially, in the same context or separately (Diller, 1970; Guttfreund, 1990). These theories suggested that people who learned a second language in a different environment are able to use both languages and the respective grammar rules independently, whereas others use their dominant language to translate into the secondarily acquired language. Current research indicates that bilingual individuals inhibit interference as they switch between languages (van den Noort et al., 2019). The cognitive benefits of bilingualism have been dubbed the *bilingual advantage*; they include cognitive control, which facilitates code switching, a journey of interchanging identities, cultures, and lived experiences.

Bilingual people may show different aspects of themselves depending on the language they are using. Research has demonstrated that people are better able to access their affective experiences in the language in which the experience occurred. People often feel that it is safer to communicate their traumatic experiences and associated emotions, such as grief, fear, sadness, and terror, in their native language because it can be difficult to express these emotions and access these experiences in their second language (Dewaele & Costa, 2013; Kokaliari et al., 2013). Similarly, a person may use their first language to convey *dichos*, colloquialisms, a feeling state, dreams, or a specific phrase (Kokaliari et al., 2013). At times, an individual might use a second language during health care treatment as a form of defense to compartmentalize trauma, distancing themselves from emotional valence and experiences when sharing. Other times, the second language has been used to discuss taboo subjects deemed unacceptable in the culture of origin, such as gender identity or sexual orientation issues. Bilingual individuals often describe feeling more trust in and attunement with care providers when they can speak in their dominant language or switch between languages.

NUESTRO CORILLO

The Latinx population in the United States continues to grow at unprecedented and substantial rates. Data from the U.S. 2020 Census indicate that there are 62.1 million Latinx individuals living in the United States, representing 18.9% of the U.S. population, making it the largest ethnic group after non-Hispanic Whites (U.S. Department of Health and Human Services Office of Minority Health, 2023). The Latinx population in the United States is projected to reach 119 million people (28%; U.S. Department of Health and Human Services, n.d.) by 2060. It is a heterogeneous group made up of Mexicans (61.6%), Puerto Ricans (9.6%), Central Americans (9.3%), South Americans (6.4%), and Cubans (3.9%), with the largest Latinx populations living in Arizona, California, Colorado, Florida, Illinois, Nevada, New Jersey, New Mexico, New York, and Texas. More important, Latinx communities encompass multiple races, ethnic groups, and languages; among these groups there exist diverse cultural practices and traditional beliefs and values.

Approximately 71.1% of Latinx individuals in the United States report speaking a language other than English, and 28.4% indicate that they are not fluent in English (U.S. Department of Health and Human Services, n.d.), yet it is important to recognize that prior to the colonization of present-day Latin America, an estimated 1,700+ native languages were spoken (Salinas & Lozano, 2021). Most of those native languages were erased because many speakers were forced into colonial rule and White European hegemony. However, several languages and language families (e.g., *garífuna*, *maya*, *náhuatl*, *quechua*) have survived, and continue to be passed down generationally. Although Spanish is a colonial and imposed language for many, Latinx communities in the United States face additional oppression as they encounter another colonial language: English. In this new context, for some, speaking Spanish can serve as a means of rebellion, liberation, identity, and pride. It is also one of the primary vehicles for conveying cultural beliefs and traditions for the Latinx diasporas in the United States (Altarriba & Santiago-Rivera, 1994; Biever et al., 2002). Spanish and native languages hold *sabiduría*, knowledge, and power.

With only 7.95% of psychologists identifying as Latinx (American Psychological Association [APA], 2022), and 5.5% identifying as Spanish speaking (Phillips Davis, 2019), achieving representative justice is paramount; to do so, deliberate efforts to diversify recruitment, retention, training, and promotion are required (Valencia-Garcia & Montoya, 2018). Furthermore, cultural humility and attunement, including consideration of language and its function for expressing and transmitting customs, values, and sociocultural beliefs, need to be addressed. Failure to recognize language differences prevents the understanding of cultural nuances, leading to misinterpretations and thus compromising the quality of psychological services (Altarriba & Santiago-Rivera, 1994; Biever et al., 2002; Santiago-Rivera & Altarriba, 2002). In the absence of proficient bilingual providers, the use of interpreters has been shown to pose many challenges, including omissions, errors, substitutions, condensation, oversimplification, and erasure of parts of communications (Vasquez & Javier, 1991). For example, when conveying *disgusto*, a Spanish speaker may use words considered profane by the interpreter, who might refuse to translate or might modify the language for their own comfort level. Although seemingly innocent, or even considered polite, such interpretation inadvertently changes the intended message and undermines the person's communication. As such, interpretation services can result in distinct barriers to providing adequate treatment to Latinx and Spanish-speaking communities in the United States.

It is important to consider the compounding impact and intersectionality of language and the health disparities that negatively affect the Latinx community. Latinxs have the lowest rates of health insurance coverage in comparison to all other ethnic groups in the United States (Macias Gil et al., 2020). The lack of preventative health care is multidetermined; it includes lack of employment-related benefits as well as fear and mistrust of medical institutions and public health services. Immigration status often poses barriers and restrictions to securing public health benefits and medical care. Lack of quality health care in one's preferred language also contributes to decreased access to care and worse health outcomes.

Long-standing structural health inequities that have historically adversely affected the well-being of Latinx communities remain salient issues and concerns, yet immigration, health care, and occupational safety and compensation policies that directly influence these disparities, for example, remain unchanged. These disparities directly affect access to mental health services. In 2021, over 18% of Latinx adults in the United States reported experiencing a mental health disorder, yet only 36% of Latinx adults in need received mental health treatment, compared with almost 52% of non-Hispanic White counterparts and with a rate of 46% as the national average (Substance Abuse and Mental Health Services Administration, 2023). Although Latinx individuals face a unique set of psychosocial stressors that result in vulnerability to mental health challenges, they continue to underutilize mental health care because of numerous unique barriers, including limited access, English-only services, lack of insurance coverage, and stigma related to mental health disorders. These barriers are compounded by the U.S. poverty rate among Latinxs, which reached 19.4% in 2016 and further exacerbate psychosocial stress (Macias Gil et al., 2020).

HISPANIC, LATINO/A/@/X/E/*, CHICANO/A/@/X/E/*, AND EVERYTHING IN BETWEEN

In the 1970s, Spanish speakers in the United States primarily identified with their countries of origin and did not believe they shared many similarities with their Spanish-speaking counterparts (Gershon, 2020). "Cuban,"

"Mexican," "Chicano/a," "Puerto Rican," and "Boricua" were terms most Spanish speakers and people from the Latin American diaspora used to refer to themselves (Blakemore, 2022). Each identity connoted a different lived experience that characterized distinctions among these groups. Such identification stressed differences over similarities and reflected diversity across many positionalities, including race, socioeconomic status, educational attainment, and sociopolitical histories, that shapes varied experiences with oppression and privilege (Gershon, 2020). However, the U.S. Census homogenized these groups as being of "Spanish" origin or as White, generating a sense of identity erasure (Noe-Bustamante et al., 2020; Villanueva Alarcón et al., 2022). After significant advocacy efforts in the 1970s by Mexican American organizations lobbying for more sociopolitical support through data collection, the U.S. government began to use the term "Hispanic." In 1980, ahead of the upcoming census, major media outlets (i.e., PBS, Telemundo, Univisión) were enlisted to disseminate knowledge and possibly propaganda using the term "Hispanic," promising that the Hispanic identity would facilitate access to resources for these communities (Villanueva Alarcón et al., 2022). This, in turn, facilitated a mass audience that could be used for marketing and advertising purposes. The success of this campaign was reflected by 2019 national survey findings that 63% of individuals preferred the term "Hispanic" (Noe-Bustamante et al., 2020).

However, simultaneous resistance to the term's connections to Spain, the colonizing entity, prompted the use of the term "Latino," which by 2000 was added to the U.S. Census (Noe-Bustamante et al., 2020). "Latino" was purported to be a more historically inclusive alternative that reflects an identity separate from—and, at times, absent of—racial, ethnic, and linguistic ties to Spain. However, both terms fail to comprehensively and accurately capture the intersection of different racial, ethnic, geographical, and linguistic demographics and identities. Systems of imperialism, colonialism, slavery, genocide, and oppression used to subjugate many in these *comunidades* permeate both terms (Noe-Bustamante et al., 2020; Villanueva Alarcón et al., 2022). Moreover, the same 2019 national survey found that in more than 15 years of surveying this community, country-of-origin labels have been preferred over pan-ethnic terms (Noe-Bustamante et al., 2020).

In the early 2000s "Latinx" was introduced as a gender-expansive and inclusive term (Borrell & Echeverria, 2022). Its popularization followed the shooting at Pulse dance club, which catered to lesbian, gay, bisexual, transgender, and queer/questioning individuals, in Orlando, Florida, during a Latin

Night in 2016. Social media, politicians, and organizations propelled Latinx to denote gender inclusivity, a trend that continued afterward (Borrell & Echeverria, 2022; Villanueva Alarcón et al., 2022). In 2018, "Latinx" was added to the *Merriam-Webster* dictionary (https://www.merriam-webster.com/wordplay/word-history-latinx), although it has not been included in *el Diccionario de la Real Academia Española*, reflecting the rebuff of the term in many Spanish-speaking circles claiming to center tradition and preserve proper grammar. Although "Latinx" was described by the Pew Research Center as a "gender neutral" (Noe-Bustamante et al., 2020, p. 5) alternative to Latino/a/e communities, many individuals have not heard of, use, or agree with the term.

"Latinx," as a term, gained traction in academia and higher education settings in 2016, and its use has propagated over time to social media platforms and activism (Salinas & Lozano, 2021), although the national survey previously mentioned observed that most people prefer not to use the term "Latinx" and find the term to be "annoying" (Noe-Bustamante et al., 2020). The survey also found that approximately 42% of individuals between ages 18 and 29 have heard the term "Latinx," yet only 7% have used it. In contrast, only 7% of those age 65 and older were familiar with the term, and 2% or fewer of those age 30 and older used it.

Vidal-Ortiz and Martínez (2018) considered the criticisms of the use of "x" in "Latinx" as representing efforts to maintain power and privilege through the denial and refusal of self-identification by oppressed groups. They pointed out how language has the power to produce and carry out the ways in which resources and privileges are unevenly distributed. The letter "x" has historically often represented resistance and uniqueness (e.g., Malcolm X, Generation X [McCrary-Ruiz-Esparza, 2022], Mexico [Bautista, 2021]). McCrary-Ruiz-Esparza (2022) observations that "the presence of x always prompts questions of identity" (para. 5) and assertion that "the same symbol capable of erasure, prohibition, and restriction is equally capable of identification, rebellion, and expansion" (para. 6) are relevant when contending with "Latinx" as a term today. Nonetheless, concerns with "Latinx" have included a lack of definition; an unclear intent motivating its use; perceptions of imposing U.S. customs, such as English; and the categorization of people. Instead, many have opted to use "Latine" as a form of resistance to both the perceived U.S. imposition of imperialism and gendered language and as reflective of Spanish phonological fluidity. "Latine," many argue, poses less grammatical and linguistic awkwardness in both English and Spanish, making it slightly more user friendly while remaining inclusive, albeit with its own challenges (e.g., *chiques, academiques*).

LATINIDAD: A SOCIAL CONSTRUCT

Much like its corresponding and continuously changing terms, *latinidad* has become the subject of examination and reconsideration in the past 10 years. The concept is not new to those traditionally excluded by *latinidad*, and its pitfalls as a monolithic term to identify a diverse community have gained a lot of attention. *Latinidad*, as a construct used contemporarily in the United States, encompasses many migrants from across Latin America seeking to have a shared cultural identity abroad. However, when the question of "*Latinidad* for whom?" is raised, factors such as religion, race, language, and even geographical location are often omitted from the discourse. Many argue that such omissions uphold marginalization and oppression by mere implication that these identities, and their sociopolitical histories, do not merit their own recognition. Such omissions imply White-ness as the default, reflecting underpinnings of White ideology and anti-Black policies that historically have benefited White, cisgender, able-bodied men (Adames et al., 2021). A construct that generates the unification of the Latinx community as a collective for some, *latinidad*, as viewed through a postcolonial lens, is posited by others as failing to recognize its colonial and White supremacist ideological foundations, as evidenced by socially sanctioned practices and beliefs such as *blanqueamiento* [whitening] and *mejorar la raza* [to better the race], which are rooted in colorism and racism (Adames et al., 2021; Flores, 2021; Garcia-Louis & Mateos-Campos, 2022; Hernández, 2003).

In the United States, *latinidad* is branded as a pan-ethnicity centered on the assumed shared features of Latin American identity, such as language and cultural practices, and is believed to transcend race, class, social mobility, gender, and nationality. However, this is not the reality of many, including Black/Afro-descendant and Indigenous individuals. *Latinidad* does not contend with histories of institutionalized racism and oppression in Latin America and the United States. Moreover, efforts towards a unified U.S.-based Latinx diaspora must also balance the inclusion of diverse Latinx identities, which are multifaceted and layered, and extend past Spanish language and White or mestizo/a/e race.

Despite the exclusionary features inherent in the construct of *latinidad*, in 2023 the U.S. government proposed including "Hispanic or Latino" as a race identifier (Office of Management and Budget, 2024), thus conflating race and ethnicity. The 2020 U.S. Census yielded a 42% increase in Latinxs choosing "Other" for race, which reportedly prompted the proposal (Franco, 2023). However, the proposal fails to acknowledge the aforementioned limitations, thus perpetuating the long-standing issues inherent in using one term for such a diverse group of individuals. Considering that U.S. census data are used for resource allocation, the implications from this conflation could be dire; many assert it will further marginalize Black and Indigenous folx (Hernández, 2023). Latine *comunidades* in the United States deserve comprehensive, intentional, and inclusive considerations that highlight their strengths and connections while also actively denouncing and dismantling the marginalization of many. Providers accompanying these communities must critically consider the impact of such policies and act in accordance with APA's (2019) Guidelines on Race and Ethnicity in Psychology as they pertain to operationalizing these constructs, identifying impacts on policy making, addressing inequities, and maintaining updated knowledge pertaining to these constructs.

CURRENT STANDARDS OF BILINGUAL TRAINING

A study conducted by Lanesskog et al. (2015) that surveyed health professionals found that providing care for the growing Latinx community required four distinct skill sets: (a) language skills, (b) cultural competence, (c) empathy, and (d) the will to act on behalf of the Latinx community. Organizations often erroneously view bilingual health professionals as engaging in translation services and rely on the employee's self-assessment of their language skills. Moreover, many institutions do not recognize the increased time, effort, and burden that bilingual health professionals must bear. Proper recognition through additional monetary compensation and supports are crucial to honor and foster this distinct skill set.

Bilingual scientists and practitioners are often faced with the moral quandary of overexerting their limits to support Latinx communities or attempting to offset the burden to systems by challenging current models and advocating for the need for more bilingual services, faculty members, staff, and support. However, both options often leave bilingual health professionals feeling exhausted, frustrated, and demoralized. The U.S. systems of care continue to face a growing demand for quality bilingual service providers yet fail to engage in the steps necessary to appropriately train, hire, and support bilingual professionals, which is ultimately an encumbrance.

The need for culturally and linguistically competent mental health professionals is an ethical issue. With respect to APA's (2017a) Principle A (Beneficence and Nonmaleficence) in its *Ethical Principles of Psychologists and Code of Conduct* (hereafter *Ethics Code*), to promote doing good (beneficence) over harm (maleficence), the need to improve psychologists' understanding of the impact of conducting research and providing services in a language in which the proper training is not available and in which language ability and fluency may be lacking, remains. The Ethics Code—specifically, Standard 2: Competence—provides guidance for competent and ethical boundaries, in particular as they pertain to social determinants as essential for effective treatment. Additional APA standards related to informed consent (Standard 3.10) require bilingual psychologists in training to disclose the extent of their training and supervision in Spanish and the source of translated documents.

As a field, professional psychology appears to be mostly not in compliance with many of the guidelines set forth by professional organizations, with no one organization regulating the multilingual abilities of mental health researchers and practitioners. The narrative that some care is better than no care (see Standard 2.01 [d], APA, 2017a,) yields the continued minimization of the need for bilingual training and appropriate standards for linguistic competence when conducting research and delivering mental health care in Spanish in the United States. As such, bilingual researchers and providers are often short-changed from receiving the required education and supervision needed to feel confident in their ability to conduct research and provide quality care. The dearth of formal bilingual training maintains systemic inequities. Many organizations and institutions minimize or flat-out dismiss the sophisticated skill set required to render quality bilingual work, thereby refuting efforts amongst bilingual scientists and practitioners for differential compensation and added supports. Many administrators diminish Spanish fluency as a soft skill and fail to recognize the magnitude of effort and courage needed to become skillful in the area of bilingualism. This dynamic breeds discomfort and low proficiency in bilingual professionals and trainees, contributing to possible maltreatment, impairment, injury, inequities, and injustice.

Higher education and training institutions in professional psychology also lack standardization for language competency pertaining to education, supervision, and training, despite APA's (1993, 2003, 2017b) guidelines and Ethics Code (APA, 2017a). There is a pressing need for more programs focused on fostering bilingual professional development in the three main areas involved in a graduate degree in mental health: (a) education, (b) training, and (c) experience (Consoli & Flores, 2020). Coursework must incorporate the support and facilitation of not only English but also Spanish language development with the goal of professionals competently conducting research and providing mental health services in both languages. In addition, curricula should include topics related to the unique experiences of Latinx communities in the United States; their sociopolitical history; and Latin American psychology, such as Liberation Psychology (emancipatory approaches to understanding and addressing oppression; Comas-Díaz & Torres Rivera, 2020) and Indigenous practices of wellness and being (Consoli et al., 2022). Last, training models should provide education, research, and supervised experiences in both languages to solidify professional language and build confidence.

Though few, there are some institutions that have successfully incorporated these elements into their programs, such as Our Lady of the Lake University in San Antonio, Texas. This university has developed a higher education curriculum focused on language proficiency, cultural competence, and service in Spanish (Biever & Santos, 2016). Biever and Santos noted unique challenges in recruiting and retaining staff who are sufficiently qualified and experienced to teach in Spanish. Faculty members often require continued support to improve their own Spanish language proficiency. Financial feasibility for both students and universities were also noted, given smaller enrollment cohorts and expenses for students. It is imperative for institutions to be responsive to these training needs if they are to have a prepared bilingual workforce and meet the demands of the growing Latinx population. Chapter 5 (this volume) provides more information about this and other bilingually focused programs.

Language Guidelines and Mental Health Professionals

In 1993, as part of its *Guidelines for Providers of Psychological Services to Ethnic, Linguistic, and Culturally Diverse Populations*, APA suggested that psychologists should provide services in the language requested by the client or make an appropriate referral to a psychologist with the requisite language skills. Over the years, linguistic matters have been included in APA's (2003, 2017b) subsequent, relevant guidelines, albeit in a limited manner. Many authors have supported and elaborated on the existing recommendations (e.g., Castaño et al., 2007; Valencia-Garcia & Montoya, 2018). The necessity for systemic change and improvement in recruitment, training, and professional development of bilingual–bicultural individuals seeking to conduct research and clinical care with this ever-growing population is critical. Bilingual mental health professionals are entering a field with increasing demands for linguistic and cultural dexterity, both of which require humility for optimal training and development in order to fulfill this requisite.

Bilingualism has been described as lying on a continuum, with one end denoting introductory fluency in a second language and the other end representing advanced fluency in both languages (Dykes, 2018). Mental health providers often fall somewhere in the middle of this continuum, requiring linguistic support and education to strengthen and expand fluency, vocabulary, and confidence in the second language. Many bilingual providers working in the mental health field report that they did not receive adequate training to provide bilingual services (Valencia-Garcia & Montoya, 2018). In addition, "psychologists with conversational proficiency in Spanish have very few resources or guidance in making the transition from social to professional levels of Spanish proficiency" (Biever et al., 2002, p. 330). Often, the mistaken assumption is that conversational fluency skills are sufficient to provide psychological services, which include professional and technical language. Instead, bilingual therapists often have developed their Spanish-language skills in the home or in social settings and are more comfortable using English when providing mental health services because it is the language in which they received professional training.

Spanish-speaking mental health providers traditionally experience overburden from the overwhelming unmet need for culturally and linguistically accessible services. This shortage and excessive burden also apply to supervision, where the availability of competent bilingual supervisors capable to supervise in Spanish is also limited. Academia is not immune to the same critical shortage, whether with respect to teaching or research; most bilingual graduate students who provide services and conduct research in Spanish do not receive professional instruction or research guidance in Spanish. Such experiences of diminished support, high demand, and increased cognitive toll contribute to intensified exhaustion.

The challenges are real, and yet so are the joy and fulfillment *que puedes lograr* in bilingual mental health training. Part of intentionality requires you to have full awareness of the both of these sides so you can move forward with preparation and determination. This comprehensive chapter was meant to facilitate your understanding of the landscape for bilingual mental health training so that you may join these *caminos* with purpose and meaning, manage expectations, and set your standards and goals for your *futuro* in this field. *¡Vamos!*

TAKEAWAYS

- *¡Sí se puede!*
- Language is central to our lives and to mental health. It influences communication, identity, and emotional experiencing.
- We need more bilingual mental health professionals to accompany bilingual populations and their unique needs.

REFLEXIONES

- What is my current level of Spanish language proficiency? (Consider taking proficiency examinations through your institution or online.)
- What is the role of bilingualism in my *camino*, and what bilingual skills would I like to strengthen?
- What are my current short- and long-term goals in my bilingual mental health training?
- Who inspires me to be part of the bilingual mental health community, and why?

¡CONSEJO!

- Join or build a network of bilingual scientists–practitioners!

RESOURCES

- Latino/Hispanic Is Not a Race: https://www.latinoisnotarace.info
- National Latinx Psychological Association's Bilingual Issues in Latinx Mental Health Special Interest Group: https://www.nlpa.ws/special-interest-groups
- Organización Panamericana de la Salud (2021). *La salud de la población afrodescendiente en América Latina* [The health of the Afro-descendant population in Latin America]: https://doi.org/10.37774/9789275323847

REFERENCES

Adames, H. Y., Chavez-Dueñas, N. Y., & Jernigan, M. M. (2021). The fallacy of a raceless Latinidad: Action guidelines for centering Blackness in Latinx psychology. *Journal of Latina/o Psychology, 9*(1), 26–44. https://doi.org/10.1037/lat0000179

Altarriba, J., & Santiago-Rivera, A. (1994). Current perspectives on using linguistic and cultural factors in counseling the Hispanic client. *Professional Psychology: Research and Practice, 25*(4), 388–397. https://doi.org/10.1037/0735-7028.25.4.388

American Psychological Association. (1993). Guidelines for providers of psychological services to ethnic, linguistic, and culturally diverse populations. *American Psychologist, 48*(1), 45–48. https://doi.org/10.1037/0003-066X.48.1.45

American Psychological Association. (2003). Guidelines on multicultural education, training, research, practice, and organizational change for psychologists. *American Psychologist, 58*(5), 377–402. https://doi.org/10.1037/0003-066X.58.5.377

American Psychological Association. (2017a). *Ethical principles of psychologists and code of conduct (including 2010 and 2016 amendments)*. https://www.apa.org/ethics/code

American Psychological Association. (2017b). *Multicultural guidelines: An ecological approach to context, identity, and intersectionality*. https://www.apa.org/about/policy/multicultural-guidelines.pdf

American Psychological Association. (2019). *APA guidelines on race and ethnicity in psychology: Promoting responsiveness and equity*. https://www.apa.org/about/policy/guidelines-race-ethnicity.pdf

American Psychological Association. (2022). Data tool: Demographics of the U.S. psychology workforce [Interactive data tool]. https://www.apa.org/workforce/data-tools/demographics

Bautista, M. (2021, November 15). *Spanish letters: How to pronounce X, or la equis*. Babbel. https://www.babbel.com/en/magazine/spanish-letters-how-to-pronounce-x-or-la-equis

Biever, J. L., Castaño, M. T., de las Fuentes, C., González, C., Servín-López, S., Sprowls, C., & Tripp, C. G. (2002). The role of language in training psychologists to work with Hispanic clients. *Professional Psychology: Research and Practice, 33*(3), 330–336. https://doi.org/10.1037/0735-7028.33.3.330

Biever, J. L., & Santos, J. (2016). Ofreciendo terapia en el idioma de preferencia del cliente: El modelo de preparación profesional calificada en dos idiomas de OLLU [Providing therapy in the client's preferred language: The OLLU model for professional competence in two languages]. In L. L. Charlés & G. Samarasinghe (Eds.), *Family therapy in global humanitarian contexts: Voices and issues from the field* (pp. 51–63). Springer. https://doi.org/10.1007/978-3-319-39271-4_5

Blakemore, E. (2022, February 10). "Hispanic"? "Latino"? Here's where the terms come from. *National Geographic*. https://www.nationalgeographic.com/history/article/hispanic-latino-heres-where-terms-come-from

Borrell, L. N., & Echeverria, S. E. (2022). The use of Latinx in public health research when referencing Hispanic or Latino populations. *Social Science & Medicine, 302*, 114977. https://doi.org/10.1016/j.socscimed.2022.114977

Castaño, M. T., Biever, J. L., González, C. G., & Anderson, K. B. (2007). Challenges of providing mental health services in Spanish. *Professional Psychology: Research and Practice, 38*(6), 667–673. https://doi.org/10.1037/0735-7028.38.6.667

Comas-Díaz, L. E., & Torres Rivera, E. (2020). *Liberation psychology: Theory, method, practice, and social justice*. American Psychological Association. https://doi.org/10.1037/0000198-000

Consoli, A. J., & Flores, I. (2020). The teaching and training of bilingual (English/Spanish) mental health professionals in the United States. In G. Rich, A. Padilla López, L. Ebersöhn, J. Taylor, & S. Morrissey (Eds.), *Teaching psychology around the world* (pp. 441–454). Cambridge Scholars.

Consoli, A. J., López, I., & Whaling, K. M. (2022). Alternate cultural paradigms in Latinx psychology: An empirical, collaborative exploration. *Journal of Humanistic Psychology, 62*(4), 516–539. https://doi.org/10.1177/00221678211051797

Dewaele, J. M., & Costa, B. (2013). Multilingual clients' experience of psychotherapy. *Language and Psychoanalysis, 2*(2), 31–50. https://doi.org/10.7565/landp.2013.005

Diller, K. C. (1970). "Compound" and "coordinate" bilingualism: A conceptual artifact. *Word, 26*(2), 254–261. https://doi.org/10.1080/00437956.1970.11435596

Dykes, R. (2018). Code-switching among bilinguals. *International Education and Exchange Research, 2,* 73–83. https://www.u-fukui.ac.jp/wp/wp-content/uploads/Robert-Dykes-2.pdf

Flores, T. (2021). "Latinidad is cancelled": Confronting an anti-Black construct. *Latin American and Latinx Visual Culture, 3*(3), 58–79. https://doi.org/10.1525/lavc.2021.3.3.58

Franco, M. E. (2023, January 31). *U.S. government considers changing how it asks about Latinos' race.* Axios. https://www.axios.com/2023/01/31/census-latino-hispanic-race-ethnicity

Garcia-Louis, C., & Mateos-Campos, J. (2022). Racial identity exploration and academic belonging: LatinX faculty navigating the counters of Latinidad. *Race Ethnicity and Education,* 1–20. https://doi.org/10.1080/13613324.2022.2154373

Gershon, L. (2020, September 15). *Where did the term "Hispanic" come from?* JSTOR Daily. https://daily.jstor.org/where-did-the-term-hispanic-come-from

Guttfreund, D. G. (1990). Effects of language usage on the emotional experience of Spanish–English and English–Spanish bilinguals. *Journal of Consulting and Clinical Psychology, 58*(5), 604–607. https://doi.org/10.1037/0022-006X.58.5.604

Hernández, T. K. (2003). "Too Black to be Latino/a": Blackness and Blacks as foreigners in Latino studies. *Latino Studies, 1*(1), 152–159. https://doi.org/10.1057/palgrave.lst.8600011

Hernández, T. K. (2023, March 16). *The new census proposal may likely undercount Black people by ignoring Afro-Latinos: We can't let that happen.* The Grio. https://thegrio.com/2023/03/16/the-new-census-proposal-may-likely-undercount-black-people-by-ignoring-afro-latinos-we-cant-let-that-happen

Kokaliari, E., Catanzarite, G., & Berzoff, J. (2013). It is called a mother tongue for a reason: A qualitative study of therapists' perspectives on bilingual psychotherapy—Treatment implications. *Smith College Studies in Social Work, 83*(1), 97–118. https://doi.org/10.1080/00377317.2013.747396

Lanesskog, D., Piedra, L. M., & Maldonado, S. (2015). Beyond bilingual and bicultural: Serving Latinos in a new-growth community. *Journal of Ethnic & Cultural Diversity in Social Work, 24*(4), 300–317. https://doi.org/10.1080/15313204.2015.1027025

Macias Gil, R., Marcelin, J. R., Zuniga-Blanco, B., Marquez, C., Mathew, T., & Piggott, D. A. (2020). COVID-19 pandemic: Disparate health impact on the Hispanic/Latinx population in the United States. *The Journal of Infectious Diseases, 222*(10), 1592–1595. https://doi.org/10.1093/infdis/jiaa474

McCrary-Ruiz-Esparza, E. (2022, May 20). *Naming the unnamed: On the many uses of the letter X.* Literary Hub. https://lithub.com/naming-the-unnamed-on-the-many-uses-of-the-letter-x/

Noe-Bustamante, L., Mora, L., & Lopez, M. H. (2020, August 11). *About one-in-four US Hispanics have heard of Latinx, but just 3% use it.* Pew Research Center. https://www.pewresearch.org/hispanic/wp-content/uploads/sites/5/2020/08/PHGMD_2020.08.11_Latinx_FINAL.pdf

Office of Management and Budget. (2024, March 29). Revisions to OMB's Statistical Policy Directive No. 15: Standards for maintaining, collecting, and presenting federal data on race and ethnicity. *Federal Register, 89*(62). https://www.govinfo.gov/content/pkg/FR-2024-03-29/pdf/2024-06469.pdf

Phillips Davis, R. (2019). How can we impact society's biggest challenges? *Monitor on Psychology, 50*(8), 6. https://www.apa.org/monitor/2019/09/pc

Salinas, C., & Lozano, A. (2021). The history and evolution of the term Latinx. In E. G. Murillo, D. Delgado Bernal, S. Morales, L. Urrieta, E. Ruiz Bybee, J. Sánchez Muñoz, V. B. Saenz, D. Villanueva, M. Machado-Casas, & K. Espinoza (Eds.), *Handbook of Latinos and education* (2nd ed., pp. 249–263). Routledge. https://doi.org/10.4324/9780429292026-24

Santiago-Rivera, A., & Altarriba, J. (2002). The role of language in therapy with the Spanish–English bilingual client. *Professional Psychology: Research and Practice, 33*(1), 30–38. https://doi.org/10.1037/0735-7028.33.1.30

Substance Abuse and Mental Health Services Administration. (2023, January). *Key substance use and mental health indicators in the United States: Results from the 2021 National Survey on Drug Use and Health* (Publication No. PEP22-07-01-005). https://www.samhsa.gov/data/sites/default/files/reports/rpt39443/2021NSDUHFFRRev010323.pdf

U.S. Department of Health and Human Services. (n.d.). *Hispanic/Latino health.* Retrieved July 16, 2024, from https://minorityhealth.hhs.gov/omh/browse.aspx?lvl=3&lvlid=64

U.S. Department of Health and Human Services Office of Minority Health. (2023, January 25). *Profile: Hispanic/Latino health.* Retrieved May 30, 2023, from https://minorityhealth.hhs.gov/node/10/revisions/525/view

Valencia-Garcia, D., & Montoya, H. (2018). Lost in translation: Training issues for bilingual students in health service psychology. *Training and Education in Professional Psychology, 12*(3), 142–148. https://doi.org/10.1037/tep0000199

van den Noort, M., Struys, E., Bosch, P., Jaswetz, L., Perriard, B., Yeo, S., Barisch, P., Vermeire, K., Lee, S.-H., & Lim, S. (2019). Does the bilingual advantage in cognitive control exist and if so, what are its modulating factors? A systematic review. *Behavioral Sciences, 9*(3), 27. https://doi.org/10.3390/bs9030027

Vasquez, C., & Javier, R. A. (1991). The problem with interpreters: Communicating with Spanish-speaking patients. *Psychiatric Services, 42*(2), 163–165. https://doi.org/10.1176/ps.42.2.163

Vidal-Ortiz, S., & Martínez, J. (2018). Latinx thoughts: Latinidad with an X. *Latino Studies, 16*(3), 384–395. https://doi.org/10.1057/s41276-018-0137-8

Villanueva Alarcón, I., Mejia, J. A., Mejia, J., & Revelo, R. (2022). Latiné, Latinx, Latina, Latino, or Hispanic: Problematizing terms often used in engineering education. *Journal of Engineering Education, 111*(4), 735–739. https://doi.org/10.1002/jee.20486

2

SUEÑOS Y LOGROS

Maximizing the College Experience and Applying to Graduate School as Aspiring Bilingual Mental Health Scientists–Practitioners

JEANETT CASTELLANOS, VERONICA FRANCO, KAREN E. GODINEZ GONZALEZ, AND ERICK FELIX

In this chapter, we provide a liberation and social justice framework for maximizing Spanish–English bilingual and culturally responsive college student preparation while completing undergraduate studies and then pursuing graduate education. We heed the urgent call for bilingual, multicultural, and culturally responsive mental health professionals; *les necesitamos* as Latinx bilingual Spanish-speaking students eager to accompany your communities. Students pursuing a graduate degree face restrictive and intentionally oppressive systems that uphold White supremacy, eurocentrism, and colonialism, and they benefit from people and spaces that empower, position, and encourage them to embrace culture, intersectionality, history, *familia*, and *comunidad* on their educational journeys. Engagement in culturally rich pedagogical opportunities, training, and cocurricular and community activities underscore the value of cultural understanding and inclusive practices. Through these experiences, prospective graduate students learn the power of culture and language in academic spaces; ways to center culture and language in training; and the value of language, *cultura, y familia* for a career in mental health.

https://doi.org/10.1037/0000481-003
Forging Caminos: *Pathways to Becoming a Bilingual Mental Health Professional,*
M. Campos, Y. Mejia, and A. J. Consoli (Editors)

Latinxs are a multiracial and multicultural collective who embody diversity with a multitude of stories and experiences (Adames & Chavez-Dueñas, 2017) and, to best serve them, it is crucial to train, mentor, and support professionals in psychology to understand the centrality of power, language, history, and culture in becoming culturally and linguistically responsive mental health providers (Godinez Gonzalez, 2022). As you progress through your educational journey (your initial steps of *el camino*), it is critical to recognize the value of your heritage, upbringing, and cultural wealth. We encourage you to engage the path of learning, unlearning, and expanding your own notions of what it means to be Latinx. This practice entails introspection, reflection on ancestral lineage and cultural wisdom, and the acknowledgment of the multitude of histories and traditions that encompass Latinx culture, with a special focus on social justice and equity.

In the sections that follow, we address the unique experiences of Latinx students in higher education, ways to embrace culture and language on the journey, and useful practices that will help you build your bilingual skills. We offer an array of directives for students considering a graduate degree while centering these directives on culture, mentoring, one's academic family, and language skill building. We, the authors, engage in bilingual services, either through mentorship, research, clinical practice, or assessment in higher education and the field of psychology. We recognize the value, the need, and the responsibility we hold as bilingual professionals in advancing, serving, and advocating within our Spanish-speaking communities.

AQUÍ ESTAMOS: AHORA, NECESITAMOS PATHWAYS TO GRADUATE SCHOOL

In 2020, 10.3% of K–12 public school students identified as English language learners (ELLs), with Texas reporting the highest percentage of ELL students (20.1%), followed by California (19%; National Center for Education Statistics, 2023). Today, Latinx students make up 20% of all postsecondary enrollments. In 2022, 3.2 million Latinx undergraduates attended nonprofit higher education institutions, and there were 600 Hispanic-serving Institutions (Hispanic Association of Colleges & Universities, Office of Policy Analysis and Information, 2024). Equally important is the fact that there were more than 2 million Hispanic/Latinx students enrolled in 451 Hispanic-serving Institutions. In a time when colleges and universities are working toward offering culturally relevant education, students of color are sharing the value of studying minoritized communities, understanding the challenges communities of color face, and learning ways to serve them (Smith et al., in press).

In relation to psychology, students of color seek graduate programs that expand their skills as culturally responsive practitioners (Santa-Ramirez, 2022). They seek to serve their communities and bridge the gap in the field. Unfortunately, the number of Latinx students who are eligible to enter graduate school is still very limited because of their academic preparation, scarce research experience, and limited mentoring (Castellanos et al., 2022). Furthermore, an examination of pathways and completion of doctoral programs reveals an underrepresentation of Latinx doctoral graduates. For example, Latinx students earned a total of 4,013 of the 24,710 doctoral degrees conferred in 2021 (Statista, 2023). Limited Latinx doctoral representation leads to lonelier paths, with less Latinx peer mentoring, role modeling, and networking along the *camino*. Further impacting the problem, Latinx academics represent only 3% of full-time faculty (National Center for Education Statistics, 2023). Prospective Latinx graduate students often select doctoral programs with Latinx faculty who are conducting research in their area. As programs seek to increase the representation of Latinx students, greater efforts are needed to train and create pathways for students of color to be ready for graduate education (Castellanos et al., 2022). In this chapter, we unveil some of the myths related to applying to graduate school, the various factors to consider in the application process, and effective means to find a good match in a program that has a demonstrated record of inclusivity and culturally responsive training practices.

LATINX COLLEGE STUDENT EXPERIENCES: *NO SOY YO—ES EL SISTEMA*

A deeper examination of Latinx students in college reveals the issue of a lack of a sense of belonging (Dueñas & Gloria, 2020), a markedly limited number of mentors of color (Bañuelos & Flores, 2021), and a disconnection between their undergraduate studies and post-bachelor's planning (Martinez, 2018). A review of Latinx college experiences showcases the impact of financial stress, unwelcoming social spaces, the role of stereotype threat, and microaggressions (Dueñas, 2021). Latinx college students likely experience imposter syndrome and limited academic self-efficacy. As you navigate the university system, you may also feel incongruent, or not fully equipped to thrive. Question these self-defeating thoughts: Where do they come from, and why are they surfacing? Many of these thoughts arise from messages minoritized students receive along *el camino*. Instead, embrace your skills, your preparation, and your abilities. Seek family support, build an academic family, and rely on peer support and mentor support to persist (Gloria et al., 2019).

Ask yourself, "Who are the people that can uplift me when I experience self-defeating thoughts?" Academic families, which comprise peers and faculty mentors, are support systems that promote and support students. Academic families create spaces where students feel validated in their experiences and find resources along the way while enhancing their sense of belonging and persistence.

Self-worth and academic self-efficacy are also key factors in your persistence, success, and acceptance in a graduate program. Recognize that you have several cultural assets. For example, many bilingual students may have experience of serving as language brokers within their family. If you were a cultural interpreter or broker, you navigate more than one language; and this skill is an asset. As you work toward a graduate degree, honor your ancestors, family, and personal goals. Build your goals and dreams around your *comunidad* and cultural values. Ask yourself, "What does pursuing a degree in psychology signify for me and my community?" "How does this degree connect with my value of social engagement within the Latinx community?" "What is the value of this degree, and what social change do I want to pursue with it?"

Latinx students have historically been first-generation college students (Martinez, 2018). This reality has led to many Latinx students feeling like they know very little about graduate school planning, ways to prepare a competitive portfolio, and the expectations of a graduate degree. On your *camino*, you may be feeling unsure of what steps to take, whom to solicit for direction, and even what resources are available. Some Latinx students openly share that they did not know there were degree options after a bachelor's degree. This lack of knowledge is based on the system's gaps, the limited exposure to educational opportunities, and the scarce number of mentors. If given the opportunity, together with academic, social, and financial support, Latinx students are more likely to pursue a graduate degree (Martinez, 2018), but limited resources and educational barriers are likely to deter such a path.

SENSE OF BELONGING THROUGH CULTURAL AND LINGUISTIC VALIDATION

Because a sense of belonging and cultural validation are key to persistence, students must engage in practices to persist and to resist unwelcoming spaces (Gloria et al., 2019; Gopalan & Brady, 2020). These practices contribute to academic success and postbaccalaureate placements (e.g., employment, internships, graduate school). For example, at the University of California, Irvine, students created the Latinx Student Psychological Association—an undergraduate organization that focuses on community, psychology, and culture. It supports students through a cultural lens, offering opportunities to assist one another and share culture, language, resources, and space. Students need community to persist (Dueñas, 2021); by being part of a community during your undergraduate years you gain a sense of connection; build a network of mentorship; and engage in cultural learning, sharing, and expansion of knowledge. If these spaces are limited at your institution, find community through professional organizations and their student groups (e.g., the National Latinx Psychological Association, the American Psychological Association [APA]). You can also find community in local organizations that are serving the Latinx community in the areas of mental health. Assess the connections that help you thrive as a Latinx student on your journey. What culturally relevant and inclusive spaces/organizations connect your education to your *gente*?

Cultural congruity and cultural validation are also critical in the shaping of a student's scholarship and professional development. As students engage in spaces that promote a sense of belonging, there is also a need for cultural validation. Students must also be encouraged to explore the history of colonization within Latinx communities and the role the Spanish language plays in ongoing colonization. Understanding the role of language in how communities have been colonized and disenfranchised offers critical insights into how systems of oppression exclude and affect communities. Reflect on your ancestral lineage, dialects, and forms of dialogue that are present within your families and communities. This reflection about your own relation to language opens opportunities for the expansion of language, dialogue, and expression. What systemic barriers have limited the transmission of language across your family/community? What does it mean to you to be bilingual? How do you want to honor and contribute to the legacy of your community?

It is also valuable to build a Spanish-speaking community as you navigate your undergraduate years. You will benefit from having spaces where you communicate with others in Spanish, both on campus and in the community. Spaces of language and cultural validation promote a sense of belonging and foster persistence; cultivate protective factors that help students engage in their native language (if an ELL); validate various identities; and promote the connection among education, community, and professional development. Most universities tend to emphasize the role of teaching students to learn how to write and communicate in English, and to develop communication skills, but little emphasis or encouragement is provided to students to speak in their native tongues and to build their skills in their native languages when possible. Universities traditionally have provided limited opportunities for students to fully express themselves academically, culturally, and linguistically. Students often feel that language expression is limited to English, and they speak in Spanish primarily to their family, or to some peers, but not to their faculty mentors. Engage in cultural spaces that encourage you to further your native language and help you use it as an asset. This will ultimately help you bridge your personal and professional identities.

Another great learning practice includes educational games in which students can build community through *diversión*. An example is facilitating a *lotería* lunch among peers to informally practice the language and facilitate engagement and a sense of belonging. Playing music in Spanish also creates a culture of joy, connection, and language affirmation; it can surface cultural memories and promote full identity expression. To facilitate these practices, join ethnic groups that promote cultural and linguistic diversity and seek internships and field placements that facilitate students' professional, linguistic, and cultural skills development. Nonprofit groups are often excellent venues given their mission to serve marginalized communities in need. These organizations often need assistance, and their staff are likely to welcome young professionals who wish to expand their skill set. Internship and field placement opportunities can be found through the university career center. On occasion, institutions offer workshops, internship days, and civic engagement fairs. Attend these opportunities! These are excellent spaces to pursue vetted organizations that have established partnerships with your university.

In the highly colonized and Eurocentric spaces of higher education, Latinx students often report experiencing cultural incongruity and imposter syndrome (Dueñas, 2021). Students have historically been given the message to assimilate, adjust to the university's culture, and adopt the norms (Durkee et al., 2019). These practices minimize the value minoritized students offer to the university's learning environment. Today, as universities aim to work toward inclusivity, there is a movement to help students live out their culture and their identities. There are new pedagogies of strength that center the role of family (Garcia, 2019) and the cultural wealth their teachings offer. Students are showing more pride in their cultural heritage, and this practice is creating a more holistic college and learning experience. What practices do you engage in to facilitate the transmission of language on your educational trajectory? How do you claim your roots? How do you reclaim the Spanish language? How do you foster Spanish language development in your preparation to serve the field?

As ELLs aim to enhance their language skills during their journey through their undergraduate years, it is powerful for students to have an understanding of and an appreciation for how communities engage in dialogue and expressions of joy, distress, resilience, and challenges. An example of how students gain insight into culture and ways of living is through *dichos*.

According to Aviera (1996), *dichos* can facilitate effective means of building rapport with clients. Their usage can enhance emotional expression through familiar sayings that resonate and have cultural roots. Similarly, the use of *dichos* in higher education can help build *confianza* and give depth to your full range of expressions while also bringing background knowledge and lessons to your everyday experiences. As aspiring bilingual practitioners, students begin to recognize the healing role of language, the value of retaining the heritage language, and its necessary role in the field. Ask yourself, "What *dichos, refranes, o frases* help me better describe my day-to-day experiences in academia?"

The following are three examples of *dichos* that often resonate for students:

1. *Flores en vida* [Bring me flowers while I'm alive]. Given that some students pursue their degrees for their families, this *dicho* reminds students of the essence of the moment and the value of doing and persisting in honor of family.

2. *Los lunes, ni las gallinas ponen* [On Mondays, not even the hens lay eggs]. This teaching reminds students it is okay to take a few days to rest, reset, and balance. Hard work and productivity are emphasized, but balance and self-care are also central processes for retention and persistence.

3. *No dejes para mañana lo que puedas hacer hoy* [Don't leave for tomorrow what you can do today]. College students have many demands today, and there are many responsibilities. It is important to cultivate the power of the moment; the value of planning; and the importance of attending to one's personal, social, academic, and community enjoyment.

Pláticas can serve as instructional conversations that build on cultural and linguistic strengths. The use of Spanish can influence and facilitate discourse and storytelling, word order, and colloquial expressions (Ernst-Slavit & Egbert, 2019). Although these experiences will not ensure proficiency, they do offer an opportunity to practice entry-level language awareness and knowledge. Students benefit from understanding that social language relies primarily on the narrative and requires basic vocabulary, but psychological assessments and therapy are more complex and demand greater grammatical and linguistic knowledge to be most effective.

Practicing and engaging in Spanish discourse are valuable; you will refine aspects of your proficiency, from informal to formal and from basic to complex skills. Through internships, working in the community, and engaging in professional roles you will acquire listening, talking, and writing skills that facilitate your language development. It is important to note that in language and in the context of psychology, multiple layers of the Latinx culture are expressed (e.g., the differences in *dichos*; in what we name certain dishes, such as *torta* vs. *pastel*; and in how we express emotion and resilience). These are all critical lessons and skills to help you gain the proficiency to best serve the community.

WORKING ON AN ACADEMIC PORTFOLIO: *LOS CINCO PILARES*

Castellanos et al. (2022) identified five educational pillars (i.e., academics, research, practical experience, leadership, and community service) to launch students on the path to successfully earning a graduate degree. The building of an academic portfolio is a central process to preparing for a graduate degree. Good preparation for a graduate degree goes beyond taking courses and attending a multitude of workshops; your work must demonstrate intentionality, good planning, and the building of skills through cocurricular activities.

Pilar 1: Academics

As you work toward graduate school admissions, expand your portfolio. For the first pillar, academics, take extra classes that show your interests and passion. Seek certificates to complement courses in your major, and find academic programs that will showcase your interests. For example, some schools offer certificates in gender studies, cultural understanding, cultural humility, and social justice. In addition, you may consider taking language courses that help you strengthen your bilingual skill set. This set of extra classes adds to your academic training and demonstrates your drive to learn and understand a specific area.

Pilar 2: Research

To augment your research skills, the second pillar, find laboratories and scholarship opportunities that will enhance your practice in this area. Because scientist–practitioner graduate programs seek students with research experience, an effective strategy is to obtain support from mentors to conduct research in an area of interest. The shaping of a research topic centered on the community and its needs often inspires students to be more engaged in the project. Cultural relevance and personal connection motivate students in their scholarship development. What is your interest in research? What do you want to understand in relation to your community, their healing, wellness, and coping? As you seek research opportunities, engage your passion, centralize your community, and find researchers who recognize the value of culture and a strengths-based approach in research design.

If you have a limited understanding of research, you will benefit from guidance on theory, approaches, and design. Find a mentor who teaches you from a strengths-based approach and who practices culturally responsive scholarship development. Such scholars account for the role of race, ethnicity, oppression, cultural values, and home cultures in their work. They use research methods that encompass inclusive perspectives and account for inequity and power differences in their conceptualization, design, and analysis (Lahman, 2018). Undergraduates find faculty mentors by taking multiple courses with a faculty member, joining a research team, or completing a research program. As a scholar, you want to be creative and innovative and find ways to contribute to the current literature. Through mentorship and guidance from faculty, graduate students, and peers you can gain insight into the various approaches that exist within research. These opportunities, in turn, will inform the development of your scholarly identity as you learn to engage in research that is guided by your cultural experiences and that offers a unique dimension to the existing research (Castellanos et al., 2022).

Pilar 3 and *Pilar 4*: Practical Experience and Leadership

To gain practical experience, completing an internship in which you accompany the Latinx community is valuable. Moreover, within this third pillar it is essential for students to give back in their educational years—learning first hand the challenges the community faces at multiple levels. Interning at a local nonprofit that serves Spanish-speaking clients often offers opportunities to learn from bilingual Latinx professionals (e.g., mental health clinical providers, community activists, *promotores*) in leadership, the fourth pillar. Working with Spanish-speaking clients and engaging in activities will help you build skills in problem-solving central issues faced by the community. Additional initiatives include pursuing study abroad and pre–health programs that entail hands-on training in Latin American countries to support community members' psychological and medical well-being. These service opportunities provide the day-to-day insights related to Spanish-speaking clients, their challenges, needs, and strengths. They may also facilitate and strengthen bilingual acquisition. It is helpful to seek guidance from peers who have participated in similar initiatives (e.g., career center, study abroad center, civic engagement office) that serve the community of which you are a part or that you are interested in serving.

Pilar 5: Community Service

During an internship, it is crucial to learn the role of intersectionality in the context of service, the fifth pillar, and the impact of socioeconomic status on help-seeking patterns. Working in low-income communities and at nonprofits will provide you with an understanding of how finances, transportation, time of services, location, language, trust, and rapport building influence the work you do. You will also benefit from learning service-related options in the context of giving back to the community in the courts, at a nonprofit, through private practice, in a hospital setting, or even through the university. Consider doing an internship at various locations to get to know your fit. Consult with your university's career center for assistance on applications, and seek support from peer mentors who are paving the way. Most universities offer academic credit for pass/no pass options to gain experience through service hours in the community. Once there, have conversations with professionals about how their various paths require different experiences and present different challenges (e.g., overhead costs, insurance and liability, personal gains, career satisfaction).

To reflect on your understanding, keep a journal in which you write about the new insights you gain related to culture, community, communication, coping, and well-being. Seek social justice–oriented work, and consider what specific movements (e.g., Border Angels, United We Dream, Black Lives Matter) you want to engage in. Can you bridge new insights between your family experiences and community placements? Do you understand communal experiences and their needs?

THE CHECKLIST: SOME UNIQUE INSIGHTS–¿Y PARA QUÉ?

The graduate school application process is one that requires time and planning. First-generation students do not always have the knowledge they need early in the process. When they learn about graduate school and the opportunities that come with graduate degrees, first-generation students often feel they are late to the start and must play catch-up in their third and fourth years in college as they work toward a comprehensive portfolio. In contrast, second-generation college students often start conversations with their parents about their professions and careers in high school (Ives & Castillo-Montoya, 2020). They dialogue about ways to maximize their college experience for the next step *en el camino*. In the following paragraphs, we offer insights into important components of the process and tips relating to these practices.

A few important components of the process include strong letters of recommendation, clear and detailed personal statements (or a statement of purpose), a curriculum vitae (CV; vs. a resume), a graduate school matrix, mentors, and a supportive community. As you review the following directives, you may know some of the recommendations, but the details provided will complement the general knowledge.

The list of tasks that you must complete when applying to graduate school may seem simple, but there is detail to the collection and creation of the materials. For example, when considering who will write your letters, ask faculty and professionals who know your work. If you ask a faculty member, they should know you beyond one class. Faculty teach many students, and you do not want template letters (i.e., generic letters that may not help you in your application process); instead, you want to select a faculty member whom you have seen during office hours, a professor you had for a few courses, and so on. They know your narrative and will likely have talked with you about your graduate plans. There will be a minimum of two to three letters required. If you have one or two faculty letters, the other letters must be from professionals who can assess your skills outside the classroom (e.g., leadership, problem-solving, listening skills).

When requesting a letter, give the person your materials and ample notice. Your materials include your transcript, a copy of the work you have done with them, your personal statement (a one-pager on what you are most proud of during your journey [brag sheet]), what you plan to do with the degree, and a list of the schools and their deadlines. If the letters are due in early December, give the faculty your packet of materials no later than mid-October. Some faculty will require 4–6 weeks for a letter of recommendation.

Consider creating a graduate school grid, a simple matrix that highlights the names of the schools and departments you are considering. This list can include various columns that highlight the faculty (including website links), their research, the specific components of the program you like, any concentrations you wish to pursue, the cost of the program, whether Graduate Record Examination scores are required, and the number of years to complete the degree. The list is meant to keep you on track and to offer a wide view of the programs—why they are a match and any unique components of the programs (e.g., Latinx counseling emphasis, Spanish-speaking population program) that align with your interests.

Last, some students create a CV for their application. CVs highlight research, leadership, practical experience, and other important training the student has pursued. Although this document is not required, some students have one and, when comparisons across the pool of applicants are made, CVs facilitate the process of distinguishing the more skilled students from those with less training and experience. Consider crafting a CV as an overview of all your activities that showcase what you did in the development of your academic portfolio.

YOU HAVE APPLIED: *¿Y AHORA QUÉ?* INTERVIEWS, VISITS, *E IMPRESIONES*

Applying to a graduate program can be psychologically demanding, financially straining, and time consuming. Given the many dimensions of the process, some students opt to not apply. For example, many Latinx students contend with application costs, timing, worries that they are not competitive candidates, mismatches with certain local programs, and limited mentoring (Santa-Ramirez, 2022). The combination of self-doubt, imposter syndrome, and setting time aside for the process are significant challenges to overcome. Find a community that will support the process, a mentor who will do periodic check-ins, and an academic family that will offer resources and a community of student scholars with similar goals. Cost is another factor that determines how many schools to consider. Students typically are guided to apply to 8–12 programs. Each application, however, has a cost ($50–$100), and universities also charge a fee for transcripts. Some schools will offer fee waivers for school applications. Be ready to solicit schools for these fee waivers to reduce the cost of the process. Do not be shy about asking because schools are ready for these requests.

Once applications are submitted, many students worry about the outcome and wonder what alternative options they will have if they are not matched with a program. Postbaccalaureate programs, internships, research experiences are all excellent alternatives if you need to apply a second time. Some students apply three times until they are happy with their match. In the process, their applications get stronger, and they refine their skills and professional goals.

For some master's programs and most doctoral degrees, if you are being considered for the program you will be invited to an interview. The interview is an important part of the process. In this stage of the process, committees are examining the match, the students' commitment to their studies, their skills, and their ability to articulate their goals and readiness. Problem-solving and leadership skills, and level of experience, are a few of the many abilities the committee assesses. They want students to express their interests and to have a strong foundation that will allow them to excel in the program.

Preparing for the interview entails talking with other graduate students about the application process and having mock interviews with professionals, mentors, and peers. You will gain from reviewing previous admissions questions that are commonly used, for example, "Why our program?" and "What do you wish to do with the degree?" When answering these questions, you want to be detailed, provide examples, and demonstrate your readiness. A good practice is to write your answers down prior to the interview to have three to four main points to respond to key questions.

The interview can take place virtually or in person. If virtual, make sure to have a private space to participate in the interview. Reserving a room at the library is helpful. In addition, make sure your internet is working without issues and that your camera and microphone will facilitate a good delivery. Have a notebook at hand to write down the questions the interviewers ask you to stay on track. Let them know you are taking notes. Also, when you respond, be mindful of your time. Be concise but detailed. Some students wonder if it is better to attend an interview in person, but cost may keep some from traveling, and some programs offer only virtual interviews. If the program is local, take the time to visit the campus, learn about the campus climate, read the university newspaper, and gain insight into the role of inclusivity at the institution.

Some programs will cover your travel if you opt to visit the campus. Some students receive multiple campus invites and select a few schools to see in person and others to tour virtually. If a school covers your travel, make the time to visit. Remember, they are assessing the match, and you can use the interview to assess how the program feels to you. Enrolled graduate students are a wonderful resource for you to learn about their experiences and the support they receive from the program and faculty. When you visit, aim to wear business attire, bring copies of your CV, and have a notebook to take notes. For all interviews, take the names of the individuals present and write a follow-up email thanking them for the time and opportunity.

CREATING PATHWAYS WITH MENTORS

Faculty mentors are central in creating pathways for Latinx students to pursue a graduate education (Dueñas, 2021). They are pivotal in helping students with articulating interests, bridging academics and social issues, identifying educational goals, and carving *el camino* that helps students achieve their aspirations. It is important that you identify mentors who are invested in helping students bridge the gap. Seek mentors who value culture, the power of community building, and the essence of a degree that could contribute to social and community change. You want mentors who understand the importance of the liberation of the mind, who will empower you and support your educational journey.

Castellanos et al. (2022) articulated a culturally responsive mentoring model (the multiracial/multiethnic/multicultural mentoring model), whereby effective mentors set goals while offering opportunities and resources for skill building. They teach mentees the inside game through networking and open conversations about oppression and racism. The model stresses cultural understanding, competence, humility, and respect. Your identities must be honored and uplifted.

Mentoring often is viewed as a formal relationship in which only academic matters are discussed. Find mentors who work toward building trust, *confianza*, and reciprocity. To feel a connection with a faculty, strive to build bonds. Find mentors who value community and seek to understand the role of family and your family responsibilities. It is also helpful when the relationship allows for the discussion of cultural pride, language, and social connections to best position you in shaping your educational dream (i.e., goals and plans). Sharing your story, the role of family, and the value of community will connect your hard work and the value of the degree. It will bring meaning to the pursuit of graduate training while helping you build clarity on the path.

Find mentors who stress networking, connections, and family-like systems. Travel with mentors to conferences that address matters relevant to Latinx and communities of color, and ask them to introduce you to other Latinx scholars. These connections will inspire you and help you build community, creating a sense of belonging both at the student level and in the field.

EXPLORING PROGRAMS AND STRONG MATCHES: ¿QUÉ BUSCO?

Because of the growing number of Spanish-speaking clients, there is an urgent need to provide training that expands students' cultural-specific skills to better serve the Latinx community. Moreover, there is a need to offer bilingual training and expertise in graduate programs (Godinez Gonzalez, 2022). Training must range from practicing professional language for practice and research to bilingual supervision and bilingual research mentoring. At present, bilingual students seeking to serve Spanish-speaking clients often report feeling the burden of not having Spanish-speaking supervisors (Godinez Gonzalez, 2022), being overloaded with extra work (Delgado-Romero et al., 2018), and receiving unique requests from their training programs (e.g., translating their sessions conducted in Spanish into English). As you aim to provide bilingual services as a future mental health practitioner, it is important that you inter-act with and meet bilingual professionals. Having interactions with Spanish–English bilingual professionals will help you gain mentorship opportunities as well as identify your ability and interest in developing as a bilingual scientist–practitioner. Again, you can have these exchanges through internships, attend-ing panels offered by your department, and even by requesting an opportunity to interview local professionals on your own. Identify top agencies that offer mental health services and see if you can visit their facilities and interview one or two professionals.

There are still only a handful of programs with a wide range of language training and Latinx-specific cultural training (see Chapter 5, this volume). As you aim to find programs that are accredited by the Council for Accredi-tation of Counseling and Related Educational Programs (CACREP) and APA that can facilitate bilingual and cultural training, keep in mind the impor-tance of cost, the role of social and cultural integration for success, the role of diversity and inclusion in the general coursework, and faculty representa-tion. Seek programs that demonstrate advocacy for the community and that implement a framework that supports Latinx communities in their strengths and challenges.

To narrow down the options, engage in opportunities to assess the pro-grams and the faculty. For example, if they invite you to the campus for an interview, get to know the other students, ask them about their experi-ences, and note how the faculty engage students of color. During the visit, observe how the program engages the local community; examine the practi-cum opportunities outside the university; and note the conversations faculty and students are having related to race, ethnicity, identity, intersectionality, power, privilege, and oppression. What explicit practices does the program engage in to help students expand their language skills and cultural humil-ity? Does the program offer an emphasis, specialization, or opportunities for development to become a bilingual scientist–practitioner? Will you have access to practicum sites with a bilingual supervisor?

In the context of retention and acclimation, recognize the role of cost, the location, the homogeneity of the community, the makeup of the faculty, their research interests, and ways students of color adapt and find community. Does the program cover your tuition, or are there assistantships? How many students will be in your cohort, and what is the racial and cultural makeup of the other cohorts? How does the program help students who have undocu-mented status? Do they provide extra scholarships if a student does not qual-ify for assistantships? Some doctoral programs may cover tuition and offer assistantships (research, teaching, or staff assistantships) to its students. It is important you get an offer letter from the program that documents the promised funding for the length of the program. Some programs and schools offer fellowships, and some mentors help students secure fellowships outside the university (e.g., APA's Minority Fellowship Program, Ford Foundation Fellowship). With respect to master's programs, it is more difficult to secure funding, but sometimes financial aid will cover some of the costs. Some programs in the Midwest seek diversity (e.g., students who are low income; first generation; and people of color) and offer funding to competitive applicants with a wide range of experiences of working with underserved communities. However, students must commit to 2 years of studying out of state. You may wonder, why should I live out of state when there are local programs? These programs can offer financial support and excellent training with top scholars that can prepare you for a doctoral degree.

Another factor that contributes to a program match is the representation of Latinx and Spanish-speaking faculty and practitioners. Having one Latinx or Spanish-speaking faculty member is not enough to create a supportive community for students seeking a culturally inclusive program committed to diversity and social justice. It is important to have Spanish-speaking faculty of color to facilitate bilingual and Spanish supervision. Identify programs with faculty who conduct research on immigrant communities, Spanish-speaking clients, and the role of language in therapy. Ensure that the program will help you in the delivery of bilingual services through research, practice, and assessment. Does the program provide workshops on developing as a bilingual provider? Does it create community among bilingual providers?

Although accredited programs follow a curriculum that is CACREP or APA approved, not all programs have the same curriculum or emphasis. Assess the curriculum in relation to cultural competency and cultural responsiveness in the program (Consoli & Flores, 2020). Programs should no longer be implementing the one-class model to address race and ethnicity; this is an antiquated and oppressive approach. All courses should address race and ethnicity and the role of equity and social justice. For example, tests and measurements courses should not only teach the various psychological assessments used in the field but also discuss the biases in the tests and ways to comprehensively assess clients. In your quest to find a program that will enhance your clinical skills in Spanish, identify programs that offer a Spanish-speaking track and include a coursework sequence in Spanish. Because some departments note that requirements for CACREP or APA accreditation are demanding, they ideally should be offering a long-term plan to work toward a fully immersive bilingual program to ensure competency and to protect bilingual trainees from exploitation. There should be Spanish-speaking practicum placements tailored to accreditation program requirements. To be specific, the placements must meet specific standards and be vetted through the program.

Students' experiences should be assessed to understand their perspective of the placements and the skills gained through these opportunities.

International opportunities will also enhance your training. Explore whether the programs you are considering have partnerships with international universities in Spanish-speaking countries to facilitate student exchanges and training opportunities. Can you receive credit for these opportunities, secure funding for the exchange program, and find ways to have ties with the exchange students? Does the program offer travel opportunities (e.g., conferences, workshops, and trainings) to Spanish-speaking countries where students can gain further understanding of language expression and Latinx cultural values and practices?

As you explore your next post-bachelor's steps, consider the existence of barriers that heighten a sense of doubt and imposter syndrome. We invite you to counter those thoughts with affirmations. Remember, you come from a lineage of ancestors that have helped you pave the way. Trust in yourself and your ancestors, and believe you have it in you to go beyond what you could have imagined.

TAKEAWAYS

- Engage in self-reflection, get curious about who you are, who you want to be, and what you want your legacy to be.
- Seek mentorship and community from faculty and peers who value and welcome you.
- Seek spaces that uplift and help deepen your identity development.
- Identify actionable forms in how you can continue your development and deepen your understanding of becoming a bilingual scientist–practitioner.
- Do a quick research search on bilingual trainees' experiences to get a sense of the initiatives in which they partake and what their experiences entail.
- Seek training opportunities (e.g., seeking a Spanish major/minor, connecting with bilingual professionals).
- Research schools that offer bilingual training opportunities (e.g., Spanish immersion graduate training).
- Engage in research opportunities that serve Spanish-speaking communities (e.g., projects that interview or collect data from the Spanish-speaking communities).
- Pursue volunteer opportunities with Spanish-speaking communities.

REFLEXIONES

- *¿Quién eres?* What are your strengths, passions, interests?

- What is the dream you envision for yourself, your family, *y la comunidad*?

- What has your experience with language been? How does language help you express yourself? What worlds do you access through language?

- How does language inform your relationship with family, community, and systems?

- Who are the people and communities within academia that you feel welcome to share your identities and aspirations with?

- What does it mean to you to share your native and/or acquired language with others who are part of an academic space?

- What comes up for you as you think about speaking your native and/or acquired language in an academic space? What similarities and differences do you notice?

- What role does switching between languages (e.g., Spanglish) play in your ability to express yourself with others?

- Who comprises your academic family that affirms your different identities?

- What specific area do you want to investigate?

- How will your scholarship contribute to the field from a cultural lens?

- What areas do you need to refine in the areas of training?

- How are the experiences shaping/solidifying your professional goals?

RESOURCES

Recommended Reading

Campoverdi, A. (2023). *First Gen: A memoir*. Grand Central.

Castellanos, J., Gloria, A. M., & Kamimura, M. (Eds.). (2006). *The Latina/o pathway to the Ph.D.: Abriendo caminos*. Stylus.

Negrón-Gonzales, G., & Barrera, M. L. (2023). *The Latinx guide to graduate school*. Duke University Press.

Online Resources

- American Psychological Association
  - "Applying to Graduate School": https//www.apa.org/education-career/grad/applying
  - "Some of the U.S. Programs That Offer Latino Behavioral Health Training": https://www.apa.org/gradpsych/2015/04/spanish-speaking-resources
  - "Cultural and Language Programs": https://www.apa.org/monitor/2018/06/spanish-speaking-programs
- American Psychiatric Association, "Mental Health/La Salud Mental": https://www.psychiatry.org/patients-families/la-salud-mental
- Cal State LA, "Resources for Applying to Graduate School": https://www.calstatela.edu/applyingtogradschools/research-prep-programs
- Big Academic Alliance: https://btaa.org
- https://ldi.apa.org/programs/minority-fellowship-program
- https://mfpapp.apa.org
- https://www.psychiatry.org/residents-medical-students/residents/fellowships
- https://www.ruralcommunitytoolbox.org
- https://ed.stanford.edu/sites/default/files/externalfellowships.pdf

REFERENCES

Adames, H. Y., & Chavez-Dueñas, N. Y. (2017). *Cultural foundations and interventions in Latino/a mental health: History, theory and within group differences.* Routledge.

Aviera, A. (1996). "Dichos" therapy group: A therapeutic use of Spanish language proverbs with hospitalized Spanish-speaking psychiatric patients. *Cultural Diversity and Mental Health, 2*(2), 73–87. https://doi.org/10.1037/1099-9809.2.2.73

Bañuelos, M., & Flores, G. M. (2021). "I could see myself": Professors' influence in first-generation Latinx college students' pathways into doctoral programs. *Race Ethnicity and Education, 27*(5), 599–619. https://doi.org/10.1080/13613324.2021.1969906

Castellanos, J., White, J. L., & Franco, V. (2022). *Riding the academic freedom train: A culturally responsive, multigenerational model.* Routledge.

Consoli, A. J., & Flores, I. (2020). The teaching and training of bilingual (English/Spanish) mental health professionals in the US. In G. Rich, A. Padilla López,

L. Ebersöhn, J. Taylor, & S. Morrissey (Eds.), *Teaching psychology around the world* (pp. 441–454). Cambridge Scholars.

Delgado-Romero, E. A., De Los Santos, J., Raman, V. S., Merrifield, J. N., Vazquez, M. S., Monroig, M. M., E. Cárdenas Bautista, & Durán, M. Y. (2018). Caught in the middle: Spanish-speaking bilingual mental health counselors as language brokers. *Journal of Mental Health Counseling, 40*(4), 341–352. https://doi.org/10.17744/mehc.40.4.06

Dueñas, M. (2021). You're not really here because you deserve to be here: How Latinx college students experience imposter syndrome (Publication No. 28650953) [Doctoral dissertation, University of Wisconsin–Madison]. ProQuest Dissertations and Theses Global. https://asset.library.wisc.edu/1711.dl/LTGOIN7G2KKSD8V/R/file-378aa.pdf

Dueñas, M., & Gloria, A. M. (2020). *¡Pertenecemos y tenemos importancia aquí!* Exploring sense of belonging and mattering for first-generation and continuing-generation Latinx undergraduates. *Hispanic Journal of Behavioral Sciences, 42*(1), 95–116. https://doi.org/10.1177/0739986319899734

Durkee, M. I., Gazley, E. R., Hope, E. C., & Keels, M. (2019). Cultural invalidations: Deconstructing the "acting White" phenomenon among Black and Latinx college students. *Cultural Diversity & Ethnic Minority Psychology, 25*(4), 451–460. https://doi.org/10.1037/cdp0000288

Ernst-Slavit, G., & Egbert, J. (2019). Integrating academic language and content in K–12 classrooms. In *Planning meaningful instruction for ELLs*. Pressbooks. https://opentext.wsu.edu/planning-meaningful-instruction-for-ells/front-matter/introduction

Garcia, G. A. (2019). *Becoming Hispanic-serving institutions: Opportunities for colleges and universities*. Johns Hopkins University Press. https://doi.org/10.1353/book.66167

Gloria, A. M., Castellanos, J., Dueñas, M., & Franco, V. (2019). Academic family and educational *compadrazgo*: Implementing cultural values to create educational relationships for informal learning and persistence for Latinx undergraduates. In J. Calvo de Mora & K. J. Kennedy (Eds.), *Schools and informal learning in a knowledge-based world* (pp. 119–135). Routledge.

Godinez Gonzalez, K. E. (2022). *A grounded theory study of the experiences of social justice committed Spanish–English bilingual Latinx clinical supervisees* [Unpublished doctoral dissertation]. New Mexico State University.

Gopalan, M., & Brady, S. T. (2020). College students' sense of belonging: A national perspective. *Educational Researcher, 49*(2), 134–137. https://doi.org/10.3102/0013189X19897622

Hispanic Association of Colleges & Universities, Office of Policy Analysis and Information. (2024, March 1). *2024 fact sheet*. https://files.eric.ed.gov/fulltext/ED662159.pdf

Ives, J., & Castillo-Montoya, M. (2020). First-generation college students as academic learners: A systematic review. *Review of Educational Research, 90*(2), 139–178. https://doi.org/10.3102/0034654319899707

Lahman, M. K. E. (2018). *Ethics in social science research: Becoming culturally responsive.* Sage. https://doi.org/10.4135/9781071878750

Martinez, A. (2018). Pathways to the professoriate: The experiences of first-generation Latino undergraduate students at Hispanic serving institutions applying to doctoral programs. *Education Sciences, 8*(1), 32. https://doi.org/10.3390/educsci8010032

National Center for Education Statistics. (2023). *English learners in public schools.* https://nces.ed.gov/programs/coe/indicator/cgf

Santa-Ramirez, S. (2022). Sink or swim: The mentoring experiences of Latinx PhD students with faculty of color. *Journal of Diversity in Higher Education, 15*(1), 124–134. https://doi.org/10.1037/dhe0000335

Smith, S. L., Ramos Martinez, M. I., Vu Xe, N. T., & Castellanos, J. (in press). Supporting the development of students' scholar activist identities: A teaching team's collaborative autoethnography. In R. Rantz & L. McNulty (Eds.), *Developing culturally responsive curriculum in higher education.* IGI Global Scientific.

Statista. (2023). *Number of doctorate recipients in the United States in 2021, by ethnicity* [Infographic]. https://www.statista.com/statistics/240150/us-doctorate-recipients-by-ethnicity

3

¡SÍ SE PUDO! NOW WHAT?

Starting Graduate School as a Bilingual Student

CRISTALÍS CAPIELO ROSARIO, GÉNESIS RAMOS ROSADO,
AND CANDICE N. HARGONS

¡Felicitaciones en ser aceptade a un programa de maestría y/o doctorado! Acceptance into graduate school is an accomplishment that can be mixed with excitement and trepidation. When you are Latinx and Spanish speaking, questions may also emerge about whether you will fit in or whether you can be your true self in graduate school. You may think, "Will I be able to use my language skills to become a bilingual clinician and/or academician?" In this chapter, we first walk you through some of the barriers, challenges, and opportunities you could encounter as a new Spanish-speaking and Latinx graduate student. These are based on the literature, our experiences as current and former trainees, and what we have witnessed from the experiences of colleagues. We also offer you a different lens that we hope can help you transform these experiences into affirmations, authenticity, and assets as you become an emerging bilingual mental health professional. Throughout the chapter, we also provide you with multiple resources and recommendations that may assist you as you prepare for and begin graduate school.

You are on your *camino* to becoming a mental health professional. When you receive your offer of admission into a graduate program, you likely feel unlimited joy because you made it in. *¡Estamos contentas* right along with you!

https://doi.org/10.1037/0000481-004
Forging Caminos: *Pathways to Becoming a Bilingual Mental Health Professional*,
M. Campos, Y. Mejia, and A. J. Consoli (Editors)

Because you are also a Spanish-speaking and Latinx student, one of your main objectives and motivations may be to become a bilingual mental health clinician and/or academician and contribute to your community. Only about 5.5% of licensed psychologists in the United States can provide services in Spanish (American Psychological Association, 2022). Obtaining a graduate degree is also exciting because you are creating economic opportunities and possibilities for yourself, your family, and your community. To many employers, your bilingualism may translate to a higher salary after graduation.

Beyond community and personal economic advancement, going to graduate school and becoming a bilingual clinician and/or academician also offers you many opportunities for individual, social, and intellectual exploration, transformation, and development. Some of the most exciting aspects of graduate education are learning and discussing new theories and developing and advancing your clinical skills. In some programs you may even have the opportunity to learn and practice supervisory skills. If your program has a research focus, you will have the opportunity to learn new research skills as you create new psychological knowledge. Another beautiful aspect of this journey will be the connections you develop with your fellow students and your faculty. You will meet like-minded individuals who share similar goals and motivations to help others. This is likely to lead to lasting friendships and circles of support. Through this journey of exploration, transformation, and development you may also have an opportunity to form a lifelong mentoring relationship with a faculty member who will continue to offer you professional guidance and support even after you have graduated.

Achieving this dream and obtaining these important benefits do not come without challenges, though. In the next section, we discuss some of the common experiences or difficulties you may encounter as you prepare and begin your graduate program. With the goal of authentic guidance, *te ofrecemos* an honest and critical reflection on what you may have to navigate in academic spaces as a Spanish-speaking and Latinx student. Although these spaces may occasionally evaluate our identities, expressions, and skills from a deficit lens, we draw on these same resources to offer you *ánimo*, *consejos*, and *recursos*.

NO HAY ROSAS SIN ESPINAS: THINGS YOU MAY EXPERIENCE AS YOU BEGIN YOUR GRADUATE PROGRAM

In this section, we explore the unique challenges and successes you may experience as a Spanish-speaking doctoral student. We focus on the emotional, cultural, and institutional obstacles you might encounter—such as distance from home, underrepresentation, and financial strain—as well as your contributions to diverse scholarly communities. We conclude by discussing how your cultural pride, resilience, sense of purpose, and commitment to advocacy can help you navigate barriers and thrive in academia.

Estar Lejos del Hogar Es Difícil

Whereas *casa* is a physical location, *el hogar* is the space where we feel we belong, are connected, and understood. The first step toward reaching the goal of a graduate degree might be to move away from your family, friends, and community. When you choose to pursue this goal far from home, you may carry the burdens of separation anxiety, fear, and isolation. You may also feel guilty and selfish for leaving your family because this may represent an additional financial stressor for them. Even when you and your family believe that pursuing this degree will help you achieve a better future, you may still struggle with feeling guilty and disconnected. Once you arrive, you will begin to adjust to a new city, region, or state, and it may take some time to learn what spaces and places are safe for you. This is especially important for those of you with historically marginalized identities within higher education, such as AfroLatinx and/or lesbian, gay, bisexual, trans, and queer/questioning Latinx students.

Depending on where you move, it may also take you some time to identify where you are safe to genuinely show up in all your identities, such as speaking Spanish, without experiencing hostility. You might want to cook food from home to help alleviate your homesickness, but you might also have trouble finding a place that sells your favorite *arroz* or *sazón*. We recommend that as you prepare to start your program and meet fellow students, you also start building connections and community outside of your program. For example, your institution, or students at your school, may have organized social or support groups for Latinx students or students of color. We have also found it helpful to find social groups through social media platforms created by and for us (e.g., *Peruanos en* Phoenix, Arizona). Such groups are an excellent source of information about cultural events in the area, meet-ups, where to find your favorite foods, or where to celebrate Latin American national holidays.

Once you start your program, you may also find that the efforts by your institution and program to support your retention and success are not as robust as their efforts to recruit other Latinx students and students who identify as people of color. This gap is palpable in the marked underrepresentation of Latinxs among psychology faculty. For example, Bichsel et al. (2019) found that only 17% of all psychology faculty represented a racial or an ethnic minority. Of that percentage, only 5% were Latinos, and 4% were Latinas.

Bichsel et al.'s report did not provide information about the race or the language(s) spoken by Latinx psychology faculty. Therefore, it is likely that you may be enrolled in a graduate program with no Latinx faculty members or a Latinx faculty member who cannot communicate with you in Spanish. It is also likely you will be the only Latinx or Spanish-speaking student in your cohort or program. As of 2017, Latinxs only made up 11.7% of all psychology graduate students in the United States (Bailey, 2020).

The markedly limited representation among the student and faculty bodies may understandably intensify your feelings of isolation, anxiety, and fear. In addition, the literature shows that we do better academically and are more likely to complete our graduate degrees when we feel represented and connected to our programs (e.g., Holloway-Friesen, 2021; Rincón, 2020). Thus, not being able to interact with others like yourself, or talk with others in Spanish, may affect your feelings of connectedness and belongingness to your program. If your goal is to become a bilingual mental health practitioner, the lack of bilingual faculty may also represent a barrier to this goal because the program may not be able to provide in-house opportunities for supervised clinical hours in Spanish. If your program includes a research component, you may be concerned about your mentor's or advisor's ability to guide you and support you through research that is relevant to your experience or to Spanish-speaking communities. Their lack of understanding may even lead them to discourage you from pursuing research topics that focus only on Spanish-speaking communities or recruit only Spanish-speaking participants for fear that you will lack the resources (e.g., measures available in Spanish) to complete the project.

The barriers that may make it difficult to reach your clinical and research goals as a bilingual mental health student require you to draw upon the *coraje, acción*, and *ganas* that you have acquired and learned through your previous experiences and from family, friends, and the community. For example, in our experience it has been this lack of representation that has, in part, fueled us to *echar pa'lante* and motivated us not only to complete our programs but also to open doors to other students like us. If available in your program or institution, we encourage you to serve on student committees that provide feedback or ideas about admission and retention procedures that seek to attract and keep Latinx and other students of color in your program. Your program may also have a doctoral student organization that advocates for student issues; this could also be a source of support and advocacy on behalf of Latinx and Spanish-speaking students. Remember, *quién no llora, no mama*. It may also be important to ask your faculty in your program to help you identify sites outside the program that may offer opportunities to train in providing services in Spanish; your program may already have a list of practicum and field placement sites that can provide training in Spanish.

Ahora bien, el trabajo compartido es más llevadero. We acknowledge that encouraging you to take actions that other students do not have to take because of their privilege is a form of cultural taxation and burden (Padilla, 1994). Therefore, we believe that it is important to have allies if you engage in actions to advocate for what you need. Your program or institution may have a designated faculty ally or a Diversity, Equity, and Inclusion committee that is charged with raising awareness, sharing concerns, and advising school leadership and faculty on diversity issues. This person or committee, along with their contact information, may be identified in your student handbook or on your program's or school's website. If this person or committee is available in your school or program, we encourage you to contact them to share your concerns. If you are apprehensive about contacting them directly, ask an ally if they would be willing to reach out on your behalf.

Many organizations outside your institution also offer support and training to emerging bilingual mental health providers like yourself. In the United States, the National Latinx Psychological Association (NLPA; https://www. nlpa.ws) has opportunities for students and professionals who would like to be bilingual mental health providers. NLPA's Bilingual Issues in Latinx Mental Health group is a special interest group that provides free training and discussions for NLPA members interested in this topic (https://tinyurl. com/52zm9k86). We also encourage you to connect with international psychological associations, such as the *Asociación Latinoamericana para la Formación y Enseñanza de la Psicología* (https://www.alfepsi.org) or the *Asociación de Psicología de Puerto Rico* (https://www.asppr.net). These organizations typically offer low-cost registration fees for students and scholarships to attend their major events. They may also offer their members free or low-cost psychology workshops, symposiums, and books in Spanish. Becoming a member of these organizations is also a great way to build community and receive support.

Loneliness and lack of representation may also influence how you approach the research requirements of your program. Faculty and programs not familiar with your methods, experiences, and communities may view your research topics and methodologies as biased, unscientific, or unviable. Consulting with other researchers within and outside of your program can help determine the appropriateness of your research work. This may also require you to engage in ongoing discussions with your research mentor or advisor about the appropriateness and manageability of your project and the skills you possess to carry it through. We also recommend that you become familiar with the research methodologies, writing styles, and topics of other Latinx and Spanish-speaking scholars. A good place to start is accessing the *Journal of Latinx Psychology* (https://www.apa.org/pubs/journals/lat) through your school's library and the *Revista Interamericana de Psicología* (https://journal.sipsych.org/index.php/IJP), which is an open-access journal. Attending conferences hosted by racial and ethnic minority psychological associations, such as NLPA and the Society for the Psychological Study of Culture, Ethnicity and Race (https://division45.org), may also provide opportunities that can support research focused on Latinx and Spanish-speaking communities. Forming connections and mentoring relationships with scholars who share your experiences and interests is also important, in particular when you need to consult someone or seek support. NLPA offers a free mentoring program for students and early career professionals (https://www.nlpa.ws/mentoring-program), and the association's conferences offer several student-centered programs and opportunities for development.

Remember that your personal stories and experiences can be tools that can help you succeed in graduate school. These experiences can spark research ideas and projects that can, in turn, have a positive impact on your communities. Relying on your knowledge of *la comunidad*, you can produce research that does not overpathologize your community. In clinical settings, the language and knowledge that you bring with you can help you establish rapport, trust, and effective communication with your clients. Therefore, we also encourage you to stay connected with your family, friends, and community and to the issues relevant to them. This connection can be a source of support for you (Matos, 2015) and, in turn, your graduate education can become an asset to them as you help increase access to culturally and linguistically responsive mental health care. If possible, take time to physically travel to your community and reestablish your connection to it.

Microagresiones

The climate of your program and institution will have an impact on your experiences with *microaggressions*: brief, subtle, commonplace, intentional or unintentional acts of racism or discrimination toward minoritized communities (Sue et al., 2007). For example, some programs have adopted concrete ways to deal with microaggressions directly and at the time they occur (e.g., seeing every instance of microaggression as a critical incident that needs to be analyzed by all involved in the incident, including witnesses). Other programs take a passive approach (e.g., making global statements via an electronic mailing list or through newsletters about the importance of respecting others). Some programs may use a combination of direct and indirect actions to respond to microaggressions. In the worst-case scenario, some programs ignore the problem. The approach your program takes could be completely disconnected from its commitment to racial and social justice. As Puerto Rican professor Dr. Melanie Domenech Rodríguez (2014) stated, even those committed to multicultural competence will commit microaggressions from time to time and hurt others despite their intentions. Regardless of the approach your program takes to confront these acts of racism and discrimination, some students and professors will unfortunately engage in microaggressions that question your competence, especially if you have an accent.

Your intersecting identities (e.g., race, gender, class, ethnicity) will influence how others in your program evaluate your level of competence across all aspects of your program (i.e., classes, practice, research). For example, if you are a White Spanish-speaking Latinx student you are more likely to be perceived as competent than if you are an AfroLatinx Spanish-speaking student. Other microaggressions that could take place are the pathologization and exoticization of your cultural values and norms (e.g., "Why are you calling me *mami*?", "I like how spicy you are!"), your designation as an expert or spokesperson for the Latinx community (e.g., "As a Latina, what do you think?"), and the invalidation of your identity (e.g., "You don't look Dominican," "You speak English so well!"), among others (Pimentel, 2015; Proctor et al., 2018).

Along with your competence, your level of professionalism will likely be attached to your tone of voice, mannerisms, and manner of dress and grooming. If these expressions deviate too much from White norms you may be considered unprofessional. In turn, this assumed unprofessionalism could affect how others evaluate your level of competence. However, being presumed incompetent or unprofessional is different from the concept of *imposter syndrome* (Clance & Imes, 1978), which is defined as a pattern in which you may think and feel that you are a fraud who does not deserve praise for accomplishments. Imposter syndrome is a problematic concept for students like yourself because it decontextualizes what you face inside and outside of academia, namely, being presumed incompetent and other racist or discriminatory acts (e.g., microaggressions, being denied academic opportunities). In other words, you may feel like an imposter in your program— not because you are incompetent or incapable but because others in your program ignore or minimize your achievements and knowledge. You may also be made to feel like you do not belong in your program if your mannerisms or your speech, for example, is erroneously evaluated as unprofessional because of someone else's bias. Nonetheless, we recognize that as a

Spanish-speaking and Latinx person you may have encountered this same epistemic violence throughout your life and indeed may experience doubts and anxiety about your competence to succeed in graduate school.

To overcome these challenges, you may feel the need to prove to others that you are indeed deserving of your spot in your program and capable of completing it. To do that, *vas a querer darle duro al programa*, perhaps by volunteering or participating in many program events or initiatives, pushing yourself to excel in your classes and always be on point, or enrolling in advanced and difficult courses to prove that you are smart (McGee & Martin, 2011). Adopting an "I'll show them" attitude can give you feelings of satisfaction and pride. You could also experience a reaffirmation of your capabilities and aptitude for graduate school. However, you need to keep track of how you are feeling and doing as you continue to face and manage these aggressions. Research points to how students of color, in particular Black and AfroLatinx students, who persistently experience microaggressions, racism, and discrimination on campus, are at risk of developing a wide range of emotional, psychological, and physiological symptoms (Quaye et al., 2020). This is often conceptualized in the literature as *traumatic stress* (Nadal, 2018) and *racial battle fatigue* (Smith et al., 2011).

In response to these *microagresiones*, you may also adopt code-switching. For example, you start dimming and modifying yourself by "sounding Whiter" (e.g., *dejas de usar jerga*), avoiding wearing certain types of jewelry, changing your interpersonal and communication style, smiling more to appear friendly and professional, or avoiding talking too much about your personal life. Depending on the location of your program, you may also have to present an edited version of yourself outside. For example, if your school is in a state with anti-immigrant laws you may want to protect yourself by changing your customs (e.g., avoiding speaking Spanish in public) and other forms of expression (e.g., removing national symbols from your car). Acquiring new ways to move through, within, and outside of academia that are based on different racial and cultural values and norms can be protective to an extent, but code-switching can also take a significant toll on your psychological health (Hewlin, 2009).

Seeking support from faculty allies, family, and fellow students can be critical in helping you navigate these challenges. We also encourage you to search for culturally competent psychological care. Your program may already have a list of community psychologists and counselors who are available to work with their graduate students. Websites like Therapy for Latinx (https://www.therapyforlatinx.com) and Therapy for Black Girls (https://therapyforblack-girls.com) also can help you find competent mental health care. Bilingual

Latinx scholars and clinicians, such as Drs. Hector Y. Adames and Nayeli Y. Chavez-Dueñas (see Chapter 4, this volume) have also produced tool kits that promote healing and well-being among people of color (https://icrace.org/our-partners/toolkits). Taking time to rest, heal, and recharge is also critical. Although it may be tempting to use school calendar breaks to catch up on research, classwork, and work, it is important to prioritize rest and fun during these breaks. Creating a plan with your advisor to tackle important research, coursework, and clinical milestones is important. For example, breaking major course- and research-related tasks into smaller components can help you feel less overwhelmed by these projects. We also encourage you to establish a check-in meeting plan (e.g., weekly, biweekly, monthly) with your mentor/advisor and set support and expectation goals for these meetings. If your program requires a research capstone or dissertation, you may also find dissertation planners and support groups helpful.

Doctoral student support groups, such as the Facebook groups Latinas Completing Doctoral Degrees (https://tiny.cc/wkmjyz) and PhinisheD/FinishEdD (https://tiny.cc/vkmjyz) at times offer free opportunities to join dissertation/thesis writing support groups. These groups are also great communities where you can share your difficult experiences in graduate school and get support from others who get it. Your school may also have additional resources or access to programs, such as NCFDD (formerly the National Center for Faculty Development and Diversity; https://www.ncfdd.org), which offers a success program each semester designed to help doctoral students work on their dissertations.

Sacrificios Financieros

Financial assistance packages will vary greatly depending on the program and institution to which you are admitted. Some programs guarantee funding through grants or assistantships, but others cannot. Other institutions may not offer any funding. Even within the same program, the funding packages may vary depending on the funding source. However, funding packages may not be enough to cover living expenses and additional costs (e.g., student fees, books, computers). Although some students can rely on family, credit, or savings to cover these expenses, these may not be options for you. In addition, student loans may or may not be available to you depending on your citizenship status. If you can take out student loans, they become available only after you have completed your move. Despite the known gap between funding and the cost of graduate school and living expenses, many programs unfortunately adopt a classist view of expecting students to see their pursuit of doctoral degrees as a full-time job, *cómo si el dinero cayera del cielo*. Because of this, it is common for students to look for part-time work without informing faculty in their programs. This is problematic because your performance will be evaluated on the basis of the unreasonable expectation of full-time effort. If you have faculty you trust in your program, we encourage you to share this concern and other financial issues you face. Depending on the institution you attend, there may be an Office of the Dean of Students that has resources and emergency funds for students facing financial emergencies. Faculty can help you contact this office. When you begin clinical practice, your work likely will be unpaid at first. However, some sites may be willing to pay bilingual student clinicians a small stipend, or pay them on a per-hour basis, after they have passed a language competence evaluation. Because this may not be openly advertised by all clinical practice sites, we encourage you to inquire.

If your program follows the scientist–practitioner model, you will also be expected to attend and present your work at scientific conferences. *Pero ir a conferencias no es gratis.* You will need to cover travel, lodging, food, transportation, and registration costs. Your program may or may not offer financial assistance for this. We encourage you to contact your institution or graduate school to inquire about potential scholarships for conference travel. Some conferences offer scholarships to help cover part of the cost. For example, NLPA has offered scholarships to student presenters and provided other ways to reduce costs if you volunteer during the conference. In addition, be on the lookout for conference attendance scholarship announcements by the American Psychological Association (https://convention.apa.org/attend/future-conventions). You may also find it helpful to use crowd-sourcing accounts, such as GoFundMe, to help you collect funds that can help you cover some conference expenses. Similar strategies can be used when you begin conceptualizing your thesis and dissertation projects and need funding for participant incentives.

Sentido de Responsabilidad

Although getting into graduate school is a wonderful personal accomplishment, you may also be doing this *por tu familia y comunidad*. Knowing that the goal to complete this degree goes beyond yourself is a wonderful feeling. It gives you pride and responsibility. You have your whole family (natural, chosen, or both) cheering you on. *¡Vamos que tú puedes!* But when *los huevos se ponen a peso* in your classes, practice, or research, that is when you may begin to feel the pressure and a fear of failure. Any one of these could be *la gota que colma la taza*, considering all the other challenges you are experiencing in your program (isolation, microaggression, financial sacrifices). After all, your family and community are counting on you, *¿verdad?*

You may also find that when you talk to family and friends, and try to explain how difficult your classes, research, and clinical work are, they are not able to offer you much *consuelo* or say the right things because *no están en tu lugar.* It is normal for you to be angry and feel somewhat resentful. This is when it is important to reach out to family and people you trust within and outside of your program to tell them what they can do to support you. Is it to let you vent and listen? Help you contact professional help? Help you identify affinity groups on campus or outside of campus? Serve as an intermediary between you and a faculty member? Report racist acts on your behalf to program leadership? Serve as an intermediary between you and your mentor? Do you have to discuss with your advisor or clinical supervisor the need to lower your clinical caseload or reduce the number of classes you take the next semester? Is it possible for you to visit your family, or for your family to come visit you? This will not only help you take actions that will have a positive impact on your mental health and your performance in the program but also focus on the dynamics that are at the root of the fear and pressure you are experiencing: academic spaces that can be lonely, hostile, and unsupportive to students like you.

No Solo Eres Estudiante

Academia is grounded in the same capitalistic norms of production and work ethics that guide labor outside of it; therefore, your program may have an underlying assumption and expectation that your primary or only responsibility is school. However, being a student is not your only identity or responsibility. Many of you are partnered; married; and/or are taking care of children, parents, or both. You may also be contributing to your family financially; therefore, you also have responsibilities as an employee. It is important to ask your family for support. For example, if you have space in your home, could your family help you create a separate study space? If you do not have the space available, is there a public library nearby where you could go for a couple of hours every week? Could family members assist with caretaking responsibilities or meal preparations during times you need to study?

It is also important to make time for family and friends. Putting off an assigned reading or paper for a couple of hours to go to a movie or a walk with your partner will not make a huge difference to the fulfillment of the assignment. Other students take a different approach. They bring their schoolwork to their children's sports games, to work on during moments when their child is on the bench during a soccer game or on time out in their basketball game. The important thing is to show up for your family. As you grow personally, you can also grow as a partner, parent, and family member. If it is difficult to do during the week, could you plan a special outing or family night once a month? Facebook pages like #DoctoralMomLife (https://www.facebook.com/groups/478383452542983/) and Working Folks' Guide to a PhD/EdD (https://www.facebook.com/groups/2455080648051393/) may offer additional tips (e.g., easy meals to prepare) and resources for graduate parents and working students.

It is important to stay organized with your schoolwork, ask for support from your program, and set appropriate boundaries with school. For example, if at the beginning of the term you notice that an examination falls on a special day for your family, you could ask the instructor whether you could take the examination before or after the special family event. When you face family emergencies, do not hesitate to ask your program and faculty for support. For example, they may be willing to work with you to give you extensions on your deadlines, offer you flexibility in attendance, or provide some other arrangement to help you meet your academic responsibilities as you also meet your family responsibilities. In terms of boundaries, it is important to communicate to faculty your time limitations and boundaries. For example, if you are collaborating with a faculty member on a research project, give them a realistic description of your availability and the amount of time you would need to complete a task. Do not overpromise.

CAMARÓN QUE SE DUERME SE LO LLEVA LA CORRIENTE: YOU HAVE TO BE ON TOP OF THINGS

In this section, we emphasize strategies you can use to help you throughout your doctoral journey, such as staying informed, organized, and connected with your faculty mentors. We also talk about the importance of understanding program policies, maintaining regular communication with faculty and mentors, and navigating academic expectations while embracing your bilingualism and cultural identity. More important, we encourage you to see your experiences, language, and authenticity as powerful tools for success as a bilingual doctoral student.

Mantente en Contacto con les Administradores

In addition to attending your classes and fulfilling all other program requirements, there are many other things you need to keep track of. One of the most important is becoming familiar with your program's student handbook. Do not assume that all faculty members know the handbook; some of them may be familiar only with a previous version that contains outdated program policies. The handbook is likely to have important information about requirements, program forms, and deadlines. Programs adhere firmly to these deadlines, many times because they also need to work within university deadlines. *Así que, ¡apunta estas fechas en todos los sitios que puedas!* The main form of communication between you and the program administration will likely be email. Program administration will send information such as forms, all kinds of deadlines, information about class registration, scholarships, and assistantship applications and opportunities. Make it a habit to check your email inbox daily.

Mantente en Contacto con les Profesores

When faculty communicate with you via email and they await a response, they will expect you to answer within 24–48 hours, even when this is not explicitly stated in the message. Unfortunately, longer response times are often incorrectly interpreted as representing a lack of professionalism. Although the program and the handbook will give you a list of deadlines, faculty may have their own set of deadlines. For example, if you are scheduling the proposal for a thesis or dissertation, and your program handbook advises that the committee members receive a copy of your proposal 2 weeks before the proposal meeting, realize that they may want to receive the proposal a month before. In addition, although some students can meet with faculty during the summer and make progress toward clinical and research milestones, other faculty members will not be available during those months. You will have to discuss with your advisor, mentor, and committee members their availability and time expectations. Faculty will also have different boundaries and expectations about communication; for example, some faculty members prefer to be called by their degree or title and last name, and others will want you to call them by their first name. Ask them what their preference is. Whereas some faculty members intentionally build relationships with their advisees/mentees (e.g., hosting social gatherings with research team members), other faculty members prefer to not establish these relationships. *A todes les profesores les cortan con tijeras diferentes.*

Mantente en Contacto con tus Mentores

One of the most important things to do at the beginning of your program is to set up meetings with your advisor/mentor/main professor to help establish the parameters of your working and mentoring relationship. Here is a list of questions and topics we suggest you discuss:

- What is their preferred mode of communication (e.g., email, phone, text)?
- What are their deadlines and expectations for research?
- What are their deadlines for writing you recommendation letters?
- What are their expectations for communication and meetings?
- What are their expectations regarding assistantship responsibilities (if this is your case)?
- How do you expect them to support you throughout the program?
- Will they support you if you collaborate with other faculty members?

Discuss specific professional goals, and ask if they have opportunities to help you reach these goals. After these expectations have been established and clarified, it is important to evaluate during follow-up meetings how these are being met or unmet and what changes need to be made. *Es una conversación continua.* Your mentor/advisor can also be your biggest ally in the program. In addition to offering you support and guidance throughout your program, they can advocate for you in the program. For example, would they be willing to work with other faculty members and the director of training of your program to help identify clinical sites that would allow you to provide services in Spanish?

DE AHORA EN ADELANTE: RETHINKING YOUR EXPERIENCES, IDENTITIES, AND BILINGUALISM

We know that as a Spanish-speaking and Latinx student, your skills and identities are tools that can help you navigate academic and nonacademic spaces. To gain admittance to graduate school, you have had to cross cultural and linguistic borders. Such crossings perhaps have taught you about loss, different racial and cultural norms, resource disparities, and oppression— but, more important, these experiences demonstrate your courage, creativity, and curiosity. To take the risk of applying to a doctoral program, perhaps away from family, where you do not feel represented, and in a language that does not always let you express what you feel and think, requires *coraje.* To thrive in a program and keep true to yourself while navigating different racial and cultural norms and values requires *creatividad.* To wonder about the possibilities that becoming a bilingual mental health professional will offer you, your family, and your community requires *curiosidad.* Therefore, our hope for you is that as you progress through your program you will question, challenge, *y les des una buena mandá para ya tú sabes dónde* to all the problematic narratives that make you feel inferior, unprofessional, or unwelcome. Instead, we want you to view your experiences, identities, and bilingualism as sources of affirmation and resources that can help you thrive in your program. For example, your experiences and identities as a Spanish-speaking and Latinx student give you knowledge and methods (e.g., migration processes; Latinx identity processes; Latinx history, cultural values, traditions, and knowledge; Indigenous and African healing practices) not fully available to others. Your skills as a bilingual student give you access to a larger community of English and Spanish speakers. You can also communicate with them in a way that is linguistically competent. More important, your bilingualism gives you the opportunity to expand access to communities that are underserved. To tap into these sources and resources, we encourage you to be authentic and creative.

Autenticidad

Autenticidad should be something you should strive for not only as a mental health professional but also as a student. It is only when you let go of the fear of being yourself that you will begin to feel that you belong, that you fit in, sort of, "*Este es quién soy, me tomas o me dejas.*" Authenticity for you may be about speaking Spanish (in classes, in clinical work, with supervisors) to others even if they do not understand it, then translating. It may be about using *jerga* or *palabras soeces*, dressing how you like, and *dándole un besito en la mejilla* to people you trust in the program. These negotiations will teach you that learning the academic language and norms does not have to come at the expense of losing yourself. You are an asset.

Creatividad

Instead of thinking of code-switching as a way to edit or hide parts of yourself, code-switching can be reinterpreted as a decision-making process about what you say, how you say it, and who you say it to, throughout your graduate training journey. For example, code-switching can transform the unserviceable language of academic training into language that is relevant to the Spanish-speaking communities with which you are working. Because you share cultural knowledge with the community, you also know which dialect, *dichos, refranes,* cadence, manners, posture, tone, volume, and interpersonal style to use when you speak with them. For example, you know that when you are working with a Spanish-speaking client, apart from having the linguistic competence you need to consider how values like *respeto* (deferential treatment towards others) and *confianza* (trust that comes from knowing that a person "is one of us") may influence their consent to participate in clinical work or research. Within the clinical setting, code-switching also allows you to communicate more easily, build connections with Spanish-speaking and bilingual clients, increase comfort when talking about personal experiences that affect your clients, and facilitate expression. In other words, code-switching helps build rapport and empathic communication by conveying to your clients, "I get you." Your language skills and cultural knowledge also give you access to places others do not have access to. For example, you can reach out to Spanish-speaking communities near your program and learn about their needs and wants, perhaps by attending cultural festivals or local organizations. As we previously mentioned, because of the lack of representation issues these communities are often ignored by academia. You can serve as a bridge.

If your program has a research component, code-switching can also take place when you determine how you share your research data. For example, will you transcribe texts and data verbatim; translate from one language or dialect to another; or omit aspects of the data, quantitative or qualitative, that align with linguistic styles excluded in academia or may harm the community if not accurately contextualized by those tasked with reading and approving your project? You could also engage in code-switching when you analyze, conceptualize, or interpret data, whether collected during research or a clinical process. When you undertake a code-switching approach to data analysis you engage simultaneously in interpretation, given the high context communication of Spanish-speaking Latinx communities. For example, if you interpret something a client told you as racist and an English-speaking White supervisor suggests that you are reading too much into it, that may represent the analytic disparity between a high-context culture and a low-context one. This is where your knowledge of the community, your language skills, and your lived experiences become valuable because you have a context that your supervisor lacks, and thus you have a more nuanced understanding and interpretation of what is happening in the case. This same approach can be practiced in qualitative and quantitative analysis and interpretation. To illustrate, at times you may have to rely on your language skills, personal experiences, and knowledge of the community to help you interpret the data.

We are proud of you, your accomplishments, and the fact that you have been accepted into graduate school. Although you may face some challenges, we are confident that you have what it takes to succeed in your program and achieve your goal of becoming a bilingual clinician and/or academician. Rely on your community, your family, your friends, allies in your program, as well as your skills and experiences. *¡Lo vas a lograr!*

TAKEAWAYS

- Seek assistance from your community, mental health professionals, faculty, support programs in your institution, and fellow students when you face challenges.

- You made it into graduate school, which means that you have the capacity and skills necessary to be successful in your program. You belong in your program!

- Learn about all the funding opportunities and resources available to students within and outside of your institution.

- Our responsibility to our communities is a source of pride and support.

- Learn program policies, and stay in contact with the administrators and faculty in your program.

- Your identity, experiences, and skills as a bilingual and Latinx student are a source of pride and resources for success.

REFLEXIONES

- What are you looking forward to the most when you think about becoming a licensed bilingual clinician or a bilingual professor? What are some resources you think you will need to help you accomplish this goal?

- Do you have specific bilingual training goals? How can your program help you achieve these goals?

- Have you discussed with your faculty advisor your training goals? How can they support you in meeting these goals?

- Do you have a plan of support you can use if or when you face difficulties?

¡CONSEJO!

- Seek opportunities to meet your bilingual training goals, and do not be afraid to reach out for support to reach these goals, or when you face barriers on your journey toward meeting these goals. Remember that your experiences and identity as a bilingual and Latinx student are resources, not deficits.

RESOURCES

Bell, D. B., Foster, S. L., & Cone, J. D. (2019). *Dissertations and theses from start to finish: Psychology and related fields* (3rd ed.). American Psychological Association. https://doi.org/10.1037/0000161-000

Burke, J., & Dempsey, M. (2022). *Undertaking capstone and final year projects in psychology: A practical guide for students.* Routledge.

Castellanos, J., Gloria, A. M., & Kamimura, M. (Eds.). (2006). *The Latina/o pathway to the Ph.D.:* Abriendo caminos. Routledge.

Negrón-Gonzales, G., & Barrera, M. L. (2023). *The Latinx guide to graduate school.* Duke University Press.

Ngetich, G. C. (2022). *The PhD journey: Strategies for enrolling, thriving, and excelling in a PhD program.* Aviva.

Reichard, R. (2023). *Self-care for Latinas: 100+ ways to prioritize and rejuvenate your mind, body, and spirit.* Adams Media.

Rodríguez, C. O. (2018). *Decolonizing academia: Poverty, oppression and pain.* Fernwood.

REFERENCES

American Psychological Association. (2022). *Data tool: Demographics of the U.S. psychology workforce.* https://www.apa.org/workforce/data-tools/demographics

Bailey, D. (2020). Enticing new faces to the field. *Monitor on Psychology, 51*(1), 60. https://www.apa.org/monitor/2020/01/cover-trends-new-faces

Bichsel, J., Christidis, P., Conroy, J., & Lin, L. (2019). Datapoint: Diversity among psychology faculty. *Monitor on Psychology, 50*(9), 11. https://www.apa.org/monitor/2019/10/datapoint-diversity

Clance, P. R., & Imes, S. A. (1978). The imposter phenomenon in high achieving women: Dynamics and therapeutic intervention. *Psychotherapy: Theory, Research, & Practice, 15*(3), 241–247. https://doi.org/10.1037/h0086006

Domenech Rodríguez, M. (2014, December 2). *No way but through* [Video]. YouTube. https://www.youtube.com/watch?v=2orqr-nOIPk

Hewlin, P. F. (2009). Wearing the cloak: Antecedents and consequences of creating facades of conformity. *Journal of Applied Psychology, 94*(3), 727–741. https://doi.org/10.1037/a0015228

Holloway-Friesen, H. (2021). The role of mentoring on Hispanic graduate students' sense of belonging and academic self-efficacy. *Journal of Hispanic Higher Education, 20*(1), 46–58. https://doi.org/10.1177/1538192718823716

Matos, J. M. D. (2015). *La Familia*: The important ingredient for Latina/o college student engagement and persistence. *Equity & Excellence in Education, 48*(3), 436–453. https://doi.org/10.1080/10665684.2015.1056761

McGee, E. O., & Martin, D. B. (2011). "You would not believe what I have to go through to prove my intellectual value!" Stereotype management among academically successful Black mathematics and engineering students. *American Educational Research Journal, 48*(6), 1347–1389. https://doi.org/10.3102/0002831211423972

Nadal, K. L. (2018). *Microaggressions and traumatic stress: Theory, research, and clinical treatment.* American Psychological Association. https://doi.org/10.1037/0000073-000

Padilla, A. M. (1994). Research news and comment: Ethnic minority scholars; research, and mentoring: Current and future issues. *Educational Researcher, 23*(4), 24–27. https://doi.org/10.3102/0013189X023004024

Pimentel, C. (2015). *The experience of microaggression against Latina graduate psychology students* [Unpublished doctoral dissertation]. William James College.

Proctor, S. L., Kyle, J., Fefer, K., & Lau, Q. C. (2018). Examining racial microaggressions, race/ethnicity, gender, and bilingual status with school psychology students: The role of intersectionality. *Contemporary School Psychology, 22*(3), 355–368. https://doi.org/10.1007/s40688-017-0156-8

Quaye, S. J., Karikari, S. N., Carter, K. D., Okello, W. K., & Allen, C. (2020). "Why can't I just chill?": The visceral nature of racial battle fatigue. *Journal of College Student Development, 61*(5), 609–623. https://doi.org/10.1353/csd.2020.0058

Rincón, B. E. (2020). Does Latinx representation matter for Latinx student retention in STEM? *Journal of Hispanic Higher Education, 19*(4), 437–451. https://doi.org/10.1177/1538192718820532

Smith, W. A., Yosso, T. J., & Solórzano, D. G. (2011). Challenging racial battle fatigue on historically White campuses: A critical race examination of race-related stress. In R. D. Coates (Ed.), *Covert racism: Theories, institutions, and experiences* (pp. 211–237). Brill. https://doi.org/10.1163/ej.9789004203655.i-461.82

Sue, D. W., Capodilupo, C. M., Torino, G. C., Bucceri, J. M., Holder, A. M. B., Nadal, K. L., & Esquilin, M. (2007). Racial microaggressions in everyday life: Implications for clinical practice. *American Psychologist, 62*(4), 271–286. https://doi.org/10.1037/0003-066X.62.4.271

4

CONSTRUYENDO A DECOLONIAL LATINX MENTAL HEALTH WITH BLACK AND INDIGENOUS LATINXS AT THE CENTER

HECTOR Y. ADAMES AND NAYELI Y. CHAVEZ-DUEÑAS

Es necesario hacer un mundo nuevo. Un mundo donde quepan muchos mundos, donde quepan todos los mundos.

—Subcomandante Marcos, *Our Word Is Our Weapon*

In this chapter, we invite readers to reimagine and rebuild a Latinx mental health that centers the experiences of Black and Indigenous Latinxs. We provide a brief overview of Latinidad within a historical context, emphasizing the colonial influences and ideologies that remain present today, including colorism and mestizaje racial ideologies (an ideology whereby everyone of Latinx descent is deemed to be of mixed race). These colonistic ideologies and practices render invisible the racialized experiences of Indigenous Latinxs and AfroLatinxs, including Latinx in mental health. In this chapter, we offer thought-provoking strategies, scenarios, and reflections to encourage scholars, practitioners, and educators to explore ways to decolonize Latinx mental health.

Envisioning and creating a world where many worlds can fit is at the heart of human rights. It is also a cornerstone of our work as professionals

https://doi.org/10.1037/0000481-005
Forging Caminos: *Pathways to Becoming a Bilingual Mental Health Professional,*
M. Campos, Y. Mejia, and A. J. Consoli (Editors)

in the field of mental health. However, translating this life-affirming stance into action is more challenging than simply talking about it. Many structures and forces, including the culture of White supremacy and its institutional policies, economic systems, and power dynamics, aim to prevent or make it challenging for many to reenvision and devote energy, time, and resources to rebuilding a dignified world for all. Still, this is just one part of the narrative. Historically, Black[1] and Indigenous communities have disrupted and resisted structures and forces designed to dominate, silence, and oppress them. Despite the obstacles they have encountered, Black and Indigenous people throughout the globe have persevered and continue to imagine and construct a world beyond the dehumanizing confines of Euro-American dominance and worldview. Let's pause for a moment and envision a world like that:

- What are your immediate emotional reactions as you visualize *el nuevo mundo*?

- What are some thoughts that come to mind?

- How does your own socialization, and the messages you have learned about how the world is structured, influence your initial reactions to envisioning a different kind of world?

Through our actions, we can uphold human rights and contribute to shaping a world that extends beyond the gaze of White supremacy culture. Although constructing such a new world is critical, it has not received the serious attention it deserves in the discipline of mental health in general and Latinx mental health in particular. In this chapter, we invite you to reimagine and rebuild Latinx mental health by centering the experiences of Black and Indigenous Latinxs. In our invitation, we intentionally use the symbol "x" in "Latinx" to express a rejection of White supremacist, capitalist, heterosexual, cisgender, patriarchal ideologies that dehumanize, marginalize, and criminalize people for simply living, loving, and thinking—for simply existing beyond the grip of the Spanish colonial language and ideals. Instead, the "x" is making space for inviting and uplifting the beingness of those being other-ized. From this stance, Latinx is disruptive, generative, and hopeful; it is a call to take a pause, to be mindful of who we were, where we are, and what we can become. It aims to (im)perfectly embrace the often complex and messy process of centering, honoring, and loving our uniqueness, our beauty,

---

[1]Throughout the chapter, we use the terms *Black Latinxs* or *AfroLatinxs* to honor the diverse ways individuals of African descent within the Latinx community choose to identify themselves.

and the collective promise of Latinidad. However, the process of reconstruction demands a strong foundation; it starts with revisiting history and elevating the silenced voices of Black and Indigenous Latinxs. It also requires us to examine our racial socialization and honestly discuss what all these parts invoke in us and how it influences our work with Latinxs. Let's build!

LATINIDAD IN HISTORICAL CONTEXT

Podrán cortar todas las flores, pero no podrán detener la primavera.
—attributed to Pablo Neruda

Latinxs in the United States can trace their ancestry to many different countries across Latin America, with its own array of cultures and unique histories. The U.S. Census Bureau (n.d.) categorizes individuals from these various Latin American communities under a single ethnic classification known as Hispanic/Latinx. Scholars have also used the term "Latinidad," which was first introduced by Felix Padilla in 1985, to describe the shared cultural characteristics of people across Latin America, invoking notions of unity and influence in politics. However, several problems exist in the conception and application of such pan-ethnic terms. For instance, scholars have described how such terms fail to recognize and center racial differences within Latinidad (Adames et al., 2016, 2021; Chavez-Dueñas et al., 2014). To illustrate, young Black and Indigenous Latinxs have described the concept of Latinidad as an "exclusionary identity fabricated by—and for the benefit of—White and Mestizo elites and the American political class" (Salazar, 2019, para. 2).

The psychology literature has also provided a race-neutral representation of the Latinx community, frequently overlooking, downplaying, and obscuring the experiences of Indigenous Latinxs and AfroLatinxs (Adames & Chavez-Dueñas, 2017; Chavez-Dueñas et al., 2022; Sanchez, 2021). The long-standing disregard and neglect of Indigenous and Black communities' unique experiences and valuable contributions to Latinidad is neither new nor accidental (Adames & Chavez-Dueñas, 2017; Soler Castillo & Pardo Abril, 2009). These omissions, often rooted in White supremacy ideologies, were first imposed by Europeans during colonization and, over time, reinforced in every part of contemporary Latin American society inside and outside the United States (Chavez-Dueñas et al., 2022; Soler Castillo & Pardo Abril, 2009). Comprehending and revisiting history is fundamental for us as scholars and practitioners if we are to place Latinidad into its proper context (Chavez-Dueñas et al., 2022).

Latin America's Preexisting Diversity and Colonization

Although often overlooked or unappreciated, the rich diversity in Latin America has always been present; its diversity is not a product of colonization. Thousands of diverse Indigenous groups have lived in this geographical region, each with its own ancient culture and traditions, contributing to the captivating tapestry of Latin America today. Thus, before the calamitous arrival of the Europeans in 1492, thousands of languages, distinct cultural practices, and spiritual traditions were practiced by Indigenous people in the Americas (Adames & Chavez-Dueñas, 2017).

The arrival of the Spaniards led to a new era, a historical period known as *La Conquista* [The Conquest]. *La Conquista* was characterized by the cruel actions of the Europeans against Indigenous and African peoples. These actions included the genocide of Indigenous populations, appropriation of the land and its resources, exploitation of Indigenous people, and enslavement of African people (Adames & Chavez-Dueñas, 2017). Ideologies rooted in White supremacy justified these barbaric actions, intentionally placing Europeans, their descendants, and their cultures at the pinnacle of the power hierarchy within the constructed stratification system. In this invented hierarchy, the colonizers dismissed the cultural richness within Indigenous and African communities; instead, they treated these communities as inferior, denying them the fundamental human rights and dignity they deserved. In other words, the Europeans established, imposed, and reinforced a racial order in which access to wealth, power, and dignity was based on dividing people on the basis of perceived race. This system was supported by the Catholic Church. Those at the top of the hierarchy, possessing white skin and other European phenotypic features, actively granted themselves land ownership, political power, and the authority to exploit and dehumanize those they deemed inferior. European dominance actively prohibited Indigenous and Black peoples from using their native languages and engaging in their cultural practices and traditions. Furthermore, despite Catholicism's purported rejection of slavery, the colonizers systematically denied Black people the fundamental human right of freedom.

Now that we have briefly contextualized Latinidad, we encourage you to reflect on the following questions:

- Do any parts of the history we described come as a surprise to you? If so, which ones?

- What were your perceptions of the concept of Latinidad prior to engaging with this section? How has your perspective on the concept changed, if at all?

- What word do you use to characterize your ethnicity or culture? What makes you inclined to choose that particular term?

- If you are Latinx, how has the history covered in this section influenced you, your family, and your understanding of the world?

- If you are not Latinx, how has the history covered in this section influenced your perspectives of Latinxs, their families, and communities?

Mestizaje Racial Ideologies

Although the racial hierarchy of power established in the Americas during colonial times remains alive today, its legacy and impact are rarely acknowledged. Stated differently, within Latinidad, people often fail to name, question, or challenge the racial inequities existing in Latin American society, in the United States, and beyond—precisely as the colonizers intended. The intention was to lead an entire population into believing that because of the assumptions that everyone in Latin America is supposedly mestizo [racially mixed], distinction in skin color had no impact on people's lives—a concept referred to in the literature as *mestizaje racial ideologies* (MRIs; Adames et al., 2016; Chavez-Dueñas et al., 2014). Today, MRIs are ingrained in many facets of Latinidad, from family gatherings to mainstream media, educational institutions, and even in our own Latinx mental health discipline. All in all, being socialized to uphold MRIs ensures that the colonizers' objective remains in place by new generations of Latinxs who continue to deny the influence of race on access to or denial of power and resources while silencing the voices and minimizing the racialized experience of Indigenous and AfroLatinxs.

In the mental health field, researchers and healing approaches often overlook racial differences within Latinidad, demonstrating how MRIs operate and influence our discipline (Adames et al., 2021), with some exceptions (see Adames & Chavez-Dueñas, 2017; Chavez-Dueñas et al., 2022; Comas-Díaz, 2021). Instead, there is an assumption that the experiences of Latinxs are homogeneous, disregarding our racialized and intersectional realities. As a field of study, Latinx mental health was established to enhance our comprehension of the well-being of people with Latin American heritage; however, it has not significantly improved much with respect to naming and addressing Blackness (Adames et al., 2021; Sanchez, 2021), Indigeneity (Chavez-Dueñas et al., 2022), and colorism (Adames et al., 2016; Chavez-Dueñas et al., 2014). Instead, much of the literature centers on shared cultural characteristics and experiences, such as traditional cultural values, bilingualism, acculturation, and adaptation to U.S. culture, with many treatments and interventions focusing on cultural adaptations (Consoli et al., 2022). To illustrate, studies that focus on language among Latinx immigrants tend to concentrate on individuals who speak English and Spanish. They seldom address how Spanish is a colonial language or consider that Indigenous Latinxs may not speak Spanish or that Spanish is their second language (Perry & Gámez, 2023; Wang et al., 2023). Nevertheless, the distinct cultures of Indigenous or AfroLatinx individuals within the Latinx community are seldom acknowledged, referenced, or considered, albeit there are a few exceptions (e.g., the Culturally Responsive and Racially Conscious Ecosystemic Treatment Approach; Adames & Chavez-Dueñas, 2017; the Intersectionality Awakening Model of Womanista Transnational Treatment Approach for Latinx women; Chavez-Dueñas & Adames, 2021). Said differently, much of Latinx mental health scholarship follows a paradigm set by the colonizers and fails to use an intersectional lens to help us understand the nuanced and complex experience called Latinidad.

Colorism

MRIs harm all Latinxs, but they have a more pronounced impact on individuals with dark skin and Indigenous or African phenotypes. MRIs also play a role in denying, disregarding, and downplaying *colorism*, which is a form of intra- and intergroup discrimination whereby people with darker skin are viewed more unfavorably than those with lighter skin, potentially leading to adverse outcomes related to racial categorization (Chavez-Dueñas et al., 2014; Maddox & Gray, 2002). Within Latinidad, the limited empirical literature on colorism indicates that having a darker complexion and appearing less European can have adverse effects on mental well-being, educational achievements, and income levels (Adames et al., 2021; Araújo & Borrell, 2006; Comas-Díaz, 2021; Cuevas et al., 2016; Montalvo, 2004; Montalvo & Codina, 2001).

Although in the Latinx community the existence of colorism is often refuted, there are numerous ways through which we, as a community, convey how pervasive coloristic attitudes are in the form of *dichos* (Spanish proverbs), nicknames, and jokes. Colorism is passed from generation to generation. Coloristic messages are initially learned within the family environment and then solidified by educational systems and the media. For instance, light-skinned children tend to be favored and perceived as more beautiful in families compared with their darker skinned siblings (Adames et al., 2016; Bonilla-Silva, 2014). Within the larger society, there is a prevalent portrayal of dark-skinned people as being less attractive (Vera Cruz, 2018), intelligent (Hannon, 2014), or trustworthy (Chirco & Buchanan, 2022). These portrayals can lead them to internalize these messages, giving rise to colorism's negative impact on self-worth. Tables 4.1 and 4.2 provide some examples of coloristic *dichos* and adjectives used as nicknames. Understanding these forms of coloristic expressions can aid scholars and practitioners in identifying, discussing, and addressing them when raised by people in therapy, clinical supervision, academic settings, and in research.

Now that we have examined the notions of MRIs and colorism, reflect on the following questions:

- Think about your racialized upbringing and the messages you were exposed to during your formative years. Do you recall learning MRIs? If so, how? Which messages did you learn, and from whom did you learn them? How have these messages influenced your view and understanding of Latinxs?

- In what ways do you observe manifestations of MRIs within the contemporary Latinx community?

- How might colorism influence Indigenous Latinxs and AfroLatinxs' well-being?

TABLE 4.1. Coloristic Nicknames

Nicknames	Translation
Negra/o, Negrita/o	A dark-skinned/African-looking person
Trigueña/o, Trigueñita/o	A person with olive skin
Morena/o, Morenita/o, Prieta/o, Prietita/o	A dark-skinned person
Cocola/o, Cocolita/o	A person with a dark skin color similar to the husk of a coconut
Aperladita/o	A person with white skin like a pearl
Jabao, Jabita	A person with white skin and coarse hair
Güero/a, Güerito/a	A person with white skin and light-color hair
Aborigen	An Aboriginal of Indigenous descent
Cenizo	A dark-skinned person; connotating the blackness of ashes
Indio/a	A person with Indigenous features with dark skin
Indio/a Lavado	A person with Indigenous features with light skin
Indio/a Canelo	A person with Indigenous features and brown/reddish skin

Note. Adapted from "Skin Color Matters in Latino/a Communities: Identifying, Understanding, and Addressing Mestizaje Racial Ideologies in Clinical Practice," by H. Y. Adames, N. Y. Chavez-Dueñas, and K. C. Organista, 2016, *Professional Psychology: Research and Practice, 47*(1), p. 52 (https://doi.org/10.1037/pro0000062). Copyright 2016 by the American Psychological Association.

TABLE 4.2. Ten Common Coloristic *Refranes* [Proverbs] and *Dichos* [Sayings]

Dicho	Translations and connotations
Hay que mejorar la raza; cásate con un blanco	We need to better the race by marrying a White individual.
Vete por la sombrita	Go into the shade (to avoid getting darker).
Le salió el Indio	The "Indian" in you came out. (Connotes negative stereotypes about the poor behavior of Indigenous people.)
No tiene la culpa el Indio, sino quien lo hace compadre	It is not the fault of the Indigenous person but of whomever trusts them.
Trabajo como un Negro/a	I work hard like a Black person. (Connotes working hard like an enslaved person.)
Indio, pájaro y conejo, en tu casa, ni aún de viejo	You don't want Indigenous people, birds, or rabbits in your house, not even in old age.
Cien Negros por un caballo	One horse is worth 100 Black individuals.
No hay Moros en la costa	There are no Moors in the coast. (Connotes the time when the Islamic Moors settled in Spain and resentment of darker skinned individuals.)
Está muy prieto/a, pero tiene buenas facciones; Está prieto/a, pero fino/a	They have dark skin, but they have European features.
Sacar lo que el Negro del sermón	Just like Black people, you did not understand anything from the sermon. (Connotes that dark skinned people are unintelligent.)

Note. Adapted from "Skin Color Matters in Latino/a Communities: Identifying, Understanding, and Addressing Mestizaje Racial Ideologies in Clinical Practice," by H. Y. Adames, N. Y. Chavez-Dueñas, and K. C. Organista, 2016, *Professional Psychology: Research and Practice, 47*(1), p. 53 (https://doi.org/10.1037/pro0000062). Copyright 2016 by the American Psychological Association.

• If you are an Indigenous Latinx and/or AfroLatinx, how have you been harmed by MRIs? If you are White (e.g., White Latinx, European American White), consider the following:

– How have you benefited from colorism and racism?

– In what ways might you have unintentionally or deliberately oppressed others because of their skin color?

– What actionable steps can you initiate within your personal and professional roles to confront and address colorism within yourself, your community, and in systems that affect Latinxs (e.g., school, health, judicial)? We invite you to review the resource, *We Must Do Better: A Toolkit for Non-Black Latinxs Who Choose to Address Their Anti-Blackness* (Adames et al., 2020) to learn about ways to avoid the trappings of MRIs and become active participants in helping to dismantle colorism and racism.

• What actions can you initiate to address colorism in your work with members of the Latinx community?

TOWARD A DECOLONIAL LATINX MENTAL HEALTH

Our radical imagination is a tool for decolonization, for reclaiming our right to shape our lived reality.
—Adrienne maree brown, *Pleasure Activism*

The ideologies and ensuing challenges originating from colonization persist within contemporary notions of Latinidad. The historical argument we present in this chapter suggests that the representation of Latinidad as raceless, a perspective that overlooks the richness of Indigenous and African traditions as well as their racialized experiences, can be linked back to the power hierarchy established by the Spaniards. Given this historical context, it is unsurprising that even today Latinxs are frequently viewed, studied, and described in homogeneous ways, including within the mental health discipline. In order to center Black and Indigenous Latinxs' mental health, adopting a decolonial approach becomes imperative.

Using a decolonial process means that we are "constantly disrupting the legacies of inequities, dehumanization, and domination (e.g., racism, sexism, gendered racism, heterosexism, cissexism, nativism, ethnocentrism, ableism) that maintains the global hierarchy of power" (Adames et al., 2024, p. 5; see also Comas-Díaz et al., 2024). Said differently, a decolonial approach to mental health involves "delinking from the colonial matrix of power" (Mignolo, 2011, p. 9). With this goal in mind, an approach centered on decolonizing Latinx mental health necessitates a purposeful practice of action–reflection–action. This practice seeks to continuously challenge colonial influences and ideologies on our work as mental health professionals while avoiding any additional harm to our Indigenous Latinx and AfroLatinx community members.

In our support for your journey to decolonize Latinx mental health, we would like to underscore the importance of countering the fallacy ingrained in the notion that Latinxs exhibit a distinct appearance primarily defined by racial characteristics. This premise is erroneous. Latinxs encompass a wide range of skin colors, spanning the entire spectrum, and our placement within this spectrum shapes our lived experiences, including encounters with racism and unearned privileges. It is essential, however, to stress and clarify that although we discuss skin color, race is not a biological construct. It becomes critical to untangle the complexities surrounding the interplay of race, biology, and society, along with its link to racism. As Helms (2008) stated,

> To say that race or racial categories are not biological designations does not mean that one's physical appearance is not biologically or genetically based. You inherited physical characteristics from your parents, and they inherited physical characteristics from your grandparents and so on. Extended family members look alike. However, White people have the power to designate which physical similarities among people are "racial," what racial label should be assigned to them, and who has the power to count categories and make laws and policies pertaining to them. Moreover, it is the assignment of personality characteristics and behaviors to people on the basis of these factitious "racial" categories that support ongoing racism in society. (pp. 1–2)

To this end, a decolonial Latinx mental health discipline is the active process of (a) acknowledging the role of Whiteness within Latinidad and addressing White privilege and its impact on the Latinx community; (b) moving beyond a sole focus on culturally centered notions of Latinidad; (c) explicitly recognizing and confronting the harm caused by colorism to dark-skinned Latinxs, both within the community and the Latinx mental health field; and (d) placing Indigenous Latinxs and AfroLatinxs histories, contributions, realities, and strengths at the core.

Practicing Action-Reflection-Action

We now invite you to apply the information provided earlier in this chapter as you read the scenarios and respond to the questions we provide after each one.

Scenario 1

Over the past 2 months, you have been working with Paulina, a 28-year-old Latina who expresses feeling "sad for no reason" and says she is "lacking the energy" to perform daily tasks or care for her kids. Paulina is a mother to a 3-year-old boy and a 5-year-old girl. In one of your sessions, she shared her desire for her children to resemble their father more than herself. She stated, "I married *un blanquito* [a White man] hoping to *mejorar la raza* [better the race]. . . . You know, so that my children have beautiful light skin. But my kids were so unlucky; they have my dark complexion *y el pelo malo* [bad hair]."

- Considering this scenario, what reactions do you notice you are having?
- What thoughts are going through your mind as your client describes her response to having darker skinned children?
- Is there anything that catches you off guard or surprises you about the physical reactions you have and the thoughts that come to you?

- To what extent has your mental health training equipped you for addressing this client's situation?
- How might you respond to Paulina?
- How do you perceive the connection between Paulina's expressed concerns and her commentary about her children's skin color and hair texture?

Scenario 2

You have recently taken on a new client. While reviewing the referral form, you observe that the client is identified as a 29-year-old female of African American descent. On the day of her initial appointment, as you escort her from the waiting area, she says, "*¿Señorita, usted habla español? Es que yo no hablo inglés.*"

- As you consider this scenario, what physical reactions do you notice you are having?
- How would you respond to this client? What would you say?
- How do you make sense of what happened?
- How would you take into account the history and context you have learned in this chapter when working with your client?

Scenario 3

As the only Spanish-speaking therapist in your agency, your caseload consists predominantly of Latinx immigrants of Mexican descent and their children. One of the new clients is Ayara, a 58-year-old asylum-seeking woman from Peru who arrived in the United States 3 months ago. Ayara describes having all sorts of traumatic experiences on the journey to the States. During one of your sessions, Ayara states, "Coming to the United States was difficult, but living in Peru was worse; being Indigenous in Peru is a death sentence."

- What reactions are you experiencing in your body as you read this case?
- What thoughts are coming up for you?
- What would you say to Ayara in response to her statement?
- How have you been prepared in your mental health training to work with clients who have experienced traumatic experiences because of their race? If this has not been part of your training, what may be some ways to fill in this gap?
- How do you make sense of Ayara's statement about how "being Indigenous in Peru is a death sentence"?

Scenario 4

You have been working with Atachi, a 22-year-old male college student activist of Purepecha descent who immigrated to the United States and has been facing isolation at his college campus for nearly half a year. Atachi initially was enthusiastic about receiving services from you and even mentioned, "I am so relieved that I found a therapist who speaks Spanish." However, he started missing and canceling appointments. During your recent session, while probing why he's been absent from therapy, Atachi remarked,

> I don't mean to offend, but I've realized you don't get me. I was excited to talk to you because you speak Spanish, and I thought you could help me, but it seems people like me aren't covered in the books you used in school.

- What reactions do you notice yourself having as you consider this case scenario?

- What is going through your mind?

- What may be some reasons why Atachi has been missing or canceling appointments?

- What are some ways you would consider responding to him?

- Would you react any differently if you are an Indigenous Latinx yourself? How about if you are an AfroLatinx, White Latinx, or a bilingual non-Latinx?

- How much of your mental health training has focused on information specific to working with Indigenous Latinxs?

Scenario 5

Because of the rising number of Latinx students enrolling at your college, your department chair requests that, given your knowledge about this community, you deliver a presentation to the faculty. Your chair wants the presentation to help your monolingual English-speaking colleagues with fundamental knowledge necessary to offer support and academic advising to Latinx students, including those for whom English may not be their first language.

- How would you determine whether you have the necessary training to make a presentation to your colleagues?

- What are some ways to help your colleagues understand the racial diversity that exists within the Latinx community and consider how it can affect students' experiences?

- Can you teach your colleagues the basic information they need to know to provide academic support and advising to Latinxs students in one presentation?

- What are some ways to advocate for the unique needs of Indigenous Latinxs and AfroLatinxs students in higher education?

Scenario 6

A colleague has invited you to work on a grant proposal. After reading the request for proposal, you learn that the funders are interested in studies that examine the impact of oppression on Latinxs' mental health. Given the information covered in this chapter, consider the following:

- What variables or experiences are you interested in exploring?

- How would you disaggregate the data to explore the racialized experiences among Latinxs?

- What theories can you use to center the experiences of Indigenous Latinxs and AfroLatinxs in your study?

- As a researcher, how would your racial positionality influence the study you are designing, and what can you do to proactively address any biases or oversights?

CONCLUSION

Although the Latinx community includes people with every shade on the skin color spectrum and other various phenotypic features, the entrenched racial hierarchies established during colonization remain in place today, shaping who is represented and who has access to power and privilege. These same dynamics extend into the mental health field, where Indigenous Latinxs and AfroLatinxs remain marginalized and underrepresented and their stories and experiences are overlooked. In this chapter, we have explored the narrative of Latinidad within a historical context, described the influence of MRIs on Latinxs, addressed the persistence of colorism, and emphasized the imperative need for decolonial Latinx mental health. These complex subjects help form a groundwork for greater comprehension and transformative change in Latinx mental health. We encourage ongoing reflection on how we can continue to work to create a new world that deeply values and respects Indigenous and Black Latinxs. Collectively, we can engage in this endeavor while remaining grounded in Rigoberta Menchú Tum's (1992) poignant reminder that: "*Nuestra historia es una historia viva que ha palpitado, resistido y sobrevivido siglos de sacrificios*" (para. 78).

TAKEAWAYS

- The term "Latinidad" was first used to describe the shared cultural characteristics among people across Latin America; it is not a racial classification.

- Latinxs exhibit a wide array of skin colors, covering the entire spectrum.

- The shared history of colonization by the Spaniards led to the creation of a phenotype hierarchy, one in which skin color figured prominently, positioning those with white skin and other European phenotypic features at the top. In contrast, individuals with dark skin and other Indigenous and African phenotypic features were relegated to the bottom.

- *Colorism*, a term that refers to the racial bias within a group, is prevalent within Latinx communities, influencing how people view themselves and treat each other.

- Skin color within the Latinx community influences access to power, privilege, and representation.

- Mestizaje racial ideologies play a role in Latinxs' tendency to deny or minimize the impact of skin color on people's lives and well-being.

- Within the field of mental health, the experiences of Indigenous Latinxs and AfroLatinxs are often ignored and excluded from research, psychological theories, and interventions.

REFLEXIONES

- What are some of the criticisms directed at the term "Latinidad"?

- What is the origin of the diverse range of skin colors and other phenotypic features within Latinx communities?

- How would you explain the meaning of mestizaje racial ideologies (MRIs)?

- Can you describe where many Latinxs acquire MRIs?

- What is the influence of MRIs on White Latinxs?

- How do MRIs affect Indigenous Latinxs and AfroLatinxs?

- How are MRIs embedded within the field of Latinx mental health?

- Can you explain colorism and its potential influence on the lives of Indigenous Latinxs and AfroLatinxs?

- What are some crucial points to keep in mind when providing mental health services to, studying, or teaching members of Latinx communities?

- How can we enhance inclusivity and create a more welcoming environment for Indigenous Latinxs and AfroLatinxs in academic and health settings?

RESOURCES

Recommended Reading

Adames, H. Y., Chavez-Dueñas, N. Y., Sharma, S., & La Roche, M. J. (2018). Intersectionality in psychotherapy: The experiences of an AfroLatinx queer immigrant. *Psychotherapy: Theory, Research, & Practice, 55*(1), 73–79. https://doi.org/10.1037/pst0000152

Chavez-Dueñas, N. Y., Adames, H. Y., & Perez-Chavez, J. G. (2022). Anti-colonial futures: Indigenous Latinx women healing from the wounds of racial-gendered colonialism. *Women & Therapy, 45*(2–3), 191–206. https://doi.org/10.1080/02703149.2022.2097593

Chavez-Dueñas, N. Y., Adames, H. Y., Perez-Chavez, J. G., & Salas, S. P. (2019). Healing ethno-racial trauma in Latinx immigrant communities: Cultivating hope, resistance, and action. *American Psychologist, 74*(1), 49–62. https://doi.org/10.1037/amp0000289

Online Resources

- Immigration Critical Race and Cultural Equity Lab: https://icrace.org/

- What AfroLatinos Want You to Know: https://youtu.be/ZX7EmIYdeKA?si=vJYTBElFtLX9Birv

- Afro-Mexicans: One of the World's Most Forgotten Black Communities: https://www.youtube.com/watch?v=Lv4xtcvJIGo

- Indígenas de América Latina, Más Reconocidos, Aún Marginados [Indigenous of Latin America, More Recognized, Still Marginalized]: https://www.youtube.com/watch?v=Ddn6s1RPdos

- Programa especial: La situación de los pueblos indígenas en Latinoamérica [Special program: The situation of Indigenous Peoples in Latin America]: https://www.youtube.com/watch?v=NP19wBoi7Ms

REFERENCES

Adames, H. Y., & Chavez-Dueñas, N. Y. (2017). *Cultural foundations and interventions in Latino/a mental health: History, theory, and within group differences*. Routledge. https://doi.org/10.4324/9781315724058

Adames, H. Y., Chavez-Dueñas, N. Y., & Comas-Díaz, L. (2024). Introduction: Decoloniality as a transformative force in psychology. In L. Comas-Díaz, H. Y. Adames, & N. Y. Chavez-Dueñas (Eds.), *Decolonial psychology* (pp. 3–11). American Psychological Association. https://doi.org/10.1037/0000376-001

Adames, H. Y., Chavez-Dueñas, N. Y., & Jernigan, M. M. (2021). The fallacy of a raceless Latinidad: Action guidelines for centering Blackness in Latinx psychology. *Journal of Latina/o Psychology, 9*(1), 26–44. https://doi.org/10.1037/lat0000179

Adames, H. Y., Chavez-Dueñas, N. Y., Jernigan, M. M., & Sanchez, D. (2020). *We must do better: A toolkit for non-Black Latinxs who choose to address their anti-Blackness*. Immigration, Critical Race, and Cultural Equity Lab. https://icrace.files.wordpress.com/2020/06/final-antiblackness-.pdf

Adames, H. Y., Chavez-Dueñas, N. Y., & Organista, K. C. (2016). Skin color matters in Latino/a communities: Identifying, understanding, and addressing Mestizaje racial ideologies in clinical practice. *Professional Psychology: Research and Practice, 47*(1), 46–55. https://doi.org/10.1037/pro0000062

Araújo, B. Y., & Borrell, L. N. (2006). Understanding the link between discrimination, mental health outcomes, and life chances among Latinos. *Hispanic Journal of Behavioral Sciences, 28*(2), 245–266. https://doi.org/10.1177/0739986305285825

Bonilla-Silva, E. (2014). *Racism without racists: Color-blind racism and the persistence of racial inequality in America*. Rowman & Littlefield.

Chavez-Dueñas, N. Y., & Adames, H. Y. (2021). Intersectionality awakening model of womanista: A transnational treatment approach for Latinx women. *Women & Therapy, 44*(1–2), 83–100. https://doi.org/10.1080/02703149.2020.1775022

Chavez-Dueñas, N. Y., Adames, H. Y., & Organista, K. C. (2014). Skin-color prejudice and within-group racial discrimination: Historical and current impact on Latino/a populations. *Hispanic Journal of Behavioral Sciences, 36*(1), 3–26. https://doi.org/10.1177/0739986313511306

Chavez-Dueñas, N. Y., Adames, H. Y., & Perez-Chavez, J. G. (2022). Anti-colonial futures: Indigenous Latinx women healing from the wounds of racial-gendered colonialism. *Women & Therapy, 45*(2–3), 191–206. https://doi.org/10.1080/02703149.2022.2097593

Chirco, P., & Buchanan, T. M. (2022). Dark faces in white spaces: The effects of skin tone, race, ethnicity, and intergroup preferences on interpersonal judgments and voting behavior. *Analyses of Social Issues and Public Policy, 22*(1), 427–447. https://doi.org/10.1111/asap.12304

Comas-Díaz, L. (2021). Afro-Latinxs: Decolonization, healing, and liberation. *Journal of Latina/o Psychology, 9*(1), 65–75. https://doi.org/10.1037/lat0000164

Comas-Díaz, L., Adames, H. Y., & Chavez-Dueñas, N. Y. (Eds.). (2024). *Decolonial psychology: Toward anticolonial theories, research, training, and practice*. American Psychological Association. https://doi.org/10.1037/0000376-000

Consoli, A. J., López, I., & Whaling, K. M. (2022). Alternate cultural paradigms in Latinx psychology: An empirical, collaborative exploration. *Journal of Humanistic Psychology, 62*(4), 516–539. https://doi.org/10.1177/00221678211051797

Cuevas, A. G., Dawson, B. A., & Williams, D. R. (2016). Race and skin color in Latino health: An analytic review. *American Journal of Public Health, 106*(12), 2131–2136. https://doi.org/10.2105/AJPH.2016.303452

Hannon, L. (2014). Hispanic respondent intelligence level and skin tone: Interviewer perceptions from the American National Election Study. *Hispanic Journal of Behavioral Sciences, 36*(3), 265–283. https://doi.org/10.1177/0739986314540126

Helms, J. E. (2008). *A race is a nice thing to have: A guide to being a White person or understanding the White persons in your life* (2nd ed.). Alexander Street Press.

Maddox, K. B., & Gray, S. A. (2002). Cognitive representations of Black Americans: Reexploring the role of skin tone. *Personality and Social Psychology Bulletin, 28*(2), 250–259. https://doi.org/10.1177/0146167202282010

Menchú Tum, R. (1992). *Nobel lecture* [Speech]. NobelPrize.org. https://www.nobelprize.org/prizes/peace/1992/tum/26034-nobel-lecture-spanish

Mignolo, W. D. (2011). *The darker side of Western modernity: Global futures, decolonial options.* Duke University Press.

Montalvo, F. F. (2004). Surviving race: Skin color and the socialization and acculturation of Latinas. *Journal of Ethnic & Cultural Diversity in Social Work, 13*(3), 25–43. https://doi.org/10.1300/J051v13n03_02

Montalvo, F. F., & Codina, G. E. (2001). Skin color and Latinos in the United States. *Ethnicities, 1*(3), 321–341. https://doi.org/10.1177/146879680100100303

Padilla, F. M. (1985). *Latino ethnic consciousness: The case of Mexican Americans and Puerto Ricans in Chicago.* University of Notre Dame Press.

Perry, J. S., & Gámez, P. B. (2023). Latino toddlers' bilingual output and their caregivers' bilingual input and acculturation. *Infant Behavior and Development, 70*, 101804. https://doi.org/10.1016/j.infbeh.2022.101804

Salazar, M. (2019, September 16). The problem with Latinidad. *The Nation.* https://www.thenation.com/article/archive/hispanic-heritage-month-latinidad/

Sanchez, D. (2021). Introduction to special issue on AfroLatinidad: Theory, research, and practice. *Journal of Latinx Psychology, 9*(1), 1–7. https://doi.org/10.1037/lat0000186

Soler Castillo, S., & Pardo Abril, N. G. (2009). Discourse and racism in Colombia: Five centuries of invisibility and exclusion. In T. A. Van Dijk (Ed.), *Racism and discourse in Latin America* (pp. 131–170). Lexington Books.

U.S. Census Bureau. (n.d.). *Why we ask questions about . . . Ethnicity.* American Community Survey. Retrieved May 13, 2025, from https://www.census.gov/acs/www/about/why-we-ask-each-question/ethnicity/

Vera Cruz, G. (2018). The impact of face skin tone on perceived facial attractiveness: A study realized with an innovative methodology. *The Journal of Social Psychology, 158*(5), 580–590. https://doi.org/10.1080/00224545.2017.1419161

Wang, L., Gonzalez, P. D., Lau, P. L., Vaughan, E. L., & Costa, M. F. (2023). "Dando gracias": Gratitude, social connectedness, and subjective happiness among bilingual Latinx college students. *Journal of Latinx Psychology, 11*(3), 203–219. https://doi.org/10.1037/lat0000227

5

EL ENTRENAMIENTO

Training Necessities and Opportunities to Advance Bilingual Mental Health Competencies

ANDRÉS J. CONSOLI, YVETTE RAMÍREZ-GUTIÉRREZ, MAIRA ANAYA-LÓPEZ, ISABEL LÓPEZ, AND EVELYN A. MELENDEZ

In this chapter, we address some of the most crucial components of graduate school—academia, research, and clinical work—while centering the bilingual scientist–practitioner as a person. We detail opportunities to enhance not only educational experiences but also cultural ones. We discuss different forms of bilingual training in the hopes of inspiring you to advocate for further training in your current program, as needed. We offer tried-and-true tips that have enhanced our graduate school years and beyond, starting with refusing to accept "no" as the final answer when it comes to supporting and meeting our bilingual professional needs. We conclude by offering takeaways, *reflexiones*, and resources.

To maximize *el entrenamiento*, we must intentionally center the acquisition of discipline-specific bilingual skills and professional language development. We need to do so throughout our academic journey and even across our multiple professional activities, including speaking, reading, writing, presenting, and publishing. We detail here the multiple concrete ways to advance and deepen our bilingual abilities during graduate school while advocating for our own involvement and that of departments, institutions, organizations,

https://doi.org/10.1037/0000481-006
Forging Caminos: *Pathways to Becoming a Bilingual Mental Health Professional,*
M. Campos, Y. Mejia, and A. J. Consoli (Editors)

and associations in fostering bilingual professional development. Bilingual fluency is not enough, and therefore we provide examples that underscore the importance of cultural humility and responsiveness. Yet, *al pan, pan, y al vino, vino*: English-centered training is Anglo-culture training. Accordingly, decolonizing the curricula, research, and practica by gaining critical awareness of Anglo culture's hegemonic presence in training creates the space for a bilingual education that is, ultimately, bicultural education. Moreover, we affirm and advance the healing role that bilingual professional education has in redressing inequities in mental health care and research.

To become bilingual scientists–practitioners, we want to mind our linguistic abilities, together with our cultural humility and responsiveness, in the multiple roles within graduate school. Racial, ethnic, and cultural identities alone are not credentials; the advanced work we have to do, and continue to do, on ourselves while in graduate school concerning privilege, cultural humility, and responsiveness is. The verticality of academia and many professional organizations in which we may participate can be disheartening for those of us who are more used to horizontal ways of collaborating and getting things done. Leaning into transforming such places through active participation can be exhausting, yet it is one important way to advocate for Latine communities. Advocacy allows us to honor the privileges associated with graduate school; therefore, we invite you to commit to changing the things we cannot accept, such as "We have no supervisors who speak Spanish, but we need you to provide services in Spanish." That is not acceptable and, as Leonard Cohen once put it, "everybody knows" that (Cohen & Robinson, 1988). This type of situation is both unethical and illegal. Ignoring the matter does not make it go away. Advocating for proper training is an important, tangible way of refusing to further minoritize Latine communities in the United States; we trust this chapter provides tangible ways of how to go about such advocacy.

ACADEMIA

While in graduate school, we are consumers of academia. Depending on the program and the institution, we may be guided by one or more advisors or mentors (see Chapter 3, this volume), and those relationships can prove crucial in the process of socialization into the mental health profession. The same can be said about our peer relationships. Therefore, the diversity, awareness, openness, and flexibility of our cohort, including our own and those of our peers, advisors, and instructors, are important in making our graduate experience a meaningful one. The extent to which languages other than English are acknowledged and celebrated in the context of training in the talking cure is an example, among others, of a given program's sound commitment to multicultural and pluralistic training. One way to assess the extent to which a given program affirms bilingual training is to engage in a bilingual audit of it. A bilingual audit involves identifying the program's strengths (e.g., undocumented, bilingual, and international students; bilingual, international, and immigrant faculty; bilingual supervisors, research projects that use Spanish in culturally affirmative and emancipatory ways) and shortcomings (e.g., no bilingual assessment tools, no bilingual clinical forms, no bilingual staff). It is important that you conduct a bilingual audit of the program before admission, as well as during your time in it.

The program of study, which comprises coursework and other requisites, must meet certain requirements if it is to be recognized within and beyond a given institution, typically in the form of accreditation. Regrettably, there are no accrediting bodies that recognize or enforce standards in bilingual mental health training—at least not yet. Neither is there a commonly agreed-upon curriculum that guides bilingual programs, despite decades of bilingual training in professional psychology (e.g., Biever et al., 2002). Meanwhile, it seems quite difficult for monolingual colleagues and administrators to appreciate the sizable demands involved in the *camino* from a bilingual individual to a bilingual professional.

As bilingual mental health graduate students, we often are expected to make use of our Spanish language skills to provide services, translate formal documents, assist faculty members, and offer a professional level of linguistic expertise that is based solely on our identity as bilingual individuals. Yet our formal training oftentimes lacks the structured support needed for proper bilingual professional development. Accordingly, you may experience mixed emotions: On the one hand, you are eager to help *a las comunidades* by providing services and conducting research in Spanish; on the other hand, you feel anxious and frustrated because of the lack of structures that support you as an aspiring bilingual scientist–practitioner–advocate. You are not alone in feeling this way; many bilingual graduate students, we included, have been in your shoes!

As bilingual graduate students, a "hidden curricula" often includes learning new words in Spanish and its various dialects, while dedicating hours to improving our Spanish reading, writing, and speaking skills. We also need to stay up to date with the latest cultural phenomena in both languages while honoring social complexities. Moreover, when all the coursework materials are in English, the acquisition of professional terminology in Spanish requires additional efforts by all parties involved, including instructors. For example, learning the importance of naming feelings and their corresponding terms in English does not help much when we are trying to deepen and broaden the ways a given client speaks of their *enojo* in Spanish. There are important differences, subtleties, and degrees between *enojo* and terms such as *molestia, encono, disgusto, resentimiento, despecho,* and then a cluster of almost-synonyms (though organized here by approximate degrees, from lower to higher) such as *rabia/ira/cólera/furia,* and more. To complicate matters, there are cultural variations in the most common meaning of certain words, such as *bronca* in Mexico (i.e., *problema, pelea*) in contrast to, for example, *enojo,* in Argentina.

Knowing the range of feeling words and other words only in English does not foster our professional development in Spanish. Therefore, access to and use of literature developed and published in Spanish by Spanish-speaking colleagues is vital. There are many Spanish language–oriented publishing houses that feature psychology in their portfolios, such as *El Fondo de Cultura Económica* (https://fondodeculturaeconomica.com), Hogrefe TEA (https://teaediciones.com), *Manual Moderno México* (https://manualmoderno.com), *Editorial Planeta* (now *Grupo Planeta;* https://planeta.es/es), and *Siglo Veintiuno Editores* (https://sigloxxieditores.com). Yet, to compound matters, there are cultural contexts to be considered, where certain words acquire different meanings, even offensive ones. Just as it is the case of a "hidden curricula" for aspiring bilingual professionals, there is a sizable amount of "hidden homework" ahead of us, although this is commonly unacknowledged and unappreciated by monolingual colleagues and administrators. We offer a word of caution: Learning constructs such as "coping strategies or skills" may not necessarily help much when working with a monolingual, Spanish-speaking client. Moreover, knowing those constructs in Spanish, *estrategias o habilidades de afrontamiento,* may not be of much use if clients do not understand the terms. And here is where we find ourselves in the most challenging yet common predicament: describing and explaining something in another language are extremely challenging tasks because they require a broad vocabulary base, together with sophisticated cultural and societal knowledge, to ensure accuracy. This is a superpower held by bilingual professionals, and it is something to be proud of; it is a skill that requires proper recognition and commensurately higher remuneration.

A significant advancement in academia that may support the growth of bilingual graduate education in mental health is the advocacy for decolonizing graduate curricula. Such advocacy has opened up *caminos* to challenge the status quo (Comas-Díaz et al., 2024). Decolonizing the curricula involves gaining critical consciousness (i.e., *concientización*) of the hegemonic discourse that dominates academia, a mostly English-only discourse that is both explicit and implicit at multiple levels. At the granular level, instructors may further neocolonization by requiring textbooks that have been written according to WASP (White Anglo-Saxon Protestant, White Affluent Schooled Person) and WHMP (White Heterosexual Male Power and Privilege, pronounced "wimp" by Dr. Janet Helms; see Betzler, 2018) standards, endorsing theories derived from research that has focused almost exclusively on highly educated, homogeneous populations (Thalmayer et al., 2021). Moreover, courses based on such theories and textbooks further the reach of racist ideas, most noticeably anti-Black racism, be it by omission or commission, all the while ignoring intersectionality.

Current educational plans are often developed by institutions and organizations with a reactive, rather than proactive, approach to dismantling oppressive power structures that marginalize individuals on the basis of their physical appearance and cultural characteristics. To complicate matters, expressions such as "vulnerable populations" have obscured the systemic forces that vulnerate communities and their members systematically and perniciously over time. It is precisely such contexts that have made it possible for programs, institutions, and accrediting bodies to be able to abscond their responsibilities in the intentional training of bilingual graduate students while resorting to such students when needs arise (e.g., "We have a caller who only speaks Spanish, could you take that?"; "Could you translate the research protocol? Oh, yes, the consent form too"; "We need to diversify the study sample; can you help with that?"). Moreover, programs, institutions, and accrediting bodies that do not center bilingual training yet expect bilingual science and service delivery are complicit with a power structure that further minoritizes and vulnerates Latine communities.

With respect to curricula, various institutions have articulated guidelines and standards that emphasize the importance of infusing inclusion, diversity, equity, and access into all coursework. Although this is laudable, concerns related to "infusion is diffusion" remains. Most poignantly, we are concerned with the diffusion of formal, discipline-specific language training among aspiring bilingual scientists–practitioners, with distancing statements such as "All courses are *covering* it"; "Besides, students are being exposed to Spanish through practica"; and so on. Academic training requires a deliberate, concerted effort reflected in specific coursework that addresses history, culture, and language, as well as the personal and professional development of the bilingual scientist–practitioner.

Although these areas for growth do exist within academia, there is hope for improvements. This is where advocacy becomes vital. Graduate students, may feel intimidated or even unsafe voicing concerns and offering suggestions given the various power dynamics that are often present. We specify here a few examples of the actions we have undertaken, and we invite you to consider them when advocating for changes within academia, be it at the systemic, department, or individual level. We have reviewed departmental student handbooks to gain insight into potential curriculum modifications. We have created anonymous surveys or polls through which students can offer suggestions, concerns, and questions. This has resulted in gaining student and faculty support for the development of an occasional, as-needed consultation group in Spanish in our department. We have participated in committees and organizations and have gained an understanding of the processes involved in curriculum development and of opportunities to voice concerns. In addition to these examples, the National Latinx Psychological Association (https://nlpa.ws) and its special interest groups offer concrete bilingual opportunities. Similarly, the American Psychological Association of Graduate Students (https://apa.org/apags) advocates for graduate student development. We encourage you to seek out and communicate with others who may have already successfully promoted changes—*juntes somos más fuertes y podemos más.*

Graduate students and faculty members alike may be wondering about their evolving language fluency and how to evaluate it. We recommend checking out the website of the American Council on the Teaching of Foreign Languages (ACTFL; https://actfl.org) and the resources offered there. In particular, ACTFL's (2024) fourth version of its Proficiency Guidelines, provides useful taxonomies and worksheets to assess proficiency and guide curriculum development. The guidelines distinguish five levels of proficiency (i.e., novice, intermediate, advanced, superior, distinguished) and emphasize the importance of cultural awareness. They also specify three modes of communication (i.e., interpretive, interpersonal, presentational) in four domains (i.e., listening, speaking, reading, writing) while offering performance descriptors throughout. Meanwhile, free language competency development apps are readily available online (e.g., Duolingo; https://duolingo.com/).

RESEARCH

We'll say it outright: We are not interested in conducting research on Latine communities; we are committed to engaging in research with Latine communities. To do this, professional multilanguage abilities and cultural responsiveness are crucial. Although conducting research in two languages may seem daunting, in this section we provide several tried-and-true tips to help us conduct research in English and Spanish. Bilingualism is an asset, a super-power, because it permits us to conduct research in the participant's language of choice while participants get a chance to express themselves more fully. Meanwhile, our research is much more likely to be meaningful, increasing the chances that it will positively influence the mental health field. However, language is just one of many other cultural elements, so enhancing our cultural humility and responsiveness are important factors that extend beyond language fluency.

Tip 1: Continue to Develop Your Bilingual Abilities and Cultural Responsiveness

We want to commit to hone our multilanguage skills and strive for cultural humility and responsiveness over time, yet the assumption that shared language and culture equates to cultural responsiveness would likely replicate structures of oppression (Delgado-Romero et al., 2018). Our bilingual and even bicultural skills are an asset when developing research questions; designing studies and their corresponding research protocols; administering questionnaires; conducting interviews; and transcribing, translating, and interpreting the data we collect. Such skills help us better understand participants' worldview, their responses, the meaning behind their responses, and even establish a stronger rapport. For example, a bilingual and bicultural Latina researcher may find it easier to understand cultural nuances, folk sayings, and *dichos* when conducting research with Latine communities. Nonetheless, we recognize that we are cultural beings with biases and attitudes about our own and other cultural groups that are highly likely to influence our interactions with research participants and the interpretation of the data (Ojeda et al., 2011). Accordingly, it is crucial to commit ourselves to an ongoing personal and professional development whereby we examine our prejudices, including *colorismo* (a form of prejudice and discrimination, often within a racial or ethnic group, that favors individuals with lighter skin tones over those with darker skin tones), and how they may manifest in the research we design, how we interpret the findings, and beyond. It takes much time, concerted effort, and resources (e.g., personal therapy) to redress our prejudices, and therefore a developmental view and a renewed commitment to these matters are necessary.

Tip 2: Be Mindful of the Fact That Language Influences How Participants Respond

As ethical researchers, we make every effort to engage participants in the language they are most comfortable using, all the while welcoming language-switching. Bilingual individuals have a dual sense of self such that they have two distinct ways of feeling, emoting, thinking, interpreting, and interacting. For example, bilingual individuals who learn Spanish at home are more likely to feel more comfortable talking about emotional and relationship issues in Spanish (Biever et al., 2002). Thus, the chosen language(s) may affect the research process, the data collected, the findings, and the interpretation of those findings (Lu & Gatua, 2014). The language(s) the participants speak and use in the study may influence how they respond and express themselves, especially given that language can prime them to their cultural-specific values and attitudes when responding (Ramírez-Esparza et al., 2006).

Tip 3: Consider Cultural Interpretation When Translating

As bilingual investigators, we are likely to find ourselves in need of translating, which inevitably involves interpreting a range of cultural expressions, including text, gestures, and customs. We must consider participants' language proficiency level, reading comprehension, and vocabulary usage, as well as the relationship between language and emotions, linguistic equivalency, regional variances, slang, and contextual factors (Delgado-Romero et al., 2018). Some challenges we might encounter when translating and interpreting include grammatical differences between languages; false cognates, (words that appear similar but are different), like "*éxito*" and "exit"; the fact that gestures are steeped in cultural norms, such as when somebody taps their own elbow to indicate that somebody else is stingy; and much more.

To ensure that a particular research study's concepts and questions have meaning equivalence in two languages, cultural interpretation rather than literal translation is a must. In fact, literal translations do not capture the implied meaning of phrases. To illustrate, the expression "*son buena onda*" might be translated literally as "they are a good wave" instead of its implied meaning, "they are cool." Similarly, the literal translation of the expression "*metiste la pata*" might be "you put the leg in" instead of its implied meaning, "you messed up." Overall, the process of translating and interpreting is quite laborious because it requires a blend of linguistic proficiency (i.e., reading, writing, and understanding); cultural competence; and subject matter expertise, such as knowledge of psychological terminology and concepts in English and Spanish. Moreover, consultation is key: Professional interpreters (check out https://atanet.org) and cultural brokers (e.g., trusted community leaders, *promotoras y promotores de salud*) can help determine the best course of action in arriving at pertinent interpretations and securing quality data.

Tip 4: Ensure the Research Is Conducted in a Culturally Appropriate Manner

The use of cultural experts, pilot studies, and member checks may ensure that cultural nuances are being considered when striving to conduct research in a culturally appropriate manner. In a pilot study, invite participants to share feedback on all aspects of the study, and use that feedback to modify and refine the recruitment efforts, the research design, the informed consent, the protocol, the analysis, the findings, and more. Cultural experts (i.e., bilingually trained professionals with specific knowledge of the subject matter) can help us identify biases, clarify questions, and provide advice on how to phrase questions in a culturally congruent manner. We can also get help from fellow graduate students who are bilingual to check that the research is culturally congruent and addresses the research questions and, in the spirit of bartering and reciprocity, offer to help them with their own research to avoid perpetuating the taking advantage of bilingual individuals. Preparing and conducting bilingual research that is culturally appropriate and relevant takes much more time than monolingual research, yet this preparation will influence the participants' experience and the quality of the data collected for the better.

Tip 5: Commit to Publish in Accessible Venues

Although the increasing number of studies that collect data in Spanish is commendable, we are concerned that most of them are then published in English, preventing monolingual Spanish-speaking participants from accessing research findings built upon their contributions. The *Journal of Latinx Psychology* (https://apa.org/pubs/journals/lat), welcomes quotes in Spanish and requires abstracts in Spanish, although it does not publish articles in Spanish. Many of the venues where the research is published (i.e., journals that are not committed to open access) sit behind increasingly taller paywalls. In the case of the *Journal of Latinx Psychology*, accessing its articles requires a subscription to the journal or membership in the National Latinx Psychological Association. Disseminating the findings in the original language can be a proactive form of engaging in social justice. An exemplary journal is the *Revista Interamericana de Psicología* (https://journal.sipsych.org). Freely available through the *Sociedad Interamericana de Psicología*'s commitment to open access, the journal publishes articles in four of the languages in the Americas (English, Spanish, Portuguese, and French, although all are colonizing languages). There are several databases where one can access professional and scientific literature in Spanish, such as Dialnet (https://dialnet.unirioja.es), Redalyc Scientific Information System (https://redalyc.org), and SciELO (https://scielo.org; the latter with many articles in Portuguese). Access to these databases and their content is free, thanks to the commitment by the institutions and organizations that manage the databases and the journals' allegiance to open access.

CLINICAL WORK

Watching an episode of *"Caso Cerrado," "Laura,"* or *"El Gordo y la Flaca"*; a telenovela; or a reality television show, we may notice that sometimes the storyline is not about the actual words being said but how the words are said. We know that if a concerned mother gasps while exclaiming *"¡Mijo!"*, what follows is drastically different than when a concerned mother enters the scene sobbing and exclaiming, *"¡Mijooooo!"* Both scenarios typically precede a classic dramatic telenovela scene. However, the gasp indicates an element of surprise and may foreshadow a *chisme* being revealed among characters. Meanwhile, a mother sobbing before exclaiming may be an indication that either she or her son have been horribly hurt. In typical telenovela fashion, the episode would end on such a cliffhanger scene for an added dramatic effect.

As mental health professionals, we understand that language is not solely verbal or written; language is also communicated through tone, body language, and gestures. Becoming a bilingual mental health professional involves more than speaking another language or speaking the language fluently; it requires a cultural familiarity that appreciates the nuances involved in communication. Such nuances are honored in cultural humility and responsiveness, where language is appreciated as one of many cultural elements. Said differently, it is not possible to fully understand a language without other elements, such as *usos y costumbres*, that give meaning to the words that constitute a language. *Para muestra, un botón:* A common synonym of the word "insect" in Spanish in one region is a slang term for male genitalia in another. Tools such as artificial intelligence translators are likely to run into trouble with implied and metaphorical meanings that frequently are lost in translation and may likely lead to potentially serious misunderstandings. Next, we explore various aspects of clinical training in which culture and language are paramount.

Dialects

It is important to keep in mind Spanish's cultural and linguistic variations. For example, if a clinician identifies as Panamanian and the client identifies as Bolivian, it may be helpful for the clinician to acknowledge that although both individuals may identify as Latine there may be moments when cultural

differences are stumbled upon. These differences may include cultural traditions, dialects, mannerisms, idioms, and expressions. The clinician may speak
a Caribbean variation of Spanish with specific phonetic uses, whereas the
Bolivian client may pronounce words differently, or even use terms in Quechua
(an indigenous language spoken in the Andean highlands). The clinician can
acknowledge cultural similarities and differences while explicitly stating their
openness to learning from the client's knowledge and worldview.

A clinician's prioritization of self-reflection will be crucial to uncover one's
implicit biases and create decolonized therapeutic spaces. Judging certain
accents as informal, uneducated, or too fast, for instance, often carries racist,
colorist, anti-Black, elitist, or classist undertones. For example, identifiers such
as *del rancho, del interior,* or *de la capital* can reference someone's socioeconomic status with negative or positive connotations. Even some therapeutic suggestions may not imply culturally congruent meanings, such as with
notions characterized by individualism, like self-care and self-compassion.
Reframing the notions to express care as a form of reenergizing the self to
better serve clients' communities may be more readily welcomed by a client
from a collectivist culture.

If the clinician is not confident in their Spanish fluency, they may want to
state so while welcoming feedback and opportunities to provide clarifications,
as well as for any cultural or ethnic assumptions made accidentally. Given
Spanish's gendered quality, we strive for inclusive language by using terms
like "your partner" or "*tu pareja.*" One may also substitute gendered terms
ending in the letter "a" or "o" with the letter "e." For example, "Latina/o" may
be written as "Latine" so as to be concise and inclusive of all gender identities.
Becoming bilingual professionals entails not only education but also personal
exploration of implicit biases and culturally learned norms, and although we
may try our best to evade miscommunications or misunderstandings in our
clinical work, these are frequently common aspects of learning. Within- and
between-group differences are reminders to lean into humble curiosity and
growth. So, do not let dialect differences discourage you from harnessing your
overall potential to connect meaningfully with other Spanish-speaking or
Latine people! *¡Síguele!*

Cultural Nuances

Expressions in Spanish do not always translate well to English. In the case
of "*desahogar,*" for example, a direct translation may be "to undo the act of
drowning," but the translation does not do justice to the complexity of the
expression. *Desahogarse* involves the desire to vent or verbalize internal
thoughts or concerns and is likely to be followed by a sense of relief. It is

different from "unburden," which in Spanish is *"me saqué un peso de encima."* In addition, there are idioms of distress unique to the Spanish language such as *"susto," "nervios,"* and *"ataque de nervios." Spanglish,* a creative, evolving combination of Spanish and English, is an informal dialect or slang worth noting when meeting with bilingual clients. *"Parqueadero,"* a Spanglish term for "parking lot," uses Spanish language grammar and spelling (the "que" for the "k" sound and the "-adero" ending) for the English word "parking." Expressions such as *"lonche"* and *"Vaporú"* are other terms we may hear a Latine client use in their conversational speech.

To illustrate, Samantha (a pseudonym) is a low-income Indigenous/ Mixtec, cisgender, Brown woman who previously lived in Mexico. She does not own a car, have access to reliable transportation, or own a computer, so she attends sessions via phone calls. Although she understands some Spanish phrases, she is fluent in Mixtec. Her Spanish–English bilingual clinician uses an interpreter. During one of the three-way calls, Samantha informed the clinician that she was sad and missing her hometown. It quickly became clear to the clinician, who had also been raised in Mexico, that although they both resided in the same state of their native country, they had very different childhood experiences. The clinician noted this to Samantha while also expressing her desire to learn more if Samantha felt comfortable sharing. With time, the therapeutic alliance strengthened, and the therapist helped Samantha get connected to resources.

This vignette illustrates some of the numerous multifaceted cases among Latine clients and Latine clinicians. Cultural humility is vital in learning about client's needs.

Selecting Clinical Sites

Providing therapeutic services is just as important as receiving guidance and support from bilingual and bicultural mental health professionals. We want you to consider this, as well as other needs you may have as a bilingual and/or bicultural trainee, when exploring field placements or clinical sites. For example, does it matter to you if most of your clients are Spanish speakers? Does the site provide supervision in Spanish? Is leading with a social justice framework important to you, to the site, or for the needs of your clientele? The answers to these questions have the potential to alter the professional development experiences you may seek. Connecting with current clinicians at prospective field placements to increase your knowledge is important, and so is dialoguing with current and former trainees at that site. Nonetheless, sites can change dramatically on the basis of personnel coming and going, and the experiences of each trainee can vary significantly.

Keep in mind the goal of becoming a bilingual mental health scientist–practitioner: If your caseload is solely in one language (e.g., monolingual Spanish speakers), or if supervision is provided in only one language (e.g., English), your bilingual training is likely to be compromised. Furthermore, many times bilingual abilities are taken for granted. Let's not allow sites to get away with that. When interviewing, ask directly: "What is your monetary supplement for bilingual professional abilities?" You will want to respectfully convey your disappointment, if none is provided, and your expectation that sites will be able to redress that. Again, as engaged bilingual professionals, we commit ourselves to change the things we cannot accept.

Supervisión of Clinical Work

¡Échale ganas! You have the power to one day become the bilingual and bicultural supervisor current supervisees may not have. There are resources to turn to, such as the multicultural developmental supervisory model (Field et al., 2010). This model integrates specific Latine multicultural counseling competencies and Latine ethnic identity theory with developmental theories of supervision. The model exposes the complex processes that influence the supervision dyad to offer guidance and support to the supervisor and the supervisee as well as the institutions in which supervision takes place (see Chapter 6, this volume).

Resources for Clinical Interventions

In addition to acknowledging, learning about, and addressing the cultural variations of Latines as clinicians, it is important to find and provide resources in Spanish for Spanish-speaking clients. Unfortunately, as graduate students opportunities for supervision in Spanish are uncommon. So, we spend time learning on our own how to express concepts such as self-compassion and mindfulness, to make them accessible to our Spanish-speaking *comunidades*, all the while staying mindful of possible neocolonizing practices. We use worksheets or activities with our clients from online resources such as Los Niños Services (https://losninos.com) or Therapist Aid (https://therapistaid.com). Moreover, a program may offer guided meditations in English, yet if our client is monolingual in Spanish, we will need to identify a culturally congruent one in Spanish. The Mindful Awareness Research Center at the University of California, Los Angeles, offers such resources in Spanish (https://tinyurl.com/2cf4zhd4) and Mixtec (https://tinyurl.com/3whakefc). For Latines without pertinent documentation in the United States, we need to identify local organizations and resources, such as *La Resistencia* (https://laresistencianw.org)

in Washington State, Siembra NC (https://siembranc.org) in North Carolina, and the Georgia Latino Alliance for Human Rights (http://glahr.org). The American Psychological Association offers a free downloadable resource guide for ethnic minority graduate students and suggests articles related to clinical training and working with ethnic minority clients (https://tinyurl.com/mrxkvpma). The American Psychological Association website contains multiple articles in Spanish that can be downloaded for free (https://apa.org/search?query=Spanish).

ENHANCING EDUCATIONAL AND CULTURAL EXPERIENCES

There are other ways to enhance our educational experiences while in graduate school. Here are some possibilities:

- Search the directory of the graduate student organizations on your campus. Some colleges and universities may have cultural centers specific to Latines, and others may have organizations that serve students of color. The Educational Opportunity Program, which provides social and cultural events for the student community as part of their primary services, is a resource offered at various universities (see, e.g., https://calstate.edu/attend/student-services/eop). The Society for the Advancement of Chicanos/Hispanics and Native Americans in Science (https://sacnas.org/) is a nationwide organization located across numerous campuses with the intention of supporting students on their academic journeys within the science, technology, engineering, and mathematics fields. Multicultural centers on campuses tend to host events, ranging from art gallery activities, to guest speakers, to film showings, related to enhancing cultural knowledge in the community.

- Search social media sites for bilingual, licensed mental health professionals and those who can offer insight into Latine culture and the Spanish language. Join a local or national group of Latine therapists, researchers, advocates, and allies such as the National Latinx Psychological Association, the Latinx Therapists Network (@latinxtherapy, https://instagram.com/latinxtherapy), or the San Francisco Bay Latinx Psych group (sfbay latinxpsych@googlegroups.com). Social media can be used to increase awareness of cultural shifts or movements, such as *nalgona* positivity, which addresses eating disorders with a body-affirmative approach for Black, Indigenous, and People of Color communities (e.g., https://nalgonapositivitypride.com). There are also commercial applications to help people learn or improve their Spanish skills (e.g., https://jiveworld. com) as well as find community practice opportunities (e.g., https:// meetup.com).

- Read, watch, listen to, and learn from those who have come before us (e.g., Delgado-Romero et al., 2017). Books to consider in our pursuit of *estar bien para servir bien* include *Rest is Resistance: A Manifesto* by Tricia Hersey (2022), the founder of The Nap Ministry (https://thenapministry. wordpress.com), and *Pedagogy of the Oppressed* by Paulo Freire (2017). Public radio stations and their corresponding programs are inspiring sources in our bilingual development (e.g., https://radioambulante.org, https://radiobilingue.org).

- Think about what our favorite cultural events, games, hobbies, and foods are. May we be able to enjoy these activities on campus or in a local community center, nearby Latine grocery store, *bodega*, or *panadería*? Maybe a concert in Spanish, a *bachata* dance group, a rodeo, or a *fútbol* game? Finding these experiences is more challenging in some areas than others. So, if we cannot find the cultural experiences we are looking for, let's create one! We can initiate and host events on campus or at local community centers, such as a game of *lotería con música y pan dulce*. It may be an opportunity to be creative. *¡No nos rindamos! ¡Sí se puede!*

Regardless of how we may choose to increase and expand our clinical experiences, we celebrate our doing so! As the phrase goes, *ponte las pilas*— we also want to cheer ourselves on with an understanding that our value and power as professionals are not derived from awards, client volume, accolades, publications, or other means of production. As clinicians, we care so much for our clients, and clients tend to benefit from the presence and clarity offered by us. Yet in order to be mentally and physically present for our clients, we must learn to prioritize caring for ourselves. To reframe the potential pressure to address other's commands or needs before addressing our own, we say *"Ponte las pilas y hazlo con cariño."*

BILINGUAL TRAINING

In this section, we review several bilingual training resources, organized under a taxonomy that comprises specialization, certification, and immersion. We do so with the goal of appreciating some of the offerings and in the hope that at wherever place in the *caminos* we find ourselves, and whatever program or institution we are in, we can use this information to advocate for the intentional, professional training of our bilingual abilities. If you found it difficult to identify programs in the United States that are intentional about bilingual professional development while you were applying to graduate school, you are not alone. It requires much time and effort.

Back in 2012, a directory of Latine behavioral health training was published by the Alliance for Latino Behavioral Health Workforce Development that also appeared on the Migrant Clinicians Network site (https:// migrantclinician.org; see National Resource Center for Hispanic Mental Health, 2012). The directory identified graduate programs with a Latine focus as well as certification programs and research opportunities with the Latine population. Of note, the National Latino Behavioral Health Association (https://nlbha.org) and the Migrant Clinicians Network sites include several training and intervention resources for addressing various mental health concerns among the Latine population. Although these resources may not necessarily specify Spanish–English bilingual training, they nevertheless center Latine communities and are a helpful supplement to current professional training. After the 2012 directory was published, Stringer (2015) discussed the sizable need for Spanish-speaking U.S. psychologists and the noticeably limited training opportunities for them. The article was accompanied by a list of master's and doctoral programs that offer Latine behavioral health training. Smith (2018) later revisited the subject and offered additional resources, as did Consoli and Flores (2020).

We are concerned about the numerous programs that have been discontinued either because their grant funding ended or because of lack of institutional commitment beyond one person's involvement. Examples include the Latino Mental Health Research Training Program, a joint effort between faculty in the United States and Mexico; the Alliant International University's Latin American Family Therapy certificate in Mexico City; and the Texas State University's Project SUPERB (Scholars Using Psychology and Education to Research Bilinguals).

Specialization

In this section, we highlight some graduate programs; they may serve as models when advocating for changes to graduate curriculum elsewhere. Perhaps the most well-known Latine-focused specialization opportunity is the Psychological Services for Spanish Speaking Populations certificate offered by Our Lady of the Lake University's PsyD in Counseling Psychology program (https://tinyurl.com/2fas982u). The program embeds Spanish courses within its curriculum for graduate students who are conversationally proficient in

Spanish, including practicum experience with a Spanish-speaking team. Similarly, the University of Oregon's Spanish Language Psychological Service and Research Specialization (https://education.uoregon.edu/cpsy/slpsr) offers graduate-level coursework and experiential requirements in Spanish. The latter includes lectures, panel presentations, and conferences in Spanish and a clinically relevant oral presentation in Spanish as a capstone project. Another example is Pepperdine University's MA in Clinical Psychology with an emphasis in working with Latine communities, which is part of Aliento, The Center for Latinx Communities (https://gsep.pepperdine.edu/aliento). The program includes experiential Spanish language development courses to practice technical Spanish.

California State University, Fullerton, offers the *Ánimo* Latinx Counseling Concentration in its MS Counseling program (https://hhd.fullerton.edu/Counsel/degree/animo.html), which focuses on applying the concepts learned in the program to Latine communities. Texas State University's Department of Counseling, Leadership, Adult Education, and School Psychology offers a bilingual track (https://tinyurl.com/4c738846) that is open to any language aside from English. It includes elective coursework and bilingual supervision in students' field placements. Another opportunity is the Latino Mental Health Program concentration offered by William James College for its master's programs in School Psychology, Organizational Psychology, and Clinical Mental Health Counseling (https://tinyurl.com/56tccta9). This program is also offered in its PsyD programs in Leadership Psychology and Clinical Psychology. The Latino Mental Health Program concentration is a combination of courses that focus on culture and clinical work and supports students of Latine descent who have various levels of Spanish fluency.

As graduate students, we can advocate for our training programs to enhance the curriculum to be inclusive of culture and language—as with the examples already discussed—to foster our professional growth as bilingual professionals. Furthermore, we can reach out to faculty and directors of model programs to inquire about ways we can propose curriculum changes and perhaps even ask for sample syllabi to inform new courses within our respective programs.

Certification

Examples of certificate programs include Denver University's MSW Certificate in Latinx Social Work, which involves an intensive Spanish language immersion component and is available to both Spanish-speaking students and those who do not speak Spanish (https://tinyurl.com/3brjs2ym). Meanwhile, the

University of Miami is in the process of securing authorization for an online, 16-week Latino Mental Health Professional Development Training Certificate.

The University of Wisconsin–Madison's *Esperanza* certificate (https://tinyurl.com/rk55k36e) is available to graduate students at that institution and includes coursework, micro skills training, and case management support.

The University of Texas Rio Grande Valley (https://tinyurl.com/bdh2h52m) offers an online and on-campus bilingual counseling certificate. The 15-hour online certificate is directed toward mental health professionals and people currently enrolled in a counseling program from all over the United States. Other options include the Online Graduate Certificate in Social and Community Psychology from The Chicago School of Professional Psychology (https://thechicagoschool.edu/programs/psychology/social-community-psychology/certificate/) and the Graduate Certificate in Bilingual Counseling at the University of Texas at San Antonio (https://tinyurl.com/muvtec45), which is available to students at the university and to non–degree-seeking licensed professional counselors. In addition to these examples of behavioral health training in Spanish, there are also general, Spanish graduate certification programs, such as the one offered by the University of New Hampshire (https://tinyurl.com/4hrxe56k), which is designed for professionals and graduate students of various disciplines to improve their proficiency in oral and written Spanish and promote cultural understanding of Spanish-speaking communities.

Nepantlah (https://nepantlah.education) is a contemporary effort that makes use of multiple platforms to train a range of bilingual students, cultural workers, and professionals. It seeks to create a professional network for bilingual and multicultural mental health service providers while deepening efforts in social justice advocacy. Nepantlah offers trainings that take a decolonial framework in the analysis of language. These trainings also qualify as continuing professional education credits for various mental health disciplines.

Immersion

Because many graduate programs are English centered, the importance of bilingualism and cultural responsiveness, which are crucial in providing quality mental health services, are often neglected. As a result, graduate students with a strong interest in offering mental health services to Spanish-speaking and Latine populations, but who lack access to bilingual and cultural training or concentrations within their programs, find themselves compelled to explore alternative opportunities beyond their current academic institutions. Immersion programs that center culture and language are great chances to obtain formal training and to build and develop personal and professional skills while becoming a bilingual scientist–practitioner.

Smith's (2018) article includes a list of cultural and language programs that notes immersion programs that center Spanish, culture, and mental health. On the one hand, most of these immersion programs are unique to students in a particular university. For example, the Williams James College's Latino Mental Health Program concentration includes a 5-week summer immersion in Ecuador and focuses on clinical, cultural, language, and field experience. On the other hand, few programs are open to students from different universities and disciplines. Pertinent opportunities include the Ecuador Professional Preparation Program (EPPP; https://ecuadorppp.com/) and the Psychology and Spanish Elective Opportunity (PASEO) program in Perú (https://paseo-program.com/). Both programs take place over the summer, when it is more convenient for students to take advantage of extracurricular trainings. The EPPP is designed for graduate students and mental health professionals alike. Its mission is for graduate students to develop and strengthen their Spanish skills to confidently provide mental health care to Spanish-speaking clients. The EPPP offers the Cultural Boost Experience for students, which lasts 2-1/2 weeks, during which they receive instruction in Spanish and the opportunity to practice it by working in a community facility that addresses mental health while receiving daily supervision in Spanish.

The PASEO program provides students and other psychology professionals with mental health training in Spanish with the intention of improving mental health services for Spanish speakers in the United States. The program goal is twofold: (a) help students build competent Spanish language skills for use in mental health settings and (b) increase knowledge and competencies in working with Latine youth and families. The PASEO program also includes training that centers ethnocultural mental health evaluations when assessing Spanish-speaking Latine families.

Immersion programs like EPPP and PASEO seek to facilitate the educational and professional development of bilingual graduate students. Bilingual students are understandably often not comfortable with providing services in Spanish because the Spanish used in everyday conversations does not typically translate into that used in clinical professional settings. This highlights the need for professional training that centers Spanish and culture. However, the limited number of existing specializations, certifications, and immersive programs for students to develop their bilingual, cultural, and professional skills underscores the need to advocate for more programs, and certainly more is desired. Unfortunately, when pursuing external opportunities, such as certification training or immersive experiences, expenses are likely borne by the students themselves, adding further financial burden. Through collective efforts, we must demand adequate bilingual training and respect for our bilingual abilities in ensuring that we are properly trained to deliver quality professional work with our Latine communities.

CONCLUSION

We acknowledge that there are many challenges to be encountered in our training as aspiring bilingual scientists–practitioners. To overcome those challenges, we should embrace the privilege of our educational journey, with its noticeable joys, and engage in disruptive and constructive actions, joining forces as a collective of bilingual graduate students and scientists–practitioners to promote transformation. Put differently, becoming bilingual scientists–practitioners in professional psychology involves overcoming sizable, systemic obstacles. In this pursuit, we should treasure our bilingual and multicultural know-how (i.e., our superpowers) and act as a group of committed people united by a cause. Our superpowers come with a tall order of responsibility: to give back to our communities through advocacy. Affirmative, transformative, emancipatory bilingual training is about changing the things we cannot accept. Remember, we are not alone in this journey, and perseverance is key. Here is to our continued growth and success!

TAKEAWAYS

- One concrete action that facilitates bilingual professional development is the advancement of curriculum decolonization.

- When committing yourself to conducting research with Spanish-speaking communities, it is important to consider how language influences participants' responses, the sizable challenges involved in translation and interpretation, and the significance of publishing findings in the language in which data were collected.

- Bilingual professional training at the clinical and research levels involves the centering of cultural humility and responsiveness.

- Training opportunities such as specializations, certifications, and immersion experiences can facilitate the development and strengthening of bilingual professional skills.

REFLEXIONES

- In the "Research" section we provided multiple tips on how to conduct bilingual empirical studies. Which tip feels the most feasible for you? What other tips would you include?

- We hope you use the resources we have provided as potential avenues for advancing your bilingual clinical skills. What are you doing now to foster your bilingual skills in clinical settings?

- We have offered suggestions for campus organizations, in addition to cultural events, that readers may seek to honor our diverse cultures. What are some cultural outlets at your institution of training, or personal pastimes, that support your personal and professional bilingual skills?

- Of the exemplar certifications discussed, which may be of interest in your own training?

RECOMMENDED READING

Peters, M. L., Sawyer, C. B., Guzmán, M. R., & Graziani, C. (2014). Supporting the development of Latino bilingual mental health professionals. *Journal of Hispanic Higher Education, 13*(1), 15–31. https://doi.org/10.1177/1538192713514611

Platt, J. J. (2012). A Mexico City–based immersion education program: Training mental health clinicians for practice with Latino communities. *Journal of Marital & Family Therapy, 38*(2), 352–364. https://doi.org/10.1111/j.1752-0606.2010.00208.x

REFERENCES

American Council on the Teaching of Foreign Languages. (2024). *ACTFL proficiency guidelines 2024.* https://www.actfl.org/uploads/files/general/Resources-Publications/ACTFL_Proficiency_Guidelines_2024.pdf

Betzler, K. (2018, February 23). Award winning professor discusses race and privilege. *The Racquet Press.* https://theracquet.org/4433/news/award-winning-professor-discusses-race-and-privilege/

Biever, J. L., Castaño, M. T., de las Fuentes, C., González, C., Servín-López, S., Sprowls, C., & Tripp, C. G. (2002). The role of language in training psychologists to work with Hispanic clients. *Professional Psychology: Research and Practice, 33*(3), 330–336. https://doi.org/10.1037/0735-7028.33.3.330

Cohen, L., & Robinson, S. (1988). Everybody knows [Song]. On *I'm Your Man.* Columbia Records.

Comas-Díaz, L., Adames, H. Y., & Chavez-Dueñas, N. Y. (Eds.). (2024). *Decolonial psychology: Toward anticolonial theories, research, training, and practice.* American Psychological Association. https://doi.org/10.1037/0000376-000

Consoli, A. J., & Flores, I. (2020). The teaching and training of bilingual (English/Spanish) mental health professionals in the US. In G. Rich, A. Padilla López, L. Ebersöhn, J. Taylor, & S. Morrissey (Eds.), *Teaching psychology around the world* (pp. 441–454). Cambridge Scholars.

Delgado-Romero, E. A., Singh, A. A., & De Los Santos, J. (2018). *Cuéntame*: The promise of qualitative research with Latinx populations. *Journal of Latina/o Psychology, 6*(4), 318–328. https://doi.org/10.1037/lat0000123

Delgado-Romero, E. A., Unkefer, E. N. S., Capielo, C., & Crowell, C. N. (2017). *El que oye consejos, llega a viejo*: Examining the published life narratives of U.S. Latino/a psychologists. *Journal of Latina/o Psychology, 5*(3), 127–141. https://doi.org/10.1037/lat0000071

Field, L. D., Chavez-Korell, S., & Domenech Rodríguez, M. M. (2010). *No hay rosas sin espinas*: Conceptualizing Latina–Latina supervision from a multicultural developmental supervisory model. *Training and Education in Professional Psychology, 4*(1), 47–54. https://doi.org/10.1037/a0018521

Freire, P. (2017). *Pedagogy of the oppressed*. Penguin Classics.

Hersey, T. (2022). *Rest is resistance: A manifesto*. Hachette.

Lu, Y., & Gatua, M. W. (2014). Methodological considerations for qualitative research with immigrant populations: Lessons from two studies. *The Qualitative Report, 19*(30), 1–16. https://doi.org/10.46743/2160-3715/2014.1035

National Resource Center for Hispanic Mental Health. (2012, February). *Directory of Latina/o behavioral health training*. https://www.migrantclinician.org/files/Directory2012.pdf

Ojeda, L., Flores, L. Y., Meza, R. R., & Morales, A. (2011). Culturally competent qualitative research with Latino immigrants. *Hispanic Journal of Behavioral Sciences, 33*(2), 184–203. https://doi.org/10.1177/0739986311402626

Ramírez-Esparza, N., Gosling, S. D., Benet-Martínez, V., Potter, J. P., & Pennebaker, J. W. (2006). Do bilinguals have two personalities? A special case of cultural frame switching. *Journal of Research in Personality, 40*(2), 99–120. https://doi.org/10.1016/j.jrp.2004.09.001

Smith, B. L. (2018, June). Spanish-speaking psychologists in demand: By learning or perfecting their Spanish, practitioners can better serve a large and growing population. *APA Monitor, 49*(6), 68. https://www.apa.org/monitor/2018/06/spanish-speaking

Stringer, H. (2015). *Se solicita: Psicólogos que hablen español* (Wanted: Spanish-speaking psychologists). APA *GradPSYCH Magazine, 4*, 32. https://www.apa.org/gradpsych/2015/04/spanish-speaking

Thalmayer, A. G., Toscanelli, C., & Arnett, J. J. (2021). The neglected 95% revisited: Is American psychology becoming less American? *American Psychologist, 76*(1), 116–129. https://doi.org/10.1037/amp0000622

6
ENSÉÑAME A VOLAR
Supervisión y Mentoría *of Bilingual Trainees*

JACQUELINE FUENTES, ECKART WERTHER,
CHARMAINE MORA-OZUNA, GEYSA FLORES, AND
EDWARD A. DELGADO-ROMERO

Supervision and mentorship are vital components of your success and development in the mental health profession. Both are long-term, relationally orientated experiences that require commitment and aim to help you achieve your goals (Mills et al., 2005). Supervision—an educational and training process that is work focused and manages, supports, develops, and evaluates your application of skills (Milne, 2007)—plays a formal role throughout your training and career. Supervisors, in addition to serving a legal and gatekeeping role (Behnke, 2005), help facilitate your development of competency skills related to assessment, psychotherapy or counseling, crises management responses, ethical decision making, identification of resources and referrals, and professional identity and orientation. Supervisors help you integrate the theoretical knowledge you have acquired in the classroom and apply it in a clinical space. Supervision is required throughout your training, such as when completing assessment and therapy practica or during your internship training experiences. Supervision is also common in various professional processes, such as acquiring licensure, seeking certain board certifications, or completing certain types of specialty training.

https://doi.org/10.1037/0000481-007
Forging Caminos: *Pathways to Becoming a Bilingual Mental Health Professional,*
M. Campos, Y. Mejia, and A. J. Consoli (Editors)

In addition to the relational, developmental, and evaluative functions generally expected of supervision, bilingual supervision helps bilingual trainees focus on the interplay of culture, acculturation, multicultural and linguistic competency skills, and the sociopolitical realities of their clients (Fuertes, 2004). Bilingual supervision is a multicultural and relational space that facilitates the understanding and appreciation of the complexities of sexuality, spirituality, class, gender, race, and language (Lugo, 2021). According to Gonzalez et al. (2015), "bilingual supervision can be said to occur when one member of the client–counselor–supervisor triad is communicating primarily in a language other than English" (p. 185).

It is equally important to acknowledge the role of bilingual *mentoría* in one's development as a bilingual scientist–practitioner. *Mentoría* may involve establishing an informal mentoring relationship with a supervisor who offers guidance, support, and serves as a role model to aid in your professional development (American Psychological Association [APA], 2012). This journey is one best forged *con el poder de nuestres compañeres y comunidades*—providing us the *apoyo* and mentorship needed to increase and assert your presence in the field. Accessing bilingual *mentoría* celebrates one's presence and helps one transcend oppressive and discriminatory gatekeeping because it offers guidance, holistic support, and overall care as you navigate the various aspects of the profession. Competent bilingual mentors are also invested in providing culturally responsive mentoring (Castellanos et al., 2022).

Bilingual supervision and mentorship have certain shared qualities and expectations that are critical to your development. First, your mentor or clinical supervisor should appreciate the merits of working with you, given your commitment to language justice (Dennis et al., 2024). Your racial/ethnic identity and bilingual skills deserve recognition, although these facets should certainly not be the sole value of your professional worth. You should not feel tokenized by your supervisor or mentor because of your racial/ethnic identity, and your presence should not be centered on your ability to serve as a translator (Valencia-Garcia & Montoya, 2018) or as a language broker (Delgado-Romero et al., 2018). Instead, your bilingualism and bicultural insights complement many other skills you possess. You have not reached this point by accident but rather through *esfuerzos, sacrificios*, and *logros académicos*. We encourage you and your bilingual supervisors and mentors to celebrate these successes throughout your training.

Bilingual supervisors and mentors should be well versed on issues relevant to Latinx communities in the United States while balancing the everyday experiences of being a bilingual trainee. This includes considerations for language and code-switching, bicultural identity, awareness of professional developmental needs, and honoring the additional workload and challenges you may experience (Gonzalez et al., 2015; Trepal et al., 2019; Valencia-Garcia & Montoya, 2018). Having a bilingual supervisor or mentor with whom you share language or cultural similarities can considerably benefit your development as a bilingual clinician. Linguistically, you can express yourself in the language or a language combination that best suits your strengths, such as talking about a particular emotion or cultural idiom in Spanish during your supervisory and mentorship meetings.

Bilingual supervisors and mentors should assist you in enhancing your professional identity and socialize you to the profession's norms. They should incorporate relevant ethical guidelines, such as those established by the National Latinx Psychological Association (2020). You may experience pressures to overextend yourself simply because you are bilingual, such as being asked to take on more cases or performing uncompensated work (e.g., translating materials). Your bilingual supervisors and mentors can support you by teaching and modeling creative strategies to accompany Spanish-speaking communities, effectively navigate stressors, create a healthy work–life balance, set appropriate boundaries, and recognize and support your growth areas.

Bilingual supervisors and mentors take the time to create spaces to discuss your experience as a cultural being. They model how to grapple with anti-Indigeneity and anti-Blackness, which you may have internalized or encountered in your training. Discussing such realities is a form of liberation for you and the Latinx communities because it promotes critical consciousness, decoloniality, and owning biases to enact change. Having access to bilingual supervisors and mentors is also crucial in unburdening the emotional load of navigating multiple systems so that we do not personalize the outcomes of oppressive conditions and remain rooted in social justice values when engaging in bilingual work (Godinez Gonzalez, 2022).

CLINICAL SUPERVISION

Bilingual supervision is unique compared with monolingual English supervision because it centers on the role and interplay of language, culture, and environment in your clinical work (Gonzalez et al., 2015). Within this space, you are encouraged to speak in *español*/Spanglish when discussing case concerns, role playing, or reviewing technical language (Trepal et al., 2019). Because language serves as the medium by which you articulate thoughts, distress, and emotions (Valencia-Garcia & Montoya, 2018), processing this clinical content in its original linguistic form is recommended (Perry & Sias,

2018). Doing so allows nuances from sessions (e.g., cultural expressions, metaphors, and changes in tone) to be captured instead of being lost in translation (Gonzalez et al., 2015). Your bilingual supervisor should strive to foster a robust supervisory alliance with you one that focuses on a collaboration that values your cultural heritage and personal experiences. This includes discussing your strengths and comfort level in providing services in Spanish and your linguistic and cultural competence.

What to Expect From Bilingual Supervision

Given the complexity of bilingual clinical work and its challenging aspects, creating a solid connection to and relationship with your supervisor will be essential to nurture your growth. When meeting with your supervisor for the first time, review the expectations of bilingual supervision. You may receive a formal or informal supervisory contract that lists your roles and responsibilities. These discussions should clearly outline aspects of bilingual supervision, such as boundaries and expectations, frequency of meetings, remediation, and grievance procedures. We encourage you to ask questions, seek clarification, and, ideally, have a chance to identify and express your training goals and needs.

The initial stages of the supervisory relationship can be an excellent time to discuss your skills with your supervisor and consider how your competencies align with your projected developmental milestone attainment. Your goals as a bilingual clinician can include opportunities to administer and interpret bilingual assessments, expand your diagnostic skills by considering cultural and contextual factors, use culturally adapted interventions, write case conceptualizations using cultural formulations while integrating liberatory and decolonial theoretical perspectives, and identifying and discussing countertransference. The more precise you are about what you need from your supervisor to feel supported, the more likely it will be that your supervisor can either meet that need or offer you alternative resources to help enhance your clinical skills. Explore your strengths and areas of growth with your supervisor, and leverage their expertise to facilitate your clinical growth and promote your clinical self-efficacy.

As is true of your monolingual counterparts, bilingual supervision should initially focus on the importance of common factors (Wampold, 2015). For example, bilingual supervisors should first help you understand the value of the therapeutic relationship, encourage you to engage in collaborative goal-setting with clients, and provide empathy. Next, you will likely begin practicing and applying therapeutic techniques, including interventions from specific theoretical orientations you have learned during coursework. As a bilingual trainee, your bilingual supervisor can help build your linguistic competency skills, promote culturally based perspectives, and offer resources in Spanish. Compiling and organizing resources in Spanish (e.g., handouts, worksheets, questionnaires) from the beginning will benefit you as you can use them throughout your career. You and your supervisor can also take the time to review specific content to help you decide how to interpret regional dialects or nuances in clients' verbal and nonverbal communication. Supervision will quickly transition to helping you integrate those theories in formulating case conceptualizations, developing treatment plans, and identifying interventions on the basis of these conceptualizations. As you become more experienced, supervision should also evolve to discuss psychotherapy and treatment progression in tandem with guidance on challenging oppressive systems.

In addition to your therapy practicum, part of your training will likely include completing assessments, conducting evaluations, or making diagnostic decisions. Bilingual supervision can provide a space to challenge mainstream conceptualizations of functioning and psychopathology. It also can help you identify appropriate psychological tests and measures normed and validated among Spanish-speaking samples. Because of the limited culturally competent test selection for Latinxs, bilingual supervisors should also ensure that the measures chosen are administered and interpreted in a culturally attuned manner. Supervisors can guide you to attend to language, bilingualism, and cultural etiologies of distress that contextualize Latinx clients' clinical presentation and performance on specific standardized measures.

Supervision should reinforce your Spanish proficiency by helping you tailor your clinical language to promote culturally attuned psychoeducation. For instance, if you are assessing or providing psychoeducation on attention-deficit/hyperactivity disorder (ADHD) to a Spanish-speaking caregiver, your supervisor could help you consider alternative terms, metaphors, or tools to ensure they understand the etiology of, presentation, and treatment options for ADHD. Simply providing the direct translation, *trastorno por déficit de atención e hiperactividad*, does not capture the depth of what characterizes ADHD. Caregivers must receive culturally relevant examples to promote a neuroexpansive understanding and access to psychiatric, educational, and familial supports. Examples of phrases that may be helpful to communicate ADHD include: *"dificultades de atención y aprendizaje," "dificultades en estar quieto,"* or *"dificultades en prestar y sostener la atención."* We encourage you to use bilingual supervision to role-play how to further explain to caregivers the neuroscience behind ADHD, to address difficulties with executive functioning, and to challenge unhelpful beliefs that caregivers may have about their children.

It is vital that bilingual supervision review culturally informed interpersonal styles to build rapport and trust among your clients. Incorporating small talk, appropriate disclosure, and authentic emotional expression are useful approaches that you might practice in supervision to facilitate the development of therapeutic relationships. Behavioral descriptors of mental health and illness provide clinicians with nuanced symptoms of mental disorders that may otherwise be missed when diagnostic terminology is used. Speak with your supervisor about how to assess behavioral descriptors within a client's personal or familial history.

While providing bilingual mental health evaluations and treatment, you may encounter complex dynamics that can often serve as barriers that affect clients and complicate service provision. Consider the following scenario, which involves a variety of compounding issues and circumstances: An agency that conducts sexual abuse evaluations refers a child for mental health services. One parent has been deported out of the United States, and the other parent is living out of state after a period of psychiatric difficulties. It is unclear who has legal custody of the child and who would be authorized to consent to treatment. To further complicate matters, the extended family's limited English proficiency has resulted in uncertainty and miscommunication among multiple service providers because of incomplete or inaccurate information regarding the child's clinical symptoms and therefore treatment needs.

When complex dynamics arise in your clinical training, your bilingual supervisor can guide you on nuanced processes such as care coordination with external systems (e.g., schools, child welfare agencies, various community providers) and the ethical and legal parameters of such collaboration and advocacy. Bilingual supervisors will name and honor that our *acompañamiento* with clients includes navigating multiple systems of oppression and requires (re)membering our *fortalezas*. To illustrate, bilingual supervisors may emphasize the importance of networking and interdisciplinary collaboration. Supervisors may also prioritize check-ins regarding your well-being and self-care during meetings; help you balance your autonomy in decision making while challenging you to step outside of your comfort zone; and acknowledge your level of external life circumstances, stressors, or sacrifices.

Bilingual supervisors promote ethical, liberatory, and multicultural competencies by acknowledging the impacts of race, racism, and power within the supervisory triad. Consider a Latinx clinician who identifies racially as White. As this clinician is conducting an evaluation with an Afro-Costa Rican client, and in supervision, the clinician states, "I do not see color, just people." A culturally competent bilingual supervisor would encourage this supervisee to self-reflect on the oppressive impact of biases and the harm the client likely will face if these biases remain unaddressed. Supervision is a time to attend to cultural and sociopolitical realities and, more so, challenge one-dimensional stances that dismiss the role of race, racism, and power within the supervisory triad.

At its best, bilingual supervision is a growth-promoting experience that supports you as a learner rather than an expert. Embracing flexibility and seeking feedback as a developing bilingual clinician will ease the pressure often felt by novice clinicians. A competent bilingual supervisor will point out your growth areas and provide feedback—not to criticize you but to promote your clinical proficiency and accountability in two languages. Therefore, having a well-developed supervisory relationship will facilitate the effective addressing of issues like these. Supervisors who model and foster an open and nondefensive posture are also crucial for your professional growth and development.

Throughout this process, you must reflect on the development of your ethnic identity. It is crucial to process internalized prejudices, *colorismo*, and privileges and understand how these aspects influence the lens through which you view yourself, your interpersonal relationships, and your clients. This is no small feat! Please embrace the reality of this discomfort, be willing to reflect with your supervisor, and acknowledge the natural defensiveness that may arise. Bilingual supervisors can also share their journeys with you, model appropriate professional behaviors, inform you of resources, and guide you toward a level of increased insight and self-awareness.

Identifying Bilingual Supervision and Training

We acknowledge that, depending on your training program or practicum sites, access to bilingual supervision is not always feasible, or an intentional practice. In this section, we highlight ways to seek bilingual supervision. To begin, we encourage you to inquire whether your training programs offer the following:

- Latinx courses that explore mental health or the interplay of culture and language;

- faculty members with experience working with Latinxs and mental health issues;

- identified opportunities for bilingual supervision by licensed program faculty or program-affiliated professionals within field placements; and

- documented evidence of bilingual training outcomes that include acceptance to internships, postdoctoral fellowships, and academic/professional appointments focused on bilingual mental health.

Knowing how your training program addresses these areas will equip you to understand their commitment to ethical, bilingual training. You can converse with advisors, training directors, program faculty, or senior students to gain a comprehensive outlook on the status of bilingual training within your program.

We encourage you to inquire, before engaging in bilingual work, about how your bilingual skills will be formally delegated, assessed, and developed. Questions one can ask include the following:

- Is there a requirement to take on additional tasks, such as translating and transcribing sessions?

- Are cases involving bilingual clients distributed fairly among bilingual trainees on the basis of clinical needs?

- Will there be expectations to explain the complexities of bilingual therapy to supervisors who are not bilingual?

Other important questions regarding bilingual training at your institution include

- How will the additional work that comes with accompanying bilingual communities be recognized and factored into one's training?

- Does the training program ensure that Spanish clinical experiences are on par with acuity compared with monolingual English clinical experiences?

- How does the program ensure bilingual trainees have equitable workloads compared with their monolingual counterparts?

- Is bilingual training a specialty or an add-on that does not contribute to the program's practicum hour requirements?

- If there is no formal process for bilingual practica and supervision, how are bilingual trainees recognized and supported within the program?

- Are resources available to seek bilingual supervision externally if it is unavailable within the program?

These questions aim to help you assess the programmatic structures so that you can make an informed decision on whether to engage in bilingual clinical work.

Ways to Prepare for and Benefit From Bilingual Supervision

Because of the complexity of and nuances inherent to providing bilingual mental health services, we acknowledge that bilingual supervision is a precious but all too often limited opportunity. Considering this reality, we encourage you to show up prepared for supervision to maximize the experience. *Por favor aprovecha* the shared cultural language by having your supervisor do live supervision or review your recordings of sessions conducted in Spanish, to obtain concrete feedback. Preparing for bilingual supervision is dependent on your developmental training level. As you become more comfortable in bilingual service provision, you will learn which information your supervisor deems essential to share about clients during each meeting. We encourage you to schedule time to complete your progress notes and score assessment materials before your supervision sessions. Although paperwork may feel like a tedious additional requirement with little clinical impact, clinical documentation and the proper scoring of materials facilitate communication about your sessions' content to maximize the supervisory hour. When creating an agenda for supervision, reflect on the type of feedback you desire from your supervisor about the previous session.

Over time, bilingual supervisory conversations can help you develop more practical, culturally based case conceptualizations of clients' presenting problems or behavioral functioning by discussing cultural values. To illustrate, you and your supervisor may explore the role and diverse impacts of *familismo* and consider family and systems theories as potential components of your work. For example, in working with an anxious, parentified adolescent who worries about their younger siblings, traditional individual treatment modalities (e.g., using cognitive-behavioral interventions to challenge irrational worries) would likely be ineffective, despite skillful application, because of their emphasis on individualism. These modalities seldom consider the backdrop of families' sociopolitical and economic realities, such as the lack of available social support, including affordable child care options. We encourage you to consult with your supervisor on ways to incorporate *familismo* in your work with Latinx clients.

Providing bilingual therapy also requires that you be trauma informed regardless of your preferred theoretical orientation or chosen intervention methods. Supervisors should include conversations about systemic oppression and racial trauma (Chavez-Dueñas et al., 2019), intergenerational trauma (Mora-Ozuna et al., 2023), and adverse life experiences (e.g., violence, poverty, family separations). Because of the oppressive and marginalized realities of many Latinxs in the United States, you may be assigned more complex and demanding cases than your monolingual English-speaking peers. Although this tends to be disguised as an opportunity, it is an unfair reality that should be acknowledged in supervision. If this delegation goes unacknowledged, we encourage you to be transparent about the impact of this with your supervisor. In turn, they may be able to advocate for you in balancing the size and difficulty of your caseload.

Teamwork and interdisciplinary collaboration, which positively affect clients' daily lives, often require considerable case management and advocacy efforts that extend well beyond the traditional psychotherapy session. Bilingual supervisors recognize the necessity of engaging with schools, the community, and health care shareholders to enhance access to care and resources for clients, diminishing the bureaucratic barriers that delay access to care (Fuentes et al., 2023). They also recognize how this is often dismissed in Eurocentric training. Your supervisor should encourage, model, support, and advocate for additional time for this work. For instance, suppose you were conducting an evaluation of an English-speaking minor who is a child of monolingual Spanish-speaking immigrants. Preparing for language-switching throughout assessment sessions takes time and begins with ensuring that caregivers and minors understand their rights and the parameters of confidentiality. Supervisors can also assist in demystifying and acknowledging the distrust or lack of understanding caregivers may experience.

We want to normalize and encourage discussions around experiencing interethnic and intraethnic transference and countertransference reactions (Comas-Díaz, 2012). One example of an intraethnic transference is feeling conflicted between embracing cultural norms versus ethical obligations. This can arise if Latinx parents with a limited understanding of legal age rights, privacy, and confidentiality demand to receive updates on their adult son's mental health treatment. The necessity to uphold ethical obligations and confidentiality may result in feeling like you are dismissing the parents' concerns. However, bilingual supervision can normalize conflicting feelings that arise as you uphold ethical responsibilities while honoring cultural values. Similarly, enforcing boundaries around lateness to sessions may be challenging in an interethnic relationship where societal power differentials in the client–therapist dyad may exist. For example, your White cisgender male patient continuously shows up 10 minutes late to sessions and expects to be seen for the full length of his session time. You find yourself acquiescing to this request for fear of being perceived as difficult or unprofessional. Using supervision as a space to explore these concerns is crucial and paramount to your professional development so you can learn to uphold boundaries and be assertive despite feeling an urge for overcompliance.

As you face challenging cases or personal stressors, recognize that graduate training is a time of rapid growth during which you will understandably experience overwhelming periods of discomfort. Being open to recognizing your limits and asking your supervisor for support are two of the best ways to manage these triggers. We want to empower you to take ownership of your training experience. Now is the time to claim your professional identity, while honoring that *respeto* and *humildad* may have gotten you this far. As you are exposed to different types of clients and different styles of supervisors, consider which styles feel most natural or particularly difficult. Recognizing your strengths and areas of growth will be a recurrent component of your training; being open to this feedback will help you benefit more quickly from supervision.

We encourage you to have transparent conversations with supervisors when personal challenges arise and affect your ability to provide therapy in an ethically responsive manner. Although we hope you can work with trusted supervisors who center these conversations, this is not always feasible. Recognizing that your actual life circumstances may influence the objectivity and effectiveness of your clinical work is not a deficit but an ethically responsible thing to do. Again, this may make bilingual supervision feel harder and require increased vulnerability on your part, but it also provides an opportunity for clinical and personal growth. We encourage you to rise to this challenge by being candid and willing to discuss your experiences and reactions in working within the Latinx community, especially during times that may feel uniquely personal. Being afraid to address difficult topics directly or indirectly is normal and should not deter you.

Your rapport with your clinical supervisor is paramount to your work (Jones et al., 2019). We urge you to evaluate your supervisory relationship and consider the following questions: Has your supervisor ever discussed personal and contextual factors that are influencing your training? Does your supervisor seem open and committed to learning about you? If the answers are no, this may indicate that your supervisor struggles to incorporate such topics into supervision. It is essential to understand that matters discussed in supervision are not confidential because supervision also serves a gatekeeping function. To illustrate, suppose you feel your relationship with your supervisor lacks a mutual emotional connection, positive regard, trust, and respect. In this case, you may need to enforce more protective boundaries for yourself by addressing matters with a mentor, peer, or someone you trust (professor, friend, therapist, etc.) outside of the supervision parameters. However, suppose the supervisory relationship is well established, and you feel comfortable having conversations about these matters.

In that case, prepare by writing down some of your thoughts or concerns before your supervision session.

Note that the focus should be on your growth and professional development; this should not feel like you are in therapy. When conversations include or affect your skill set as a clinician, supervisors should create a collaborative effort to support your growth. We hope you experience a supportive bilingual supervision space that does not dismiss your concerns yet shares the onus of responsibility when applicable. Although supervisors need to validate your feelings, we want to remind you that their role is to help you grow. Thus, a good supervisor may respectfully challenge you if needed. Conversations about supervisory difficulties or conflicts are most helpful when integrated as an ongoing aspect of your supervisory experience and when they focus on your well-being and development. Depending on the training program and site, recognize that it may be appropriate for your supervisor to encourage you to seek personal therapy on the basis of the impact it may have on your clinical work. This must be communicated with respect and value.

It is important to note that bilingual supervisors may not have all the answers, requiring one to extend grace and compassion. In addition, the notion that getting along personally with one's supervisor is a must is unrealistic and not always the case. Seeking a supervisor's approval is not necessary. What is necessary is understanding that supervisor–supervisee matches can be imperfect regardless of shared race, ethnicity, and language. Even when sharing intersectional identities, the pressure to get along is often put on by programs or institutions that dismiss challenges as ordinary professional dynamics and expect supervisory relationships to succeed solely on the basis of shared heritage. Acknowledging that supervisory experiences are influenced by racial/ethnic socialization, critical consciousness levels, and differing values or goals that orient one's commitments within the profession is imperative (Field et al., 2010). Another essential factor to consider is the respective developmental stages of the supervisor and supervisee because these stages have a bidirectional impact on providing and receiving feedback.

Becoming a Bilingual Supervisor

Given the specialization of bilingual training and the limited access to bilingual supervisors, we encourage you also to identify bilingual supervisory experiences within your training—to lift you as you climb. Recognize that your bilingual mental health clinician training positions you to create your own supervisor identity. Supervision training may be embedded within your graduate program, or it may available at some internship sites, where you can supervise other students at earlier developmental stages. If supervisory experiences are not readily available, you can discuss how to access supervision didactics from your training director or advisor. Another way of building bilingual and bicultural competence includes connecting to the National Latinx Psychological Association's Bilingual Consultation Special Interest Group, which provides programming on bilingual issues. Nevertheless, we strongly advise you not to pursue bilingual supervisory experiences without appropriate training and support.

MENTORÍA OF BILINGUAL AND STUDENTS OF COLOR

Bilingual mentoring is key in providing bilingual trainees with the tools and skills to promote their growth and development. Bilingual mentors may model how to claim one's presence and encourage authenticity unapologetically. Because of its nonevaluative and non-gatekeeping role, mentorship is different from supervision. *Mentoría* highlights *comunidad y apoyo*, accompanying bilingual trainees as they learn about the various professional trajectories that are available. It creates a space to gain psychosocial support during challenging circumstances and encourages you to celebrate all wins, regardless of how small they may seem. It provides psychosocial support, which is essential when navigating the multifaceted realities of the profession. Bilingual mentorship can take many forms through your educational and professional journey and can help you center your values and commitments. A culturally responsive (Castellanos et al., 2022) relationship with bilingual mentors addresses the gaps in bilingual training infrastructures while expanding and multiplying our presence and growth in this field.

From Supervision to Mentorship

Although bilingual supervision can include mentoring qualities, distinguishing these relationships promotes a comprehensive understanding of the factors *mentoría* comprises and the necessity of seeking mentoring spaces outside of supervision. The limited but growing presence of bilingual mental health professionals has resulted in supervision and mentorship often overlapping. Mentoring provides an all-encompassing relationship that focuses on various professional or personal aspects of your life. For bilingual mentors serving in both mentoring and supervisory capacities, or bilingual trainees experiencing such, we encourage having conversations about these distinctions to determine these interrelated dimensions.

In addition, mentorship is not bound by licensure and accreditation standards in one's respective mental health discipline but rather is an experience whereby one can obtain cross-discipline mentorship from other mental health fields (e.g., social workers, marriage and family therapists). By stepping outside of the silos of our respective fields, we can learn from each other's expertise and create interdisciplinary mental health networks.

Accessing and Benefiting From Bilingual Mentorship

Given the distinct qualities that comprise bilingual therapy, bilingual mentoring aims to provide critical support for bilingual trainees in a manner that is rooted in culturally responsive mentoring because it aims to "empower mentees to recognize their skills and embrace their personal power" (Castellanos et al., 2022, p. 228). The multiethnic multicultural mentoring model (Castellanos et al., 2022) outlines five stages ([a] relationship building; [b] a game plan: articulating the dream; [c] opportunity building: purpose, opportunities, and skill building; [d] learning the inside game: networking, more mentors, and positioning; and [e] letting go: colleagues and role reversal) and unique processes that are relevant to mentoring students in higher education. We lean on this model to highlight the essential characteristics of a bilingual mentor: an investment in understanding one's life trajectory and how it has inspired one's commitment and dreams toward becoming a bilingual scientist–practitioner.

Bilingual mentors, who know your aspirations, provide psychosocial and professional support as you work toward reaching your professional and academic goals in a manner that aligns with becoming authentic and operating from a place of authenticity. From reviewing curriculum vitae and personal statements to encouraging you to apply for scholarships or awards, bilingual mentors will encourage you to pursue opportunities and can provide accountability for following through. This is especially important for first-generation, low-income students, who may often find themselves burdened to have it all figured out. Bilingual mentors instead will foster your self-efficacy and agency to *hacer el camino al andar* by leaning on *comunidad*.

Mentors are critical in teaching you how to use your agency and decide your capacity to engage in bilingual work (e.g., research, therapy, consultation, assessments, advocacy). They can provide psychosocial support that can range from meeting off campus to have a *cafecito* to discussing critical negotiation skills for job offers involving bilingual responsibilities

(Castellanos et al., 2022). They can also provide support on the importance of self-respect and dignity when faced with microaggressions, discrimination, or exploitation. Bilingual mentors can model the development of professional boundaries and help you balance multiple stimulating opportunities that are presented or expected by ensuring that your capacity and bandwidth are at the forefront. You can lean on your bilingual mentor to practice turning opportunities down, delegating tasks, or asking for support.

Conversely, mentors can model self-advocacy by teaching the importance of collaborative decision making to counteract the exploitation or lack of understanding of the totality of providing bilingual services. Suppose your monolingual supervisor requests that you administer an assessment with which you have no training or practice simply because you are the only bilingual provider. It may be challenging to balance wanting to gain experience while also ensuring in-depth understanding. A bilingual mentor can support you in vocalizing your request for comprehensive training before administering such an assessment. Bilingual assessment proctoring skills are especially important to enact in programs, cohorts, or clinical practica that have limited bilingual training infrastructures. Unfortunately, these practices normalize the hegemony of English and the lack of intentionality to promote language justice in bilingual training spaces.

Competent bilingual mentors will caution you against taking on unfair workloads and help you decipher unaccounted and uncompensated work that extend beyond your training and professional responsibilities. They can impart wisdom on developing healthy work–life practices and professional boundaries to offset burnout and prevent secondary traumatic stress. Mentors can model taking paid time off for intentional self- and community care. Although mentors cannot eliminate inequitable systems, they can increase your access to essential relationships, experiences, and platforms so you can thrive when navigating these systems (M. Kanagui-Muñoz, personal communication, October 17, 2023). They also can instill the importance of broaching conversations about power, privilege, oppression, and how to enact your social responsibility. Mentors equip you with the appropriate language to confidently navigate professional interpersonal dynamics in situations characterized by significant power differentials. To illustrate, they may help you explore your goals and values to strategize a decision, prioritizing what is most important to you.

Mentors can expand your connection to other bilingual mentees, professionals, and networks, thus reinforcing the cultivation of additional mentoring relationships to support your goals. These connections will continue to build across professional stages and can foster multigenerational mentoring experiences and emphasize *valores de la colectiva*. Through academic families (Castellanos et al., 2022), mentorship will challenge isolating academic spaces by empowering you to lean on your *comunidad* for support, motivation, and guidance. The creation of academic *familias* can be beautiful and empowering; they provide *sabiduría, conexión, y apoyo*.

Academic *familias* can consist of a wide range of individuals, including peers who can provide mentorship and are mutually reciprocal of one another. Peer mentors may provide personal and professional growth possibilities ranging from direct guidance (e.g., shared learning and skill development) to ongoing empowering experiences (e.g., support, motivation, networking opportunities). Examples include providing support as you apply to graduate school, preparing for graduate interviews via role plays, and accessing practical or leadership opportunities. Bilingual peer mentors may provide you with graduate school application materials (e.g., curriculum vitae, personal statement, graduate school examination preparation materials, programs to consider). They may also support you in considering important personal, familial, or professional factors when selecting a graduate school program. Bilingual peer mentors may share similar backgrounds and experiences, thus providing in-depth conversations about financial support opportunities, the campus climate and culture, or connecting you to spaces and places where you can be culturally affirmed.

For those of you who have already entered graduate programs—*¡felicidades!* We encourage you to connect with senior people in your program who are also bilingual. Peer-to-peer bilingual *mentoría* in graduate programs can provide you with various benefits. These individuals may graciously share their knowledge and experiences with you, including lessons they have learned to help make your journey easier. They may advise you about and model ways to approach professors, provide materials to prepare for developmental milestones, or inform you of upcoming professional opportunities. For example, when you are taking comprehensive exams, bilingual peer mentors can help you request language accommodations to grant you extended time, given the cognitive load of being a heritage Spanish speaker. Bilingual peer mentors may provide you with tangible examples of how to showcase your bilingual skills. They may also share opportunities, such as connecting you to compensated bilingual training opportunities or making you privy to employee benefits you can access in Association of Psychology Postdoctoral and Internship Centers internships or postdoctoral training (e.g., tuition and training reimbursement). We hope you find yourself in spaces *para colaborar, compartir,* and *apoyar,* and ultimately foster your academic *familia*.

Cultivating Bilingual Mentorship Opportunities

Cultivating bilingual mentorship requires leaning on one's cultural strengths, such as *personalismo, colectivismo,* and humor, to overcome possible anxiety when seeking a bilingual mentor. Those pursuing or in graduate school may inquire about formal or informal mentoring opportunities with bilingual Latinx faculty members and professional training staff. Reviewing programs or institutional websites may also provide information about established peer and faculty mentoring opportunities. State associations and national organizations, such as the National Latinx Psychological Association and APA, offer established mentoring programs that can benefit bilingual trainees in various ways. For example, APA funds graduate training mentorship programs, including the APA Minority Fellowship Program (https://ldi.apa.org/programs/minority-fellowship-program) and the APA Interdisciplinary Minority Fellowship Program (https://www.apa.org/about/awards/imfp-fellowship). Both programs aim to enhance the presence of diverse professionals committed to serving communities of color. Trainees are provided mentoring relationships with diverse professionals practicing nationwide, along with supplemental training and professional development opportunities.

Attending culturally informed networking opportunities and joining student-led organizations and professional Latinx organizations are avenues to build relations with bilingual mental health professionals. We have found support at the National Latinx Psychological Association's *conferencias,* highlighting the power of *comunidad* invested in working with and mentoring the next generation of mental health professionals. For these reasons, we recommend joining county, state, or national professional associations (e.g., American Counseling Association, Association for Multicultural Counseling and Development, Association for Counselor Education and Supervision, American Association for Marriage and Family Therapy, National Association of Social Workers, Latino Social Workers Organization). Active participation in professional and leadership capacities (e.g., training, volunteering at conferences, reviewing manuscripts for journals) can also expand your network to find the support you desire, deserve, and need. These opportunities foster access to *una red de comunidad,* surrounding you with essential sources of *apoyo* during your training and professional journey (Crisp et al., 2020).

Bilingual *mentoría* is highly valued and also hard to come by. Recognizing the limited bandwidth of bilingual professionals requires that one advocate against the unrealistic expectation that one individual can provide mentorship in all areas of bilingual mentees' development, especially in settings where they are limited in numbers. Instead, acknowledge that bilingual professionals may be transparent in their inability to mentor you because of their maxed-out capacity but may still try to connect you to other people in their circle or direct you to resources related to what you need. For these reasons, we encourage you to have multiple mentors. By doing so, you can gain a network of people who support different facets of your journey. We also encourage you to intentionally foster such relationships. This includes maintaining connection and communication across developmental stages to foster a genuine connection.

We also want to acknowledge the growing presence of Latina-led virtual counterspaces (Gomez & Cabrera, 2023) that name and explain the intricacies of higher education (e.g., the Instagram handles @BecomingDoctora, @Foosinmedicine, @Gradlifegrind, @Gradconmigo, @AcademicLatina, @LatinaGradGuide) and the various trajectories one can take as a bilingual clinician (e.g., the Instagram handles @Thefirstgenpsychologist, @Oaxacantherapists). These virtual spaces serve as mentoring pathways through events, scholarship opportunities, and information about academic journeys. We encourage you to lean on these types of platforms as you embark on your academic *camino*. To expand the reach and increase the presence of bilingual trainees, we encourage creating virtual communities and harnessing the power of social media.

Becoming a Bilingual Mentor

Becoming a bilingual mentor is a layered experience that encompasses various networks that support your growth and fan your flame to begin and succeed on this journey. The development of one's network is equally dependent on the ability to rise to the occasion and share one's skills and experiences by becoming a mentor. We encourage you to create or engage in mentoring opportunities to uphold the value of interdependence. Our *comunidad* has sustained us through our long training experiences, and we must also intentionally reach out and increase the presence of bilingual and bicultural mental health professionals. If you are a doctoral student, one way of mentoring is by intentionally recruiting a research team of undergraduate, postbaccalaureate, and master's-level students to develop a bidirectional working and compensated relationship. This will allow them to access knowledge about your dissertation while engaging in a space to demystify and decolonize academia. If your program allows, you can invite mentees to attend your dissertation defense so they can witness the final stage of the doctoral process. You can similarly turn other connections with bilingual individuals into a mentoring relationship. To illustrate, suppose you are working with a colleague who is considering pursuing an internship that focuses on bilingual training. On the basis of your transparent professional experiences with this organization, you can offer them guidance and support to help them make an informed decision. Because mentorship is an investment that takes time and *corazón,* we urge you to reciprocate the relationship with your mentors, and we ask you to continue to build our professional specialization.

CONCLUSION

Your presence as a bilingual therapist is vital in dismantling barriers that are preventing access and the use of resources while restoring trust between health professionals and the Latinx community. Moreover, you are part of the creation of a more robust workforce dedicated to continuing the expansion of services and providers alike. The limited number of faculty and clinicians who hold intersectional identities within academia and training sites challenges the ability to fulfill the current mental health needs of the Latinx community. There are not enough of us, money, or time. Understanding these systematic barriers is essential if you are to temper your expectations of your supervisor and acknowledge how such realities may overburden people and result in negative interpersonal dynamics. Keeping this in mind endorses healthy longevity and a sustained impact.

Although bilingual supervision and *mentoría* are conduits to the promotion of professional development, there are important systemic changes that can create the infrastructure for bilingual trainees in mental health fields. To build infrastructure, institutions and training sites can hire bilingual faculty, supervisors, and staff. Similarly, they can establish practicum sites that offer training in bilingual therapy. We encourage training programs to recruit cohorts of professionals who are intentionally focused on developing bilingual graduate trainees.

Becoming a bilingual and bicultural clinician is an experience that allows us to support Spanish-speaking communities as they access services that promote their healing journeys. Our training and personal trajectories facilitate a heightened level of empathy, motivating us to pursue this profession while providing bilingual services that empower us to bridge the gap and promote more holistic care. We welcome more people to join us in this beautiful work. We also recognize that bilingual training is a long and intricate process, but you are not alone. Bilingual supervision and *mentoría* will give you the *alas para volar.*

Supervision and *mentoría* are critical to your development, and this chapter has centered on various ways to advocate for both. Despite the growing acknowledgment of bilingual mental health training, we highlight the dire need for more recognition and *colegas* ready to embark on this social justice endeavor. To do so, we invite you to expand your worldview from "imposter to an infiltrator" (Tran, 2023, p. 187) and embrace yourself as a change agent who is ready to show up as your authentic self and disrupt oppressive conditions. *¡Pa'lante mi gente!*

TAKEAWAYS

- Your bilingual skills and cultural insights are critical for advancing social justice and antioppressive mental health interventions.

- Bilingual supervisors, who are well versed in the Latinx diaspora, can help you refine your clinical skills while honoring your experiences as a bilingual trainee.

- Bilingual mentorship can provide you with the critical insight you need to center yourself as you embark on your professional journey and determine opportunities that best fit you.

- Bilingual supervision and mentorship are critical components of developing a healthy bilingual mental health workforce while challenging the exploitation of bilingual clinicians and academics.

REFLEXIONES

- What motivates you to continue your educational journey toward becoming a bilingual mental health professional or academic? In learning more about the unique aspects of bilingual supervision, how does having a bilingual supervisor support your goals and skill development?

- How can your supervisor or mentor help you overcome some challenges of being a bilingual clinician in a capitalist system?

- How can seeking bilingual clinical supervision and mentorship training help address language injustices and oppression while developing the next generation of bilingual clinicians and academics?

- Identify a bilingual supervisor or mentor with whom you do not have a relationship and seek to initiate one.

RESOURCES

Recommended Reading

Adames, H. Y., & Chavez-Dueñas, N. Y. (2016). *Cultural foundations and interventions in Latino/a mental health: History, theory and within group differences*. Routledge.

Comas-Díaz, L. E., Adames, H. Y., & Chavez-Dueñas, N. Y. (Eds.). (2024). *Decolonial psychology: Toward anticolonial theories, research, training, and practice*. American Psychological Association. https://doi.org/10.1037/0000376-000

Delgado-Romero, E. A. (Ed.). (2023). *Latinx mental health: From surviving to thriving*. IGI Global. https://doi.org/10.4018/978-1-6684-4901-1

Websites

- Latinx Therapy: https://latinxtherapy.com
- Therapy for Latinx: https://www.therapyforlatinx.com
- Latinx Therapists Action Network: https://latinxtherapistsactionnetwork.org
- Bilingual Supervision: https://www.therapyforlatinx.com/therapist/supervision-for-therapists
- American Psychological Association Minority Fellowship Program: https://ldi.apa.org/programs/minority-fellowship-program
- National Latinx Psychological Association: https://www.nlpa.ws
- National Latinx Psychological Association Bilingual Issues in Latinx Mental Health Special Interest Group: https://tinyurl.com/msennbf4
- National Latinx Psychological Association Mentoring Program: https://www.nlpa.ws/mentoring-program

REFERENCES

American Psychological Association. (2012). *Introduction to mentoring: A guide for mentors and mentees*. https://www.apa.org/education/grad/mentoring.aspx

Behnke, S. (2005). The supervisor as gatekeeper: Reflections on ethical standards 7.02, 7.04, 7.05, 7.06 and 10.01. *Monitor on Psychology, 36*(5), 90–91. https://www.apa.org/monitor/may05/ethics

Castellanos, J., White, J. L., & Franco, V. (2022). *Riding the academic freedom train: A culturally responsive, multigenerational mentoring model*. Routledge. https://doi.org/10.4324/9781003446873

Chavez-Dueñas, N. Y., Adames, H. Y., Perez-Chavez, J. G., & Salas, S. P. (2019). Healing ethno-racial trauma in Latinx immigrant communities: Cultivating hope, resistance, and action. *American Psychologist, 74*(1), 49–62. https://doi.org/10.1037/amp0000289

Comas-Díaz, L. (2012). *Multicultural care: A clinician's guide to cultural competence*. American Psychological Association. https://doi.org/10.1037/13491-000

Crisp, G., Doran, E. E., Carales, V. D., & Potts, C. (2020). Disrupting the dominant discourse: Exploring the mentoring experiences of Latinx community college students. *Journal for the Study of Postsecondary and Tertiary Education, 5*, 57–78. https://doi.org/10.28945/4510

Delgado-Romero, E. A., De Los Santos, J., Raman, V. S., Merrifield, J. N., Vazquez, M. S., Monroig, M. M., Cárdenas Bautista, E., & Durán, M. Y. (2018). Caught in the middle: Spanish-speaking bilingual mental health counselors as language brokers. *Journal of Mental Health Counseling, 40*(4), 341–352. https://doi.org/10.17744/mehc.40.4.06

Dennis, M., & Hung, P. Uribe, R., Lopez, T., Nieto, C. (2024, January 7). *Language justice.* Move to End Violence. https://www.movetoendviolence.org/resources/language-justice

Field, L. D., Chavez-Korell, S., & Rodríguez, M. M. D. (2010). *No hay rosas sin espinas*: Conceptualizing Latina–Latina supervision from a multicultural developmental supervisory model. *Training and Education in Professional Psychology, 4*(1), 47–54. https://doi.org/10.1037/a0018521

Fuentes, J., Rodriguez, V. J., Rodriguez, M. L., & Ordaz, A. C. (2023). *Juntos resistimos y sanamos*: The strength of Latinx families. In E. A. Delgado-Romero (Ed.), *Latinx mental health: From surviving to thriving* (pp. 211–227). IGI Global. https://doi.org/10.4018/978-1-6684-4901-1.ch012

Fuertes, J. N. (2004). Supervision in bilingual counseling: Service delivery, training, and research considerations. *Journal of Multicultural Counseling and Development, 32*(2), 84–94. https://doi.org/10.1002/j.2161-1912.2004.tb00363.x

Godinez Gonzalez, K. (2022). *A grounded theory study of the experiences of social justice committed Spanish–English bilingual Latinx clinical supervisees* (Publication No. 29320705) [Doctoral dissertation, New Mexico State University]. ProQuest Dissertations.

Gomez, V., & Cabrera, J. (2023). Theorizing virtual counterspaces: How Latina graduate students build community online. *Race Ethnicity and Education*, 1–17. https://doi.org/10.1080/13613324.2023.2292509

Gonzalez, L. M., Ivers, N. N., Noyola, M. C., Murillo-Herrera, A. C., & Davis, K. M. (2015). Supervision in Spanish: Reflections from supervisor–trainee dyads. *The Clinical Supervisor, 34*(2), 184–203. https://doi.org/10.1080/07325223.2015.1058208

Jones, C. T., Welfare, L. E., Melchior, S., & Cash, R. (2019). Broaching as a strategy for intercultural understanding in clinical supervision. *The Clinical Supervisor, 38*(1), 1–16. https://doi.org/10.1080/07325223.2018.1560384

Lugo, B. L. (2021). Spanish–English bilingual supervision. In m. polanco, N. Zamani, & C. D. H. Kim (Eds.), *Bilingualism, culture, and social justice in family therapy* (pp. 61–68). Springer. https://doi.org/10.1007/978-3-030-66036-9_9

Mills, J. E., Francis, K. L., & Bonner, A. (2005). Mentoring, clinical supervision and preceptoring: Clarifying the conceptual definitions for Australian rural nurses. A review of the literature. *Rural and Remote Health, 5*(3), 410. https://doi.org/10.22605/RRH410

Milne, D. (2007). An empirical definition of clinical supervision. *British Journal of Clinical Psychology, 46*(4), 437–447. https://doi.org/10.1348/014466507X197415

Mora-Ozuna, C., Rodriguez, I., Vazquez, M., & Fuentes, J. (2023). *Rompiendo cadenas*: Breaking down intergenerational trauma in the Latinx community. In E. A. Delgado-

Romero (Ed.), *Latinx mental health: From surviving to thriving* (pp. 196–210). IGI Global. https://doi.org/10.4018/978-1-6684-4901-1.ch011

National Latinx Psychological Association. (2020). Ethical guidelines of the National Latinx Psychological Association. *Journal of Latina/o Psychology, 8*(2), 101–111. https://doi.org/10.1037/lat0000151

Perry, V. M., & Sias, S. M. (2018). Ethical concerns when supervising Spanish–English bilingual counselors: Suggestions for practice. *Journal of Counselor Preparation and Supervision, 11*(1), Article 10.

Tran, N. (2023). From imposter phenomenon to infiltrator experience: Decolonizing the mind to claim space and reclaim self. *Peace and Conflict, 29*(2), 184–193. https://doi.org/10.1037/pac0000674

Trepal, H., Tello, A., Haiyasoso, M., Castellon, N., Garcia, J., & Martinez-Smith, C. (2019). Supervision strategies used to support Spanish-speaking bilingual counselors. *Teaching and Supervision in Counseling, 1*(1), 19–32. https://doi.org/10.7290/tsc010103

Valencia-Garcia, D., & Montoya, H. (2018). Lost in translation: Training issues for bilingual students in health service psychology. *Training and Education in Professional Psychology, 12*(3), 142–148. https://doi.org/10.1037/tep0000199

Wampold, B. E. (2015). How important are the common factors in psychotherapy? An update. *World Psychiatry, 14*(3), 270–277. https://doi.org/10.1002/wps.20238

7

LA INVESTIGACIÓN

Conducting and Publishing Bilingual Research

YESENIA URIBE, ALBERTA M. GLORIA, AND
JEANETT CASTELLANOS

In this chapter, we address what is meant by and included within bilingual research as it relates to your research skills development. We address core considerations to conduct bilingual research. In particular, we contextualize the larger systems of influence that have informed ways of knowing and knowledge production for bilingual research training. We provide research consejos and directives to conduct bilingual research.[1] These consejos include owning your positionality as a bilingual scientist–practitioner engaging with Latine communities (e.g., relationship to bilingualism), centering the knowledge you seek to explore (e.g., scoping literature reviews and community consults, theoretical framing to inform bilingual research questions, approaches to research methods, participant recruitment processes), tapping into your ancestral cultural wealth y sabiduría (e.g., analyzing and interpreting your data, publishing your data), and cultivating your academic familia to enhance a bilingual research agenda (e.g., joining professional organizations, pursuing fellowship and award opportunities,

[1]As a form of advocacy, instances of Spanish text are not italicized in this chapter.

https://doi.org/10.1037/0000481-008
Forging Caminos: *Pathways to Becoming a Bilingual Mental Health Professional*,
M. Campos, Y. Mejia, and A. J. Consoli (Editors)

finding research mentors who engage in sentipensante). Finally, we specify key takeaway points and offer reflection questions as you enact the consejos we have suggested to advance your bilingual research skill development. We suggest resources to survive and thrive entre fronteras as bilingual researchers engaging with Latine communities. Paso corto, camino largo. We hope this chapter both excites and encourages you to embrace your bilingualism and identities as bilingual researchers.

VIGNETTE: A BILINGUAL RESEARCHER

Demi is a bilingual Latine graduate student in the midst of her research (i.e., she is creating a developmental skill set, conceptualizing a process to refine her research questions, and building a structure to help inform how to answer them). While attending a predominantly White institution, she is motivated to engage Latine populations in linguistically affirming research and clinical practices. Informed in part by her personal and academic experiences, she is interested in Latine college students' sense of belonging and its influence on their well-being. Because she had some research experience as an undergraduate, she is looking to build her bilingual research skills in a way that is meaningful and allows her to engage her bilingualism fully. Following a racially based hate incident on campus during which Latine culture and language were disparaged, Demi feels an increasing sense of ganas y responsabilidad to gain the needed research skills to assess Latine undergraduates' psychological distress regarding language disparagement and to contextualize the incident's impact on Latine students' sense of belonging on campus.

As Demi began to conceptualize the project, her main sentipensantes were the following:

- How does she go about this research in a culturally and linguistically congruent way?

- How does she ask, measure, and conceptualize sense of belonging specific to Latine communities?

- How does she dismantle or move away from a universalistic (etic) approach in research and center Latine values and bilingualism (an emic approach)?

Demi, who mentors undergraduate students interested in pursuing research opportunities, wonders how she can support emic-based research that is anchored in cultural wisdom, bilingualism, and values and whether she can talk about bilingual research with her faculty advisor, particularly because she is uncertain about her advisor's relationship to bilingualism. Knowing that several of her research mentors (e.g., faculty advisor, peers in different programs, professionals whom she has met at conferences) recommend engaging in multiple research experiences, Demi excitedly initiates discussions about projects that would support her increased bilingual research skill set. As part of Demi's ongoing training and identity development as a bilingual researcher, she is building a repertoire of bilingual research skills that are informed by bilingualism and steeped in cultural context.

CONSEJOS EN PRÁCTICA: CONDUCTING BILINGUAL RESEARCH

Opportunities to engage in bilingual research remain scarce. Moreover, the structured training and support networks to assist bilingual scientists–practitioners with their professional identity development are limited. There exists a plethora of research on bilingualism (i.e., individuals who speak two languages), the linguistic processes involved (e.g., psycholinguistics, language acquisition, cognition), and bilingual education (e.g., teaching and learning, classroom processes), yet relatively less research has addressed how to conduct or publish bilingual research. Although bilingual research is frequently defined as research with individuals who speak two languages (in this instance, English and Spanish), the depth and complexity of what constitutes bilingual research is not fully portrayed within academia.

Both systemic and structural systems surrounding research (i.e., racism) perpetuate universalistic approaches and limit access to ways of knowing (Miles & Fassinger, 2021; Thompson, 2004). *Systemic racism* addresses whole-system involvement or entities that uphold these processes (e.g., political, legal, education), whereas *structural racism* emphasizes the structure's framework (e.g., laws, policies, practices, or norms), with the terms often used synonymously (Braveman et al., 2022). Particular to research and training, methods courses often use universal methods and etic conceptualizations, inaccurately deeming bilingual research a specialty topic or approach. Colonial hegemony informs how research is developed and what constitutes research from start to finish (i.e., how research is developed, funded, deemed valid, and published). Given the interconnecting network of systemic and structural systems informing bilingual research (Miles & Fassinger, 2021; Thompson, 2004; Uribe & Gloria, 2023), como primer paso we provide specific tasks, methods, and skills for your bilingual research development through consejos. Although the following consejos are not an extensive list, they provide a foundation to conceptualize and scaffold your bilingual research development. After presentation of the consejos, we highlight how Demi can apply them to her bilingual research.

Own Your Positionality as a Bilingual Scientist–Practitioner Engaging With Latine Communities

Owning your positionality as a bilingual researcher is critically important to resist the systemic and structural racism that informs research conceptualization, development, implementation, knowledge production, and publication (Thompson, 2004). The voices of many historically marginalized scholars continue to be silenced (i.e., academic institutional violence; Cueva, 2014), so naming and owning your identities as a bilingual researcher will serve to recognize your power to challenge the status quo (i.e., systemic racism) and engage in cultural resistance in academia. Awareness of our positionality and access to power and privilege as bilingual researchers includes identifying, exploring, and challenging assumptions and expectations we may have about the vastly different lived experiences within Latine communities.

Association to Bilingualism

Within our broader positionality, our specific relationship to bilingualism must also be a focus of reflection to determine what training, support, and advocacy are needed. To be specific, bilingual researchers hold dynamic and complex positionalities because Latine-focused bilingual research remains decentered, unstructured, and unstandardized (e.g., lack of required units on bilingual research skills) in training programs (including methods courses and assessment; Delgado-Romero et al., 2018). Knowing your culture and language-based positionalities requires that you critically assess your bilingual language capacities (fluency, code-switching); cultural linguistics (understanding the values that inform the meanings of various words and expressions); and associations with bilingualism (use of language in your home or professional spaces, use of Spanglish, trainings), including your social and cultural assumptions about bilingualism (Danjo, 2017; Holmes, 2016). Such self-reflexivity includes naming the contexts of when and how bilingualism gets acknowledged, recognized, or validated within academia. Put more specifically, un gran paso is the value-informed action of naming one's positionalities and relationship to bilingualism as reflected through theoretical frameworks, methods, and approaches for bilingual research development (Holmes, 2016).

Center the Knowledge You Seek to Explore

As part of owning your positionality as a bilingual scientist–practitioner engaging with Latine communities, we provide an overview of the key components of the bilingual research process. These span from your active engagement with your literature review to the return of your findings to assist and uplift Latine communities. Pa'lante!

Comprehensive Literature Review and Community Consult

Knowing the literature is important in all research endeavors; however, for bilingual research, taking an interdisciplinary approach to understand your topic more comprehensively is a fundamental practice. To do this, we suggest conducting either a scoping or systematic review of the literature that is relevant to your area of interest (e.g., Arksey & O'Malley, 2005; Munn et al., 2018). As a general overview, you would first identify the question of interest. You then would identify the relevant studies by determining key search terms in both Spanish and English databases. Broadening the databases you use to capture interdisciplinary studies will expand and deepen your perspectives of the concept you are exploring. A range of potential studies will result. Thus, the third step—determining the selection of studies that reflect different disciplines that best inform your research agenda—is critical. Although it may seem like the literature review is complete, next is implementing the fourth and fifth steps—charting the data and summarizing the results, respectively. Charting and summarizing the pertinent results will allow you to explore across disciplines and theoretical approaches as you conceptualize and frame your bilingual research questions. At the same time you conduct your literature review, consult with community members who can provide perspectives on what questions and needs are most relevant within the community to guide your literature search (Thompson, 2004). An equally important process is to determine the theoretical approach that frames your bilingual research question.

Theoretical Framing to Inform Bilingual Research Questions

There is a direct connection among your positionality, your beliefs, and the way in which you pose research questions. Your research question functions to deepen, broaden, confirm, and refute information about Latine communities. Academia and training spaces hold accountability to provide the resources and training necessary for bilingual research if equitable services for diverse communities is to be achieved (American Psychological Association, 2017). However, not all current research methods courses provide a range of theoretical frameworks, so the onus remains on you to find and determine which approaches can advance your positionality as a bilingual researcher.

Although not an exhaustive list, we offer several frameworks that highlight the community's fortaleza para sobrevivir y prosperar to assist in the development of your research question. The theory you select serves as a form of advocacy to dismantle colonial epistemologies and address systemic and structural racism (e.g., Latina/Latino critical race theory [LatCrit; Solórzano & Bernal, 2001], the LatCrit Racist Nativist framework [Pérez Huber, 2009]); honor cultural histories (e.g., a psychohistorical approach; Arredondo et al., 2006); center person–environment interdependence (e.g., a psychosociocultural approach; Gloria & Rodriguez, 2000); integrate sociocultural identity intersection (e.g., mujerista psychospirituality; Comas-Díaz, 2016); advance Chicana feminist epistemology (Calderón et al., 2012); or fuse mind–body–spirit integration (e.g., an ELLA-SANA approach; Herrera & Gloria, 2021). These and other Latine-centered, strengths-based theoretical approaches can frame your research questions as a form of advocacy.

We can use our power within our roles as bilingual scientists, practitioners, and advocates to advance Latine wellness by asking simple or easily understood bilingual research questions (the simpler the question, the better the research). It is through our actionable and integrated roles as scientists–practitioners–advocates that we can be guided by our "cultural intuition" as bilingual researchers (Delgado Bernal, 1998, p. 556). For example, enacting Latine values (e.g., personalismo, respeto, equilibrio, familismo) that directly inform cultural linguistics is a way to tap into your bilingual cultural intuition. Bilingual researchers who are still in their graduate training must balance how to get needed support while simultaneously being asked to be experts given their bilingual capabilities (Uribe & Gloria, 2023).

Ultimately, all researchers are responsible for ensuring that bilingual research development and language skill acquisition engage in advocacy and intervention at the individual and system levels both for and with the well-being of Latine communities (Uribe & Gloria, 2023). By integrating the different sources of knowledge (e.g., theories, literature, community wisdom), your research questions will reflect an expanded bilingual researcher positionality and set the foundation for your study's methods.

How to Approach Your Methods
The ways in which you select the methods to answer your study's question must be culturally framed and linguistically accurate and nuanced for bilingual research. There are many important methodological components of bilingual research. Two central and closely related tasks are (a) translation–back

translation and (b) assessing for cultural equivalence. Translation–back translation ensures accuracy in determining the linguistic, conceptual, functional, and metric equivalence of concepts of inquiry as they move between English and Spanish (Burlew et al., 2019), whereas cultural equivalence focuses on the relevance of cultural, sociopolitical, and contextual nuances and significances of terms within translations (Brown & Torres-Harding, 2021). For example, when identifying scales that will help answer your research question, assessing for whom (e.g., individuals similar to your intended participants and their sociocontextual factors) and how the scale was created (e.g., guiding theory and values, use of translation, back translation) are ways to enhance your study's validity. Similarly, review whether words/statements (on scales) or the way your question is asked (in interviews) hold the intended cultural meaning or equivalence for the population of study. For example, reviewing the cultural loading of a scale's items relative to different linguistic communities can ensure the increasingly accurate and effective use of measures (Burlew et al., 2019; Mercado & Venta, 2022).

If either measurement or cultural equivalence is unclear from your review (Mercado & Venta, 2022), this is a key indicator that you may need to create a new scale or engage a pilot study of a newly translated–back translated scale. For example, conducting a confirmatory factor analysis can help you determine whether your newly developed scale or (re)translated scale items reliably and validly convey your study's constructs (Burlew et al., 2019). Although this recommendation involves a large time commitment and has an ambitious aim, such rigorous statistical and methodological approaches are often necessary tasks for the accurate selection and use of bilingual scales (Zea et al., 2003).

Along with key methodological processes, thoughtful and substantial preparation is required for implementing linguistically accurate bilingual methods. Given the lack of consideration of bilingual research methods in methods courses, we suggest taking a mixed-methods approach to bilingual research that can center core Latine values and ways of being through quantitative (e.g., culturally grounded surveys) and qualitative methods (e.g., charlas, pláticas, focus groups, auto historias y cuentos, testimonios). A mixed methods approach allows you to obtain a more comprehensive and nuanced understanding of concepts. In both approaches, culture is a contextual factor of bilingualism that specifically informs both proximal variables (e.g., identity processes or psychological constructs) and distal variables (e.g., demographic characteristics) of a study. For example, discussing differentiating proximal and distal variables with your study participants can deepen and foster a more accurate understanding of their cultural and phenomenological processes

(Mercado & Venta, 2022). Asking about participants' Latine-specific central identities (e.g., ethnicity, race, immigration, college generation, language) also acknowledges and validates the vast within-group differences and reflection of lived experiences among all Latine communities.

Recruitment Processes

There are, unfortunately, ongoing valid reasons why bilingual and Latine communities might distrust academia and researchers from the university/college setting. It is in this context that bilingual researchers must collaborate with community members, such as Latine elders, to build trusted partnerships. Your positionality as a bilingual researcher must be considered relative to fostering connections to and relationships with the community. For example, creating culturally tailored and communal collaborations to engage with community advocates are key to building trust and conducting research with and for Latine communities (Delgado-Romero et al., 2018).

A variety of recruitment methods need to be implemented to build trust. In response to various sociocontextual identities, such as immigration status, income, or language identities, a first approach would ideally include partnering with promotores de salud or trusted community members and liaisons who have a deep understanding of the communities they accompany (Flores et al., 2022). Having them tell others (i.e., word of mouth or nonparametric sampling) about the study builds trust by association. Consulting with "promotores–researchers" (Johnson et al., 2013, p. 638) or other individuals who have community knowledge can also provide perspectives with respect to concept development and implementation (Elder et al., 2009).

A second approach would be spending time in community as an active member (i.e., becoming a known entity), as a key task for recruitment. Showing up at community centers, fairs, or community events, or even posting flyers at a local venue (e.g., a panadería or bodega) to talk with local community members are a few of many ways to become a known entity. By becoming known, you are directly letting community members understand that you honor and respect them. In this same way, providing monetary and resource or education (*plática* on a specific topic) incentives for participants directly conveys that you value them. Your knowledge of cultural linguistics as a bilingual researcher sets the context for interpersonal exchange associated with familismo, respeto, personalismo, and engagement that facilitates partnerships steeped in trust.

Tap Into Your Ancestral Cultural Wealth y Sabiduría

When academia tries to quiet or silence your ways of knowing by means of your insider and outsider connections with bilingualism, lean into your linguistic sabiduría and pedagogy of the home (Garcia & Delgado Bernal, 2021) to challenge what constitutes knowledge. During these push–pull encounters, allow your bilingualism and cultural linguistics to be your foundation of your positionality as a bilingual researcher. Your engagement of positionality becomes even more salient when analyzing, interpreting, and publishing your data in ways that embrace your bilingualism and role as a bilingual researcher.

Analyzing and Interpreting Your Data

As part of developing your identity as a bilingual researcher, you must learn to trust and lead with your cultural wealth, intuition, and home cultural pedagogies (Garcia & Delgado Bernal, 2021). It is imperative that you bring your whole self and familial/community sabiduría into your analysis and interpretation of your data. Center and hold Latine elders as experts of their own cultural and contextual experiences throughout studies to engage in respeto and personalismo; that is, collaborate with Latine elders and let them assist with data interpretation and making meaning of the study's findings (Delgado, 1997). A mixed methods approach to bilingual research allows quantitative and qualitative data to work collaboratively for a fuller understanding of one's lived experiences.

With respect to quantitative data, remember to emphasize and distinguish each level of significance (i.e., practical, relevance significance) to provide a fuller and more holistic understanding of your study's findings. Although practical significance is informative, do not overlook the role relevance significance has with respect to the real world impact, creative understanding, and meaningfulness of findings (Mohajeri et al., 2022) for Latine communities. Given the different types of significance, involving community members in the conceptualization, implementation, analyses, interpretation, and distribution of the study's methods and data will enhance the cultural relevance and applicability of its constructs. With respect to qualitative data, engage in multiple translation discussions; this includes translating narratives from Spanish to English and coming to a consensus about their linguistic, functional, conceptual and metric equivalence. You can enhance this process by returning your translations to the community (e.g., a counsel of experts and participants) so that you can ensure cultural equivalence and accuracy of translation. Participants are often more than willing to provide clarity about and insights into their statements (e.g., a participant audit) as ways to take ownership of and have pride in how they too are advancing their community. Integrating the voices and insight of community partnerships ensures that the needs of the community are being honored by and centered within your research agenda over the demands of academia.

Publishing Your Data

Without doubt, el proceso de publicación es difícil. The process calls into question the systems (or the who) that determine who is given credit for the creation and production of knowledge (i.e., authorship) and what is ultimately deemed as worthy, accurate, and meaningful for publication. Have open conversations about authorship with mentors in addition to communal partners, such as Latine community members and consultants (e.g., promotores, elders, advisory boards), when discussing authorship and author lineup (Thompson, 2004). Because authorship within the academy is determined by the person who originates an idea and assumes intellectual property rights, you must consider that Latine community members value culture-informed experiences as "collective or cultural property" (Thompson, 2004, p. 40). As you determine your author lineup, use a collective approach to normalize that community knowledge is not owned by a particular discipline or academic institution. Ultimately, there is a need for open and clear discussions about authorship, collective ownership, and representation and distribution of knowledge while negotiating the balance of systems.

This balance extends to your decision of whether to italicize Spanish text given that first-time use is required for manuscript submission and final publications (American Psychological Association, 2020). Although italicization requirements vary by publication style (e.g., Chicago, Harvard, Modern Language Association), many journals direct that Spanish words must be italicized. Latine and language scholars argue that italicizing Spanish language in text emphasizes differences from the norm and perpetuates a sense of foreignness, and thus they advocate for change (Torres, 2007; Trnka, 2016). This advocacy and academic resistance are important for bilingual qualitative research because participant narratives would be italicized in accordance with current American Psychological Association (APA, 2020) style guidelines. Bilingual research participants' words (e.g., testimonios, dichos, cuentos) should not be marginalized given that "reading or hearing comes from the minds and the thoughts of Spanish-speaking people" (Torres, 2007, p. 80). Know that you may be challenged by reviewers to conform to this standard; however, pushing back and naming your positionality and rationale in your author response to queries letter is how you enact change. Likewise, asking to include both an abstract and resumen as part of your scholarship is a component of returning knowledge to our communities. Furthermore, bilingual researchers can provide bilingual newsletters, research infographics, tool kits, Spanish local radio interviews, and informational or psychoeducation conversations at community centers or at local community clinics as ways of returning knowledge to communities.

Part of the publishing process is also being aware of the interwoven complexities of journal outlets and their related acceptance rates and impact factors. Keep in mind that these indicators of importance (e.g., impact factors) are reflective not of journal content or quality of reviews but rather of the average number of citations (Sharma et al., 2014). Because emic-focused journals highlight the deep-structured complexities and varied diversities of Latine communities, consider these as strong publication outlets for your work. For instance, the *Hispanic Journal of Behavioral Sciences* and *Aztlán* have been continuously published since 1979 and 1970, respectively, with newer journals also available, such as the *Journal of Latinx Psychology*, the *Journal of Latinos and Education*, or the *Journal of Latino-Latin American Studies*. Échale ganas, recuerda that publishing is difficult, but you can do it! The publication process is not reflective of your capacities but rather of larger challenging systemic and structural processes that you are actively navigating.

Cultivating Your Academic Familia to Enhance a Bilingual Research Agenda

Knowing that you are connected to a larger bilingual research community, and having a sense of belonging to and comunidad within the academic setting, are key to surviving graduate training. To build a bilingual research academic familia y comunidad means emphasizing the collective to advance your bilingualism and skill development as a bilingual researcher. It is important to find spaces where you can practice your professional language skills and connect with fellow bilingual researchers and mentors who hold similar positionalities and share experiences, expertise, and opportunities.

Joining Professional Organizations

Finding a professional familia is a way for you to have collective empowerment and liberation. The structural foundations of professional organizations that are steeped in Latine-centered advocacy and advancement can uplift your identity as a bilingual researcher. These organizations include the National Latinx Psychological Association (NLPA [https://www.nlpa.ws/], which has a mentoring program); the American Association of Hispanics in Higher Education (https://www.aahhe.org/); and Section III of APA Division 35—the Society of Latinx Womxn in Psychology. Joining organizations that are grounded in social justice and multicultural competencies propels dialogue and frameworks that support antiracist research methodologies and continues to call in the realities and linguistic experiences of diaspora for all Latine communities. Furthermore, finding opportunities for professional identity development and mentorship means attending, presenting, and engaging in leadership roles in local, national, and international professional associations. When you attend or present at a conference, you can create relational networks with others who are conducting similar bilingual research via formal (e.g., poster, symposium papers, roundtables) and informal (e.g., bailes, impromptu gatherings) spaces to discuss ideas and gain support. It is often from these collaborative experiences that you can refine your research questions and expand your scholarly area of inquiry (e.g., create bilingual research teams or consultation groups of peers from across the country and the world). Likewise, you will have access to resources such as grants, scholarships/fellowships, training programs, and workshops to help support your bilingual research initiatives.

Fellowship and Award Opportunities

Apply for resources to support and fund you to conduct your research (e.g., laptop/computer, participant incentives, team stipends, conference travel). There are a few possible awards you can access to support your ongoing training and the implementation of your bilingual research. These resources include:

- the NLPA Cynthia de las Fuentes Dissertation Award (https://tinyurl.com/f4zm5ktn),

- the NLPA Outstanding Dissertation Award,

- the NLPA Stephen C. Rose Award (https://tinyurl.com/f4zm5ktn),

- the American Educational Research Association Outstanding Dissertation Award (https://www.aera.net/SIG168/Awards/Outstanding-Dissertation-Award),

- the American Educational Research Association Minority Fellowship Program (https://tinyurl.com/8mhr2ub5),

- the APA Division 35 Section III Latinx Student Scholar Award (https://tinyurl.com/3f3m38xb),

- the APA Committee on Ethnic Minority Affairs Jeffrey S. Tanaka Memorial Dissertation Award in Psychology (https://www.apa.org/about/awards/tanaka-award),

- the American Association of Hispanics in Higher Education–Educational Testing Service Outstanding Dissertations Competition (https://www.aahhe.org/about-aahhe-ets-outstanding-dissertations-competition),

- Ford Foundation Dissertation Fellowships (https://www.nationalacademies.org/our-work/ford-foundation-dissertation-fellowships), and

- the APA Interdisciplinary Minority Fellowship Program (https://www.apa.org/about/awards/imfp-fellowship).

Finding Research Mentors Who Engage in Sentipensante

Find your academic familia to support your bilingual research by working with mentors who can engage in collective thinking/feeling processes (i.e., sentipensante; Rendón, 2023) by using their cultural knowledge, intuition (wealth of senses), and sabiduría. Seek research mentors from across your relational networks; these can include your faculty advisor, professional connections, or community experts who engage in reciprocal research relationships that foster confianza and awareness building (Ramírez Stege et al., 2017) through "reciprocal research relationships" (Diaz Solodukhin & Orphan, 2022, p. 207). Such relationships will encourage you to recognize and access your "funds of knowledge" and value your "skills, expertise, and relational networks cultivated . . . by [your] families and communities" (Diaz Solodukhin & Orphan, 2022, p. 207). Research mentors who place your experiences within sociocultural contexts will

- work to dismantle restricted notions of how knowledge is defined,
- confirm the language in which knowledge is validated, and
- seek to decrease harm of misdirected and colonized perspectives regarding mentorship and your research processes.

Similarly, drawing on mentors' relationships to bilingualism and experiences of bilingual research production and publication can support you in centering the knowledge you seek to explore; owning your positionality as you frame your research questions; selecting your study methodologies and recruit participants; and tapping into your cultural linguistics while you analyze, interpret, and publish your study. Given the central role of research advisors and mentors in your professional development as a scientist–practitioner–advocate who conducts bilingual research, consider whether your mentors

- take a personal and professional assessment of knowledge and awareness regarding systemic and structural processes, cultural concepts, and ways of knowing with Latine communities;

- apply a strengths-based conceptualization and implementation of Latine research that incorporates culture, cultural linguistics, and sociocultural identities;

- model, through research conversations and programmatic agendas, the production of bilingual research;

- determine how to engage in a reciprocal mentoring relationship to empower you to embody your expertise and wealth of knowledge of your communities;

- reframe the conceptualization of authorship as communal and recognize that the author lineup will prioritize the community;

- empower you to submit and present your work at professional conferences to advance the scholarly discourse;

- identify core research courses where bilingualism can be integrated into the training curriculum and programmatic discussions;

- advocate for in-program/department trainings to address bilingual research so as to foster an integrative and dynamic bilingual research practice;

- submit strong reference letters for scholarships/fellowships to support your research; and

- identify and connect you to professional organizations that can promote your understanding and practices of bilingual research.

APPLICATION TO DEMI

Conducting bilingual research requires critical consciousness (e.g., awareness of needed training, self-initiative, advocacy for support), confidence in the methodological processes used, and an understanding of cultural linguistics (Uribe & Gloria, 2023). These requirements allow us to conceptualize and complete research that is anchored in congruency and resistance within collective advocacy in the achievement of Latine empowerment. As we return to Demi's narrative, we encourage you to acompañar her in developing our collective narrative interconnected through our struggles and successes as bilingual researchers; specifically, we encourage you to identify and name how you will apply Demi's points of research processes to your engagement with research. We identify practical actions to model conceptualizations, methods, implementation, analyses, interpretation, publication, and mentorship as reflected in Demi's mixed-methods bilingual research to understand Latine undergraduates' sense of belonging, needs, and lived experiences.

Conceptualization

Demi first considers her experience and understanding of bilingualism in academia, which has at times been negative and has resulted in her capacities as a student being challenged. She holds a strengths-based belief about the systems of wealth and capital that are inherent to her identity as a bilingual Latina, and she considers the context of systemic and structural racism and academic violence as part of Latine students' educational experiences. From her bilingual positionality, she identifies her study's theoretical framework to include systemic and person–environment informed approaches (e.g., psychosociocultural and LatCrit) to guide her study.

Methods and Implementation

Demi's research questions are then embedded within Latine cultural values, bilingualism, and theory (e.g., a LatCrit approach to what it means to belong on campus for Latine students). First, by conducting a scoping review, she identifies the gaps in understanding related to belonging as a cultural process that is emotionally, linguistically, behaviorally, contextually, socially, and communally informed and engaged. For example, she asked what is a sense of belonging that is centered within the context of bilingualism and Latine undergraduates in higher education. She used EBSCO's databases to search, specifically using key journals, such as the *Journal of Counseling Psychology* and the *Journal of Latinx Psychology*, and Google Scholar. Upon initial review, she expanded outward to include "Latine communities," "Spanish/English," and "graduate students" as appended key terms. She included peer-reviewed articles and books that specifically addressed Latines' sense of belonging in higher education and bilingualism with no date restriction. Last, she sorted the articles by their specific research focus on a sense of belonging, elements, and practices.

Although it took time and poniendo ganas, Demi determined that most scales that assess belonging were not developed for, normed on, or assessed for cultural equivalence with bilingual Latine undergraduates. As a form of advocacy, she selected an etic belonging scale and conducted a confirmatory factor analysis to assess its broader utility in relation to her study and determined that a new scale needed to be developed and piloted. In doing so, she focused on the scale's cultural equivalence (translation–back translation of cultural nuances), interaction of identities (generation to college, immigration status, language), context or space (predominantly White institution, geography), time (sociocontextual history, policy), and change over time (acculturation). She collaborated with promotores académicos (e.g., a trusted Latine academic advisor, a known Latine student leader) to spread word of her study and increase participation in pláticas de comunidad. She also consulted with Latine undergraduate mentees in the form of an advisory board as well as other faculty experts who study Latine college students' belonging so she could tap into their cultural expertise through charlas, pláticas, and testimonios and access their funds of knowledge regarding the study's conceptual final interpretations of the data. To triangulate the needs and the provision of resources, she connected with advisors; student organizations; cultural centers; Latine faculty association; advocacy initiatives; and programs for Latine undergraduates.

Analyses and Interpretation

Demi sought out her cultivated relational networks to ensure the linguistic accuracy and cultural nuances of her findings. She addressed the statistical, practical, and relevance significance of her findings to provide nuanced meaningfulness and narration of experiences for Latine students. Her culturally informed meaning-making underscored Latine generational wealth (e.g., familismo, sabiduría, culture, history, language) and a sense of belonging within the larger sociopolitical and educational structures. She engaged with her relational networks to deepen her Spanish fluency and accuracy so she could engage in professional discussions and enhance her nuanced cultural linguistics for practical discussions of the study's findings and applications (e.g., returning findings to community).

Publication Considerations

To return knowledge to the community, Demi sought a journal outlet that took a strengths-based approach to address sociocontextual systems and processes in an effort to advance the multilayered understanding of how familismo and colectivismo are steeped in Spanish language engagement, such as how cultural code-switching (e.g., individualism vs. collectivism) informs Latine students' sense of belonging. She took a collaborative authorship approach that included community partners as authors who plan to implement the findings in community-based programming. As part of her equitable working relationships, she consulted with her faculty advisor about her process of sharing community knowledge. She needed to engage in multiple rounds of responding to the journal editors' queries, defending her culturally informed guiding framework, discussing the relevance significance, her decision to not italicize Spanish language text, and her inclusion of a resumen. With every rework of her manuscript, she remained ardent about her values-aligned approach, which was grounded in advocacy to publish her work.

Mentoring Others in Bilingual Research

At each team meeting, Demi had ongoing discussions about team members' positionalities (race, ethnicity, language, college generation, immigration) and how their working assumptions/biases were informing their research process. She openly discussed the power dynamics to demystify and dismantle previous approaches to research and mentorship. She also addressed their positionalities relative to methodological trustworthiness, which centered and validated the team member's cultural wisdom. Demi focused on each member's cultural intuition and sabiduría to empower their scholarly identity as students who are capable of conducting bilingual research. The team presented the study's findings at a professional conference where they met other Latine scholar activists who were conducting bilingual educational and community-based research. Demi also now plans to apply for a scholarship for two team members so they can complete their bilingual senior theses.

TAKEAWAYS

- Use your bilingual positionality and strengths when you are working in institutions to create spaces for bilingual research when there is a struggle to have it named, recognized, and valued.

- Center your conceptualization of bilingual research as the cultural linguistics of knowing and embodying the direct, attitudinal, experiential, negotiating, and meaning-making of Latine lived experiences.

- Name the systemic and structural oppressions that overshadow the role, function, and specific methods as you conduct, and conceptualize your bilingual research study for and with Latine communities; specifically, use your bilingual capacities and positionality to empower Latine communities to share their narratives and community expertise to advance well-being.

PARA REFLEXIONAR

- What does it mean to you to be a bilingual researcher? What is your association to bilingualism? What resources or supports are available to you to support your bilingual research? Who do you need to find or create relational networks to support your research (from conceptualization to publication)?

- How will you tap into cultural linguistics of Latine communities to survive, thrive, and guide you through the academy that is impacted by systemic and structural oppressions?

- Where will you engage in conversations of confianza that allow for critical reflection and the dismantling of universalistic and colonialized notions of bilingual research?

- How can you stay strong and écharle ganas to engage in the difficult work of creating bilingual and culturally meaningful research in settings/spaces that may directly and indirectly invalidate or support your process?

RESOURCES TO SURVIVE AND THRIVE ENTRE FRONTERAS

When you experience questioning, backlash, or moments of doubt, we encourage you to turn to processes of resistance to live out and live through your valores, cultural processes, and connections (Gloria & Castellanos, 2016) that can support you through your bilingual research scholarship. Honor the sacrifices, strengths, joys, and creative energies that emanate from bilingualism and the strengths-based connections and ways of knowing it offers. Paso a paso, we offer the reminder that we each hold the following resources to bolster/fuel and advance your ganas as bilingual scientists–practitioners–advocates:

- Concientización: Claim your ancestral wisdoms and ways of knowing through circles of compromiso (see Soto et al., 2009).

- Sabiduría: Write with your bodymindspiritsoul to navigate as a nepantlera and poderosx (see Herrera & Gloria, 2021).

- Conexión: Find familia académica (see Gloria et al., 2019) colleagues, comxadres, and mentors who can engage in culturally responsive mentoring (see Castellanos et al., 2023).

- Ánimo: Connect broadly with other bilingual Latinx students who are conducting bilingual research via social media and virtual professional sites to create academic family and connection (e.g., @latinx_womxn).

REFERENCES

American Psychological Association. (2017). *Ethical principles of psychologists and code of conduct (including 2010 and 2016 amendments)*. https://https://www.apa.org/ethics/code
American Psychological Association. (2020). *Publication manual of the American Psychological Association* (7th ed.). https://doi.org/10.1037/0000165-000
Arksey, H., & O'Malley, L. (2005). Scoping studies: Towards a methodological framework. *International Journal of Social Research Methodology, 8*(1), 19–32. https://doi.org/10.1080/1364557032000119616

Arredondo, P., Avilés, R. M. D., Zalaquett, C. P., del Pilar Grazioso, M. P., Bordes, V., Hita, L. C., & Lopez, B. J. (2006). The psychohistorical approach in family counseling with Mestizo/Latino immigrants: A continuum and synergy of worldviews. *The Family Journal, 14*(1), 13–27. https://doi.org/10.1177/1066480705283089

Braveman, P. A., Arkin, E., Proctor, D., Kauh, T., & Holm, N. (2022). Systemic and structural racism: Definitions, examples, health damages, and approaches to dismantling. *Health Affairs, 41*(2), 171–178. https://doi.org/10.1377/hlthaff.2021.01394

Brown, N. H., & Torres-Harding, S. (2021). Reliability and validity of a Spanish translation of the Racial Microaggressions Scale (S-RMAS). *Journal of Latinx Psychology, 9*(4), 269–283. https://doi.org/10.1037/lat0000190

Burlew, A. K., Peteet, B. J., McCuistian, C., & Miller-Roenigk, B. D. (2019). Best practices for researching diverse groups. *American Journal of Orthopsychiatry, 89*(3), 354–368. https://doi.org/10.1037/ort0000350

Calderón, D., Bernal, D. D., Pérez Huber, L., Malagón, M. C., & Vélez, V. N. (2012). A Chicana feminist epistemology revisited: Cultivating ideas a generation later. *Harvard Educational Review, 82*(4), 513–539. https://doi.org/10.17763/haer.82.4.l518621577461p68

Castellanos, J., White, J. L., & Franco, V. (2023). *Riding the academic freedom train: A culturally responsive, multigenerational mentoring model.* Taylor & Francis.

Comas-Díaz, L. (2016). *Mujerista* psychospirituality. In T. Bryant-Davis & L. Comas-Díaz (Eds.), *Womanist and* mujerista *psychologies: Voices of fire, acts of courage* (pp. 149–169). American Psychological Association. https://doi.org/10.1037/14937-007

Cueva, B. M. (2014). Institutional academic violence: Racial and gendered microaggressions in higher education. *Chicana/Latina Studies, 13*(2), 142–168. https://www.jstor.org/stable/43941436

Danjo, C. (2017). Reflecting on my positionality as a multilingual researcher. In J. Conteh (Ed.), *Researching education for social justice in multilingual settings: Ethnographic principles in qualitative research* (pp. 105–120). Bloomsbury Academic. https://doi.org/10.5040/9781350002661.ch-006

Delgado, M. (1997). Interpretation of Puerto Rican elder research findings: A community forum of research respondents. *Journal of Applied Gerontology, 16*(3), 317–332. https://doi.org/10.1177/073346489701600307

Delgado Bernal, D. (1998). Using a Chicana feminist epistemology in educational research. *Harvard Educational Review, 68*(4), 555–579. https://doi.org/10.17763/haer.68.4.5wv1034973g22q48

Delgado-Romero, E. A., Singh, A. A., & De Los Santos, J. (2018). *Cuéntame*: The promise of qualitative research with Latinx populations. *Journal of Latina/o Psychology, 6*(4), 318–328. https://doi.org/10.1037/lat0000123

Diaz Solodukhin, L., & Orphan, C. M. (2022). Operationalizing funds of knowledge: Examining a reciprocal research relationship between a White faculty member and a Latino student. *Journal of Diversity in Higher Education, 15*(2), 207–217. https://doi.org/10.1037/dhe0000286

Elder, J. P., Ayala, G. X., Parra-Medina, D., & Talavera, G. A. (2009). Health communication in the Latino community: Issues and approaches. *Annual Review of Public Health, 30*(1), 227–251. https://doi.org/10.1146/annurev.publhealth.031308.100300

Flores, I., Consoli, A. J., Gonzalez, J. C., Luis Sanchez, E., & Barnett, M. L. (2022). "*Todo se hace de corazón*": An examination of role and identity among Latina *promotoras de salud. Journal of Latinx Psychology, 10*(1), 5–24. https://doi.org/10.1037/lat0000194

Garcia, N. M., & Delgado Bernal, D. (2021). Remembering and revisiting pedagogies of the home. *American Educational Research Journal, 58*(3), 567–601. https://doi.org/10.3102/0002831220954431

Gloria, A. M., & Castellanos, J. (2016). Latinas *poderosas*: Shaping *mujerismo* to manifest sacred spaces for healing and transformation. In T. Bryant-Davis & L. Comas-Díaz (Eds.), *Womanist and* mujerista *psychologies: Voices of fire, acts of courage* (pp. 93–119). American Psychological Association. https://doi.org/10.1037/14937-005

Gloria, A. M., Castellanos, J., Dueñas, M., & Franco, V. (2019). Academic family and educational *Compadrazgo*: Implementing cultural values to create educational relationships for informal learning and persistence for Latinx undergraduates. In J. Calvo de Mora & K. J. Kennedy (Eds.), *Schools and informal learning in a knowledge-based world* (pp. 119–135). Routledge. https://doi.org/10.4324/9780429022616

Gloria, A. M., & Rodriguez, E. R. (2000). Counseling Latino university students: Psychosociocultural issues for consideration. *Journal of Counseling and Development, 78*(2), 145–154. https://doi.org/10.1002/j.1556-6676.2000.tb02572.x

Herrera, N., & Gloria, A. M. (2021). Latina students' post-IPV healing: A bodymind-spirit approach using the ELLA-SANA Model. *Women & Therapy, 47*(1), 89–108. https://doi.org/10.1080/02703149.2021.1982537

Holmes, P. (2016). Navigating languages and interculturality in the research process: The ethics and positionality of the researcher and the researched. In M. Dasli & A. R. Díaz (Eds.), *The critical turn in language and intercultural communication pedagogy* (pp. 115–132). Routledge. https://doi.org/10.4324/9781315667294

Johnson, C. M., Sharkey, J. R., Dean, W. R., St John, J. A., & Castillo, M. (2013). *Promotoras* as research partners to engage health disparity communities. *Journal of the Academy of Nutrition and Dietetics, 113*(5), 638–642. https://doi.org/10.1016/j.jand.2012.11.014

Mercado, A., & Venta, A. (2022). *Cultural competency in psychological assessment: Working effectively with Latinx populations.* Oxford University Press. https://doi.org/10.1093/med-psych/9780190065225.001.0001

Miles, J. R., & Fassinger, R. E. (2021). Creating a public psychology through a scientist–practitioner–advocate training model. *American Psychologist, 76*(8), 1232–1247. https://doi.org/10.1037/amp0000855

Mohajeri, K., Mesgari, M., & Lee, A. S. (2022). Conflating relevance with practical significance and other issues: Commentary on Sen, Smith, and Van Note's "Statistical Significance Versus Practical Importance in Information Systems Research." *Journal of Information Technology, 37*(3), 305–311. https://doi.org/10.1177/02683962221087449

Munn, Z., Peters, M. D. J., Stern, C., Tufanaru, C., McArthur, A., & Aromataris, E. (2018). Systematic review or scoping review? Guidance for authors when choosing between a systematic or scoping review approach. *BMC Medical Research Methodology, 18*(1), 143. https://doi.org/10.1186/s12874-018-0611-x

Pérez Huber, L. P. (2009). Disrupting apartheid of knowledge: *Testimonio* as methodology in Latina/o critical race research in education. *International Journal of Qualitative Studies in Education, 22*(6), 639–654. https://doi.org/10.1080/09518390903333863

Ramírez Stege, A. M., Brockberg, D., & Hoyt, W. T. (2017). Advocating for advocacy: An exploratory survey on student advocacy skills and training in counseling psychology. *Training and Education in Professional Psychology, 11*(3), 190–197. https://doi.org/10.1037/tep0000158

Rendón, L. I. (2023). Sentipensante *(sensing/thinking) pedagogy: Educating for wholeness, social justice and liberation* (2nd ed.). Routledge.

Sharma, M., Sarin, A., Gupta, P., Sachdeva, S., & Desai, A. V. (2014). Journal impact factor: Its use, significance and limitations. *World Journal of Nuclear Medicine, 13*(2), 146. https://doi.org/10.4103/1450-1147.139151

Solórzano, D., & Delgado Bernal, D. (2001). Examining transformational resistance through a critical race and LatCrit theory framework: Chicana and Chicano students in an urban context. *Urban Education, 36*(3), 308–342. https://doi.org/10.1177/0042085901363002

Soto, L. D., Cervantes-Soon, C., Villarreal, E., & Campos, E. (2009). The Xicana Sacred Space: A communal circle of *compromiso* for educational researchers. *Harvard Educational Review, 79*(4), 755–776. https://doi.org/10.17763/haer.79.4.4k3x387k74754q18

Thompson, A. (2004). Gentlemanly orthodoxy: Critical race feminism, Whiteness theory, and the *APA Manual. Educational Theory, 54*(1), 27–57. https://doi.org/10.1111/j.0013-2004.2004.00002.x

Torres, L. (2007). In the contact zone: Code-switching strategies by Latinola writers. *Melus, 32*(1), 75–96. https://doi.org/10.1093/melus/32.1.75

Trnka, K. (2016). *Foreign word alert, foreign word alert*: Rethinking editorial approaches to the italicization of foreign terms [Unpublished master's thesis]. Portland State University.

Uribe, Y., & Gloria, A. M. (2023, October 26–28). *Latinidad-centered and integrative approaches: Latinx scholar's perspectives of bilingual research* [Poster session]. National Latinx Psychological Association Annual Conference, Chicago, IL, United States.

Zea, M. C., Asner-Self, K. K., Birman, D., & Buki, L. P. (2003). The Abbreviated Multi-dimensional Acculturation Scale: Empirical validation with two Latino/Latina samples. *Cultural Diversity & Ethnic Minority Psychology, 9*(2), 107–126. https://doi.org/10.1037/1099-9809.9.2.107

8

ADVANCED *CAMINOS*

Navegando *Internship and Postdoctoral Programs as a Bilingual Trainee*

MACIEL CAMPOS AND YESSENIA MEJIA

Lo que está pa'ti, nadie te lo quita. Internship and postdoctoral training are traditionally considered to be the final steps in graduate school before one officially transitions into the workforce full time. Other disciplines follow similar patterns of training, such as internships for social work and fellowships for psychiatry. In this chapter, we focus on the intentional pursuit of opportunities for bilingual professional development at this advanced level of doctoral and postdoctoral training. We begin by reviewing the history of advanced training opportunities while exploring salient themes such as systemic inequities in higher education, training site–applicant ratios, and the furthering of an affirming path toward your personally defined success in bilingual mental health. Our recommendations and tips are intended to facilitate your application process and navigation of bilingual interviews. Our points of discussion here are a call to action for improvements in advanced training in bilingual mental health. Our lived experiences as former trainees and current supervisors inform how we provide guidance on affirming, attuned, and authentic approaches for maximizing crucial professional development requirements and milestones. This is the chapter we wished had been written for us; *lo escribimos para ti.*

https://doi.org/10.1037/0000481-009
Forging Caminos: *Pathways to Becoming a Bilingual Mental Health Professional,*
M. Campos, Y. Mejia, and A. J. Consoli (Editors)

THE RACE TO THE FINISH LINE

Podrán cortar todas las flores, pero no podrán detener la primavera.
—Pablo Neruda

¿*La ves*? Yes, we see it too—the (faint) *luz* at the end of the tunnel! *Ya casi completas* a large portion of this journey. Internship and postdoctoral fellowships are unique milestones deserving of additional and nuanced *consejos*. The number of Latines and students in higher education who are Black, Indigenous, and People of Color has steadily grown over the years. Despite this upward trend, systemic barriers, such as the markedly limited access to quality education, role models, and employment opportunities, persist, further marginalizing Latine communities. This educational marginalization is perpetuated by way of higher student-to-counselor ratios, low-resourced schools, and low academic expectations by administration and is intricately linked to economic marginalization (Pietrantonio & Llamas, 2020). Unsurprisingly, these minoritizing mechanisms and marginalizing dynamics continue at the graduate level.

There is a dearth of graduate programs that are properly staffed and designed to provide education and training to equip students with the *herramientas* needed to work with *las comunidades latinas* (see Chapter 1, this volume). This is illustrated by the relationship between a trainee and an unpaid practicum site where the student receives training, supervision, and mentorship; in return, the practicum site has an added stream of revenue and is able to outsource patients because of staffing shortages throughout mental health service systems. For bilingual and Latinx students who accompany Spanish-speaking people, however, this contract does not always include intentional considerations of the adequate supervision and guidance that are essential in delivering culturally and linguistically attuned care.

With ongoing tuition inflation, the pursuit of higher education is resulting in students from lower socioeconomic status (SES) backgrounds, students of color, and women being priced out or taking on insurmountable levels of student debt (Wilcox et al., 2021). Hidden costs, such as college life expenses, fees not associated with tuition, and technology needs (i.e., laptop, cellphone, reliable high-speed internet access), significantly affect low-income and economically marginalized students. Moreover, training requirements necessary for doctoral programs also include the cost of accepting unpaid practica, transportation, business attire, internship application expenses, membership fees in relevant associations, and attending professional conferences. The cognitive and emotional strains caused by the financial stressors related to higher education significantly affect economically marginalized, first-generation students in a way that is not experienced by students from higher SES strata, who are also more likely to have educational capital. At times, students from lower SES backgrounds will have to take on other jobs to ease the financial burden, exposing them to the professional cost of diminished time for studying, research, publishing, and other related activities.

The purported symbiotic relationship between the unpaid trainee and the practicum site is not as simple for students from lower SES backgrounds who do not have the generational wealth or financial support to offset the cost of free labor. In addition, although an internship is a funded position, the stipend offered is not enough to cover basic living expenses. Meanwhile, those with access to economic resources have the privilege to withstand low wages for the sake of learning. Calls to action include fair and equitable compensation for students of marginalized backgrounds for their unique labor contributions via practica (Kawaii-Bogue, 2020) to specialized fields like bilingual mental health. An examination of the history of psychology training programs will help you understand how requirements and expectations were determined for such programs, which are meant to provide hands-on training and experience for students while they continue their coursework.

HISTORY OF TRAINING PROGRAMS

In 1968, the Association of Psychology Internship Centers (APIC) was established to organize the internship selection process (Erickson Cornish & Baker, 2023). In 1971, the first directory of internship programs was published and made available for purchase, and in 1973 APIC established Universal Notification Day, otherwise known as "Match Day." Despite all the efforts to streamline the internship application and decision-making process for students, it was not until 1978 that the American Psychological Association (APA) recognized APIC as the principal institution for regulating internship training. APIC established the precedents for internship training requirements with their policy, set forth in 1987, indicating that internship training, with funded positions available, should occur over 2 years, with one predoctoral year and one postdoctoral year. It also recommended that internship take place after the completion of coursework and a dissertation at an accredited program. By 1991, APIC became the Association of Psychology Postdoctoral and Internship Centers (APPIC; https://www.appic.org/), to include postdoctoral training, and joined the Council of Chairs of Training Councils (https://www.cctcpsychology.org/about/) to foster relationships with other regulating bodies, such as APA and the Association of State and Provincial Psychology Boards (https://asppb.net/). Over the course of 50 years, APPIC has established an online directory, a standardized electronic application, the use of a national match system algorithm, multiple listservs, and a research committee.

The Internship Selection Process

In the early days of the internship selection process, the application forms and the extension of offers varied from program to program, making it an even more stressful and chaotic process. Over time, APPIC standardized this process and limited the match to students from doctoral programs accredited by APA or the Canadian Psychological Association. As of 2023, candidates complete a universal application and online rankings, which are then entered into a computer system that runs the national match system algorithm, ultimately matching the highest ranked site to the highest ranked doctoral student (Erickson Cornish & Baker, 2023). For students who are not matched in Phase I, there is a Phase II (i.e., the Post-Match Vacancy Service; https://www.appic.org/Internships/Match/Post-Match-Vacancy-Service), which allows students to apply to programs with openings available. There is currently an imbalance between students and available sites, which has made it more difficult for students to match in Phase I.

Internship Imbalance

In 1983, there were equal numbers of applicants and available internship positions. However, over time the number of applicants steadily increased, creating an imbalance that persisted for several years (Erickson Cornish & Baker, 2023). By 2012, at the peak of this imbalance, 29% (1,245) of applicants did not match with an internship site. This motivated APA to invest $3 million to assist in the development of accredited internship positions and APPIC to invest $500,000 to support the program accreditation process. Erickson Cornish and Baker noted that in 2017, this imbalance began to shift because of added positions and a decrease in applicants, and by 2019 there were 15 more positions than applicants. However, there were still few accredited positions available. Then, in 2021, APPIC required programs to be part of APPIC's membership to be included in the internship match process. Between this new requirement and the impact of the COVID-19 pandemic, the imbalance once again shifted, with 620 more students than accredited sites available. As of 2023, there are 646 accredited sites and 121 unaccredited sites across the United States, with a commitment from

APPIC to increase the number of accredited positions to meet the demand of applicants (APPIC, 2023; Erickson Cornish & Baker, 2023).

Health services in the United States, such as medicine, psychology, physical therapy, and dentistry, are controlled by state governing authorities; psychology is the only health service profession that allows licensure eligibility for graduates from a nonaccredited internship. Should this change, it would pose a significant barrier for graduates from nonaccredited internships seeking to directly provide mental health care to the public because current industry standards require providers to have doctoral-level degrees and state licensure. Given these specifications, graduating from an accredited graduate program and internship site provides students with the widest variety of licensure and career opportunities. On a related note, the APA Center for Workforce Studies (https://www.apa.org/workforce) has projected that by 2030, to meet the demand of underrepresented populations, including older adults, children, and Latinx populations, there will be a need for 20% more doctoral-level mental health providers than are currently in a program of study (Erickson Cornish & Baker, 2023).

A PONERSE LAS PILAS: APPLYING FOR AN INTERNSHIP

Although this chapter is based on experiences specific to psychology doctorates, we anticipate that many of the tips and considerations we share here can be generalized to other disciplines and degrees, including social work, psychiatry, and terminal master's degrees. If you are a psychology doctoral candidate and have successfully met APPIC criteria for match eligibility (see https://tinyurl.com/3juuux9z), then *ha llegado la hora* to actively pursue the internship application. Be sure to familiarize yourself with your graduate program's requirements for authorization to apply for an internship, such as the required amount of progress on your dissertation. The APPIC website on match policies (https://tinyurl.com/y3xaudsy) is a helpful resource to consult regularly. *Repasemos* the preparation steps and considerations before and during completion of your APPIC Application for Psychology Internships (AAPI; https://www.appic.org/Internships/Internship-Application-AAPI-Portals). The AAPI is a detailed and lengthy application and the first component of your internship application process that will showcase your identity as a bilingual mental health professional in training. For this chapter, we have curated a beginning-to-finish application approach *para que sientas que ¡esto es un mamey!* We want you grounded in your identity and values, prepared to complete this initial phase of the process. *Así que, a ponerse las pilas*; *¡manos a la obra* and to your keyboard to complete your AAPI!

Although you will do this continuously throughout your academic and professional careers, now is an important time to reflect on your past training and academic experiences and to review your personal and professional goals as a bilingual mental health professional seeking an internship. Consider a self-assessment of your bilingual competencies, including bilingual skills you would like to continue to develop, and any overall exposure that is missing from your bilingual mental health training. Reflect on core memories and formative experiences that have shaped and informed your identity as a bilingual mental health professional today, and consider what this identity means to you and the role you imagine it will play in your career. The intersectionality among your identities, your bilingualism, and your professional development goals will be crucial to explore as you refine the next *pasos* in your career. Your goals and envisioned future as a bilingual mental health scientist–practitioner will help guide your internship site search.

We recommend that you develop a timeline and a schedule to decrease the chances of feeling overwhelmed because due dates are very important in the internship application process. APPIC has a step-by-step timeline available on their website (https://tinyurl.com/y2xdneah). *Camarón que se duerme se lo lleva la corriente,* so give yourself ample time to complete your application at a pace that contributes to feelings of efficacy and satisfaction. Because most internship applications are due between November and December, our strongest recommendation is that you begin to dedicate time to organizing and goal-setting no later than the summer before you plan to submit your applications. You can create this timeline during the aforementioned reflective process.

In the United States, you will probably locate most internship sites with access to bilingual training in the Northeast, south Florida, Puerto Rico, the Southwest, Midwestern states, and the West coast. However, as the Spanish-speaking population in the United States increases, so does the diversification of their geographic locations. Some bilingual training sites will provide ready access to clinical experiences and research with bilingual English-/Spanish-speaking populations without a formalized bilingual training program. Other bilingual training sites will offer more formalized and comprehensive programming that includes clinical and research supervision in Spanish, training in a range of treatment models that are culturally and linguistically attuned to Spanish-speaking Latinx populations, and professional development and mentorship as a bilingual mental health professional.

The National Association of Latinx Psychology (NLPA; https://www.nlpa.ws) has made efforts to create a directory of Latinx focused predoctoral psychology internships. NLPA currently has a comprehensive list available on their website that reviews predoctoral programs and provides details about the bilingual support, services, and training opportunities available. Acquaint yourself with the possibilities as well as with your vision for your bilingual training so you can apply to sites in a way that increases your chances of success. APA's Division 53 (Society of Clinical Child and Adolescent Psychology) Bilingual Psychologists Special Interest Group also compiles a list of internship sites with bilingual training for its members. Consult with your program training director, fellow classmates, and alumni to learn and share more because programming at sites is in flux due to changes in staffing and funding. Remember, *cuando gana une, ganan todes*. The hoarding of resources is characteristic of oppressive ideologies (Jones & Okun, 2001; Okun, 2023) and misaligned with the liberation and social justice core of this book. *Aquí se comparte.*

Bring notes from your self-reflections, and complete your applications along with your *compañeres*. This is a great way to obtain feedback and *apoyo*, socialize, and make space for *desahogo*. We recommend engaging in this process with a study buddy/*compa* who understands your values and the role bilingualism plays in your identities and professional development. Taking care of yourself is also paramount to being successful in this process. Channel your ancestors' wisdom, and eat foods that nourish your body, mind, and soul. Engage in spirit-enhancing practices and maintain good *compañía*. Although some of these activities might generate a sense of guilt, we encourage you to make space for enjoying yourself during this process. Laugh! Think about curating a motivational and grounding bilingual music playlist or baking your favorite *pan dulce*. Aside from nourishing your *pancita y alma*, these activities can inspire brilliant themes for your applications or interviews.

We strongly recommend you familiarize yourself with the AAPI before you start to complete it. Emphasize your demonstrated commitment to become a bilingual professional and your intersectional identities at all opportunities on the AAPI. The major components of the AAPI, which include the cover letter, the four essays, and the case write-up/psychological assessment allow you to do this. Your cover letter is an opportunity to succinctly highlight your skills and goals in bilingual mental health and to emphasize your compatibility as a bilingual mental health professional with the internship site's mission and values, especially as they pertain to bilingual training. Similarly, obtaining letters of recommendation from mentors who can speak to your professional acumen and the values you encompass is another opportunity to highlight your merits and linguistic expertise. As of 2023, applicants include four essays that address their autobiography, diversity, theoretical orientation, and research interests. These essays are an excellent opportunity for you to create a memorable application. The autobiographical statement is likely your best platform for contextualizing your *camino* in psychology thus far. Authentic experiences that apply to the skills and values of bilingual mental health are the best subjects for the personal statement. We also acknowledge the fine balance of showcasing your lived experiences in ways that are authentic and genuine to you without feeling exploitative of your identities (Colon Hidalgo & McElroy, 2021). You are more than your struggles.

To further illustrate this point, we share an example from Maciel's AAPI. Finding herself 1,500 miles away from her native Brooklyn, New York, for the first time, Maciel used a lyric from Frank Sinatra's song "New York, New York" as the central focus of her autobiographical statement. She recalled how her father quoted this lyric to her when she relocated to Chicago, Illinois, for her doctoral program (ancestral *sabiduría*). She used this memory and song to highlight her attachment to her beloved city and family values as part of her identity; emphasized themes of resilience, acculturation, and diversity; and connected this all to her goals as a psychologist. In writing this statement, Maciel kept in mind a few priorities for herself: returning to New York City, working with historically excluded communities, and remaining her true authentic self.

The remaining essays, as well as the case write-up/psychological assessment report, offer plenty of opportunities to center your bilingualism as you reflect on your theoretical orientation, diversity issues, and research interests. We recommend that these materials highlight themes of language, bilingualism, Latinx culture, and acculturation as well as your culturally and linguistically humble and attuned approaches. Think about including Spanish throughout your application, much like you have observed us do throughout this chapter. There is no guarantee that a Spanish speaker will read your application, so consider including translations. Last, highlight strengths in bilingual and bicultural mental health and avoid tropes that present mental health practitioners as saviors; instead, center the wisdom of the communities we accompany.

The second essay will ask you to focus on your theoretical orientation. We recommend that you present a de-identified case that is not only reflective of the theoretical orientation you use to practice but also one that showcases your commitment to accompanying bilingual and Latinx communities. Highlight the linguistic and cultural nuances, adaptations, and considerations in your interventions, and be sure to present these as embedded in your orientation as opposed to an add-on. There are many identities that can be addressed in the diversity essay, and language/bilingualism can definitely be included. Our tip for this essay is that you keep in mind the dynamics of diversity in relationship to individuals, communities, and yourself. We recommend a social location that anchors you in awareness of your own proximity to power and privilege. Last, there are so many areas of bilingual mental health yet to be explored that would make excellent contributions to your research essay! If your dissertation or research topic is not focused on bilingual mental health, don't fret—highlight your expertise and *creatividad*.

We encourage both native and nonnative Spanish speakers to be transparent in your AAPI about your fluency level and experiences speaking Spanish within your academic training. Being accurate about your Spanish fluency on your AAPI will help the evaluators prepare for your interview. Refer to Chapter 2 in this volume for more tips on centering your immersion experiences to highlight your commitment to bilingual mental health. We also encourage you to acknowledge any privilege and positions of power you hold in the context of accompanying Spanish-speaking Latinx communities. As supervisors and interviewers, it has been our experience, and that of our colleagues, to share a mission to recruit applicants who demonstrate commitments to advancing their own skills within bilingual mental health as well as advancing the field.

As you complete your AAPI, remember that your skills are not limited to your professional experiences. Many of us have lifelong experiences in translating and brokering that are reflective of skills in liaising, multitasking, and team building. These shared experiences facilitate our connection with bilingual communities. First-generation applicants, and in particular first-born *hijas*, tend to have histories of *kinkeeping* whereby they assume responsibilities to ensure the success of their family system. These experiences can be translated to managerial, problem-solving, time management, and team building skills (Guzman, 2024; Rosenthal, 1985). Stories of immigration, acculturation, and navigation of systemic oppression illustrate your resilience, persistence, and determination. "You are your ancestors' wildest dream" (Brandan Odums) *pa' que lo sepan*.

LUZ, CÁMARA, Y ACCIÓN: TIME FOR YOUR INTERVIEW

The interview process can feel like a long string of performances in different arenas, all in the hope that the interviewer can see the magic that is you. When the ratio of students to training sites favors sites, each interview can feel like a make-or-break situation. Intricate beliefs and values rooted in White supremacy permeate messages about how professionalism manifests in different spaces. As a result, it can feel as though you need to be someone else in order to "wow" the interviewer. Masking your true self behind a power suit, blown-out slick hair, and muted colors for the sake of fitting into such a mold of professionalism is likely to deny you the opportunity to be your authentic self for fear that you will not be accepted, valued, or understood. Oftentimes, expressions of authenticity are met with discrimination, microaggressions, and racism.

If it is safe, we encourage you to consider ways to embody your authentic self with confidence and self-empowerment. We understand that White-dominant and English-centered spaces are intentionally and insidiously designed to pressure Black and Indigenous folx and people of color to hide and make ourselves small for the sake of self-preservation, yet this is done at the expense of our authentic selves. Society reinforces and rewards this behavior, opening doors when we conform with White and English-centered dominant culture. Think about safe ways to show up authentically on interview day, celebrating your identities in various ways. This can be a public display of *sabor*, such as a bold lip color or *estrenando* a snazzy tie or shirt. It can also be more subtle, such as signing your name with an accent. We all need to challenge anti-Black and anti-Indigenous practices disguised as professionalism and create safety for our colleagues to keep our natural hair and protective styles, wear attire that is reflective of our cultures, and rock our favorite hoop earrings or the decorative nose ring that adorns our face. Celebrating who we are promotes confidence and boldness, sprinkling swag into your strut. Your ancestors' strength and *sabiduría* runs through your veins. You belong, and so do your clients, your research participants, and our *causa*.

Keep in mind that as of 2023, many internship sites offer virtual options for their interviews. Although they are more affordable than in-person interviews, virtual interviews bring unique nuances, such as testing your devices and checking battery charges ahead of time. Try to ensure access to a quiet space with minimal interruptions, which might require trying your best negotiation skills with your roommates (and *sí*, your *abuelita* can count as a roommate!) or using a space in your school. Check out these fun tips for maximizing your on-camera appearance (see https://tinyurl.com/4dk964nn). If you find yourself struggling to find absolute quietude because of the many structural barriers reviewed at the beginning of this chapter, *no pasa nada*. We find that a good joke can always deflect from a passing car playing *reggaetón* or a beloved Mister Softee ice cream truck. Repurpose these moments to highlight your resilience and *humildad*.

Preparing for Interviews

As the field begins to acknowledge the importance of assessing linguistic fluency and competency, more sites are including bilingual assessments as part of their interview process. This allows sites to determine the range of your bilingual fluency, vocabulary, and comfort level when speaking Spanish, which helps gauge how much support, supervision, and training you will need depending on where you are in the bilingual spectrum. Although some people experience this practice as gatekeeping by some, it allows for the transparent and accurate determination of necessary resources to support both the trainee and the community the trainee will accompany. Evaluators who engage in this interview practice are ideally mindful of the linguistic spectrum, language evolution, and variability; they aim to determine applicants' foundational fluency for providing Spanish-language services. Ground yourself in the reminder that the goal for committed bilingual supervisors is to provide pertinent support and scaffolding for trainee language development so as to facilitate future professional practice in Spanish.

When considering interviews involving a Spanish-language assessment, be prepared to answer interview questions in Spanish and code-switch between both languages as needed and as appropriate. Review clinical and professional vocabulary, including vocabulary pertaining to equity and diversity. Practice your Spanish with family members; other cohort members; or mentors/supervisors, if you have any who speak Spanish. Seek out opportunities to participate in consultation groups in Spanish, like those hosted by NLPA. Listen to scholarly presentations from colleagues in Spanish-speaking countries to help expand your exposure to professional language. Remember, you do not have to know it all! Language acquisition, including bilingualism, is a developmental process that continues throughout our lives and our professional careers, so go easy on yourself!

Keep culture in mind! It is important to weave the thread of demonstrated commitment throughout all our interactions, especially in interviews. When interviewing for internship sites that accompany the Latine community it is important to understand cultural considerations, including values such as *familismo, respeto, y personalismo*. Be prepared to speak to the roles of acculturation, immigration, the intergenerational transmission of trauma, and racism in Latine communities. Before the interview, educate yourself on the community that the internship site accompanies. Become well acquainted with the history, diversity, strengths, resources, and barriers of that particular community. What are the challenges this community faces when trying to access education, quality care, and *apoyo*? Who are the cultural brokers or *les promotores de salud* in the community? What are the cultural and dialect nuances that may come up if you were to work with this community? To get ready, practice your responses to the following questions *en español*:

- *¿Qué significa ser proveedores bilingües de servicios en salud mental?*
- *¿Cuáles son algunos de los valores más importantes a considerar cuando se está acompañando a la comunidad latina?*
- *¿Qué servicios o tratamientos haz provisto en español en tu entrenamiento? Cuáles han sido los aspectos más difíciles al hacerlo?*
- *¿Por qué quieres acompañar a la comunidad latina, ya hispanohablante, ya bilingüe?*
- *¿Qué tipo de supervisión bilingüe has recibido en tu entrenamiento hasta ahora? ¿Qué aspectos de tu desarrollo profesional bilingüe quisieras mejorar como parte de tu supervisión?*

Case Presentation

As part of the interview, many sites are likely to ask for a case presentation of a current or recent patient with whom you have been working. There are many factors to consider when presenting a case. As part of this case presentation, centering the patient, their social location, and intersecting identities are crucial pieces that are most often underrated or missed. Most important, this case presentation should highlight your demonstrated commitment to your professional values, the communities you accompany, and the importance of cultural humility when working with clients. Here are some questions to reflect on as you develop a case presentation:

- Who is this person, and what is their (relational) story?
- How did they arrive here: in this country, in this place of *bien y malestar*, in care with you?
- What are their social location and intersecting identities? What are yours?
- What are the cultural and linguistic nuances that are pertinent to your work together?
- How do their identities intersect with the systems of which they are a part?
- What are their strengths, their hopes, their aspirations?
- What is your therapeutic relationship like with them? Are there matters of transference or countertransference that arise in your work with them?
- What has supervision of this case been like? In what ways has it been useful and pertinent, and in what ways were there gaps in supervisory support?

No Todo lo que Brilla es Oro

One of the questions we often forget to ask ourselves in this process is whether this site is the right one for me. When there are fewer sites than applicants, you might be thinking *a buen hambre, no hay pan duro*, feeling an urge to settle and be happy with what is provided. Challenge those urges, *pos* we are no longer accepting crumbs from the proverbial table. We have value, and the programs you are considering should be reciprocal in their appreciation and desire to have you join their program. Some programs talk the talk without walking the walk, *poniendo un* show. They present themselves as social justice advocates who are woke to injustice, racism, and oppression in the mental health field. So, are they really about it, or are they just running their mouths? Be prepared to recognize when your interviewer responds with platitudes and virtue signaling. Here are some questions to assess a program's commitment to their own decolonization and integration of antiracism and social justice:

- How is your program/institution decolonizing its practices, policies, and procedures?

- What areas of training focus on antiracism within the mental health/ medical system?

- Do faculty, providers, and leadership represent the community accompanied? How many Black, Indigenous, and People of Color, and Spanish-speaking supervisors, are on the team and in leadership positions?

- How is trainee feedback received, incorporated, valued?

EL QUE NO ARRIESGA, NO GANA: MATCHING AND NOT MATCHING

¡Wepa! ¡Felicidades on matching for internship! The previous 6–8 months of your life have likely been consumed by anticipation of this moment, and the next several months will focus on preparing to start internship. This will include navigating all of the *mandados* necessary to onboard at your new employment site and relocate, if need be. Amid these transitions, start thinking about what you anticipate, intentionally creating community and channels for support. A common experience among bilingual and bicultural interns, in particular those who match out of state, is seeking support around belongingness during this transition. For example, we have experienced the meaningfulness of directing a trainee where to find beauty and hair products commonly used

in their communities. These moments are integral to the feelings of stability, comfort, and groundedness that are so needed during a whirlwind year of milestones. "Only" one year can feel quite long if you do not have the appropriate support. You are worth every minute of that year, so make it count! *Del dicho al hecho hay mucho trecho*, and the most supportive mentors are those with a demonstrated commitment to bilingual mental health whose actions are aligned with the amplification of bilingual Spanish-speaking communities, bilingual training, and bilingual staff. Furthermore, the demonstrated commitment of the site where you will be interning is quite likely to promote your sense of visibility and fulfillment with your training experiences.

Mentors can include your co-interns and professionals from other disciplines; they can also be identified outside of your internship site. If you matched in a setting with limited access to supervision and mentorship from bilingual psychologists, or where you are the only bilingual person (see Chapter 6, this volume) creatively consider ways of strengthening your bilingual training when resources are limited. Efforts exist to connect a vast bilingual Spanish-speaking community across this nation and to justify the provision of appropriate resources to bilingual professionals such as you. Options for external mentorship might include the NLPA Mentorship Program (https://www.nlpa.ws/mentoring-program).

The predoctoral internship year is the first time many of you will work full time as a mental health provider. In addition, as bilingual mental health professionals we sometimes forgo our own needs to provide quality services for our *comunidades*, especially when resources are limited (Lanesskog et al., 2015). You might simultaneously experience doubt about and insecurity in your skills and success; these are often triggered by external pressures to achieve, insufficient institutional support, financial instability, or a lack of sense of belonging (Le, 2019). First-generation and racialized students in higher education contend with increased financial stress in the context of historical exclusion from generational wealth (Wilcox et al., 2021). Internship stipends do not approximate a livable income for any psychology intern, in particular interns with diminished financial support (Kawaii-Bogue, 2020).

Despite this stress, many of us who share lived experiences with the Spanish-speaking communities we accompany continue to do double the *esfuerzo* to assist our *comunidades*, at times prompted by a desire to leverage our access to new privileges (Teran et al., 2017). In addition, as you continue to learn and implement psychology concepts not normed for or centering our *comunidades*, you might notice internal tensions with continuing to disseminate such practices that risk perpetuating oppression. For example, you may notice discomfort in introducing various parenting techniques that are inconsistent with Latinx parenting norms, styles, and preferences. This tension can be overwhelming and trigger feelings of sadness, rage, and disillusionment. Although traditional psychology would recommend a discussion of countertransference, a more comprehensive conceptualization would include exploration of themes of systemic oppression and related vulnerabilities, power, privilege, hegemony, culture, and language. This level of unique stress, sense of responsibility, and tension will warrant equally unique and comprehensive self-care practices that replenish you and foster your boundaries and self-preservation.

Burnout, vicarious trauma, compassion fatigue, and moral injury are prominent in bilingual mental health given the nature and toll of the work. Bilingual trainees have reflected that two languages equate to double the work (Verdinelli & Biever, 2009), in the same amount of time and, to add insult to injury, for the same compensation as a monolingual English-speaking trainee. The math does not add up and, sadly, this usually remains true as you progress through your career. To combat general burnout and remain committed to our mission, we like to involve groundedness and connection with our heritage, roots, and spirituality (Teran et al., 2017). Other ways to ground and honor your body, mind, soul, and spirit are to respect your boundaries, process your experiences in trusted spaces, and *confiar y tener fe* that in spite of these challenges the community you accompany has many strengths and, in the words of Kendrick Lamar, is "gon' be all right." Tap into your cultural senses and try making a morning *licuado*; keep familiar scents, such as *palo santo*, at hand; cry in Spanish à la the viral Itatí Cantoral meme, engage in body work, wear clothing reflective of your identities, and remember that this connection is self-care. It is, as Audre Lorde (1988/2017) reminds us, resistance, thus holding you in sacredness to continue to care for your *comunidad*. Because training leadership and program development remain English centered, intentionality and considerations that affirm the nuances of additional deliberate workload in bilingual mental health continue to be minimal. Your work and efforts are worthy of that acknowledgment by way of compensation, accolades, recognition, and resources, for true advances in equity, justice, and liberation. As current and future bilingual mental health advocates, we are paving the *camino* to this long-overdue appraisal.

As an intern, you can address systemic oppression and racism. This will require you to engage in your own social location to better assess your positions of privilege and power, experiences with oppression, and worldview. "Intern" will be a salient identity given that it exists on a continuum of power in relation to supervisors and is contextualized by the evaluative process that is used to determine your eligibility to complete your graduate training. Discomfort, futility, and survival mode might thrive, in particular for Latinx and other racialized interns for whom cultural values might emphasize *respeto, simpatía,* and hierarchy, and speaking out might be risky. We see you, we understand you, *y estamos contigo.* If and when you choose to address systemic oppression issues related to your work as a bilingual psychologist this year, know that your experience is valid and your voice has power. Return to self-care and connect your concerns with the collective wisdom of the bilingual mental health field; with organizational policies; with diversity, equity, inclusion, and justice initiatives; and with competencies and ethics. Affirm your needs and highlight how this facilitates more respectful and equitable environments.

As if these milestones and experiences did not suffice for internship year, many of us ultimately must also juggle dissertation completion throughout the internship year. We encourage you to complete as much of your dissertation as possible before beginning your internship. An internship consumes a lot of your energy. Imagine dedicating your free time on evenings and weekends to your dissertation. Is this reasonable for your specific life circumstances? If your dissertation topic includes bilingual mental health, we recognize that factors such as translations and cultural attunement and humility may require more resources and affect your ability to finish prior to beginning internship. Outline a plan of communication and timeline with your dissertation chair, especially if you match for an internship that is out of state. We champion any timeline that works best for you, and we want you to be aware that completing your dissertation after your internship might delay next *pasos,* such as accepting a staff position or postdoctoral fellowship. *¡Ánimo!* With a solid plan and timeline, you can tackle this too!

Si te caes siete veces, levántate ocho. So, you did not match the first round. It's okay. *Le echaste ganas,* and that is commendable. You might notice sadness, disappointment, jealousy, and frustration with this entire process, which feels like jumping over hurdle after hurdle all so you can follow your passion and support *tu gente.* You are not the first to get rejected, and you will not be the last; you are not alone, you are in community. You are worthy; do not let this process define your value. *¡Lo que está pa' ti nadie te lo quita!* So, take a second to feel those feelings and pause to breathe. Before jumping back into the process, take a break. Give yourself time and space to heal. When you are ready, it is time to *reflexionar. Dios/el universo aprieta, pero no ahoga.* Use this experience to consider factors that could be different in a future application and whether you have control over handling it differently.

Remember that APPIC's match system has two phases, with Phase II being for applicants who do not match in Phase I. Because Phase II offers only sites with available positions, this heightens factors such as location, finances, and clinical fit. The sites that are available may not be aligned with the clinical experiences you are looking for, or they may be geographically distant. Consider a cost–benefit or pros–cons analysis that factors in important questions about choice, training experience, professional goals, priorities and values, and your future in bilingual mental health. There is no "right" answer! Depending on the available predoctoral internships, you may decide to apply in Phase II for many reasons, such as the desire to move forward in this process or financial constraints. On the other hand, you may decide to take another year before applying, to finish or publish projects, such as your dissertation, or to gain further clinical or teaching experience. This is not a sign of defeat; instead, it demonstrates the value you place on making sure this process is right for you. In addition, all options afford you opportunities to continue working toward growing as a bilingual mental health professional. *A mal tiempo, buena cara.* When faced with disappointment, we like to wrap ourselves in our favorite *cobija*, watch stand-up comedy, and take time to tap into some of your other talents. Most important, *¡no te des por vencide!* Reach out to your community; invoke your *ancestres*; and remember you are worthy as you are, regardless of when or where you match.

¿CHAPULÍN COLORADO . . . ?

By the end of your internship, you might be mentally chanting *"e' pa' fuera que voy"* on your way to picking up your diploma. *Mereces pachanga*, and part of the celebrations can include reflecting on everything you have accomplished this year and elucidating the next steps in your *camino*. Endings are really beginnings, and this ending offers you the opportunity to create scripts for being a bilingual mental health professional who is imbued with your prioritized values. This radical acceptance of the ups and downs of your training experience can facilitate data collection you can use to push yourself *pa'lante* and ensure fulfilling experiences. Consider how you can continue to cultivate meaningful relationships you have developed over the past year, or how you can center qualities from these relationships when you transition into supervisory and mentoring roles.

¿Y ahora qué? is the question many of us face on our graduation days. If you are considering a postdoctoral fellowship, you can follow many of the recommendations we have already reviewed. Although postdoctoral fellowships were included in APPIC as of 1991, at this time the postdoctoral application and selection process is not as standardized as the internship match

process, especially given that many fellowships are varied and do not adhere to the same internship accreditation requirements. APPIC currently offers to include postdoctoral programs in online standardized applications and on the universal notification day, free of charge (Erickson Cornish & Baker, 2023). Although the number of postdoctoral fellowships is growing, fewer individuals are seeking them, especially since the APA Model Act for State Licensure of Psychologists (APA, 2010) does not specify the need for a formalized postdoctoral training, resulting in states removing postdoctoral hours for licensure requirements.

Unique considerations at this juncture in your postdoctoral training include a range of possibilities, including a postdoctoral clinical, research, or combined fellowship or a staff position in a clinical or academic setting. *Ojo*, you will likely need to get to work on these applications early because postdoctoral applications tend to be due in the midst of the first half of your internship year, and applications for positions in academia tend to be due almost as soon as you start your internship. Your internship site might have one or more postdoctoral fellowships available. If it does, learn more to inform your decision-making process. You might feel a sense of pressure to have your next steps determined. We continue to emphasize self-care practices for grounding yourself during this uniquely stressful time. Systemic oppression factors, such as debt, contribute to this pressure, and although we understand that the rent is due (!), we highly encourage you not to rush yourself.

Remember to set timelines and to use your network of fellow trainees, mentors, advisors, or supervisors to connect with others in the field and learn about potential opportunities. Because the postdoctoral application process is not as formalized as the internship application process, you might learn of opportunities and receive offers simultaneously, creating a complicated decision-making process. Should you find yourself in a quandary over receiving offers from sites eager to fill their positions while you are still waiting to learn more or hear back from other potential sites, don't panic! Remember your value and worth, have a clear understanding of what you are looking for, and consider what you are or are not willing to negotiate. You can also transition into a staff position as a limited-permit professional, so long as you can receive supervision from a licensed professional. Pros and cons include more opportunities for formal ongoing training in a postdoctoral fellowship versus a permanent position and higher pay as a staff member. Both options will foster the development of your bilingual mental health provider identity. Always remember, there is no *right camino*; all roads lead home!

TAKEAWAYS

- Plan ahead, setting timelines and using goal-setting.
- Hone your self-care practices.
- Grow from losses.
- Build your community.

REFLEXIONES

- What are my bilingual training goals for my internship year?

- Who can be my internship exploration *compa*? In which parts of the application process will I discuss bilingual mental health and my bilingual identity?

- What are my self-care practices, and how can I maintain a desired connection to specific ancestors and my culture during this process?

- What benchmarks in bilingual mental health will I want to accomplish by the end of my internship year, and what opportunities can I pursue after completion?

¡CONSEJOS!

- Practice doing case presentations and discussing bilingual mental health in both English and Spanish.
- Practice code-switching between languages.

RESOURCES

Please keep in mind one resource will likely lead to another!

Organizations

- Association of Psychology Postdoctoral and Internship Centers: https://www.appic.org/

- Association of Psychology Postdoctoral and Internship Centers Quick Start Guide and FAQs: https://tinyurl.com/dyh3k7x2

- Association of Psychology Postdoctoral and Internship Centers Step by Step: https://tinyurl.com/3z8k4kyd
- National Latinx Psychological Association Mentorship Program: https://www.nlpa.ws/mentoring-program
- American Psychological Association Division 45 (Society for the Psychological Study of Culture, Ethnicity and Race): https://division45.org

First Generation

- Home Girls Unite: https://homegirlsunite.com
- American Psychological Association Division 45 (Society for the Psychological Study of Culture, Ethnicity and Race): #PsyGradWishList @psychgradwish
- Melanated Social Work Podcast: https://melanatedsocialwork.buzzsprout.com
- Marvin Toliver, LCSW: https://www.marvintoliver.com
- Black Therapists Rock: https://blacktherapistsrock.com
- Dr. Mariel Buqué: https://www.drmarielbuque.com
- Dr. Bettina Love: https://bettinalove.com
- Project Diversify Medicine: https://projectdiversifymedicine.org

Music (Instrumentals)

- Karim Kamar: https://www.karimkamar.com
- Vianney Lopez: https://www.vianneylopez.com
- Sarafina: @sitwithsarafina (Instagram, YouTube, TikTok)

Games

- *Crucigramas*
- *Lotería*

Media

- *Telenovelas*, movies, and series with Spanish dubbing

Cultural and Spiritual Practices

- Cooking a comfort meal, creating *altares*, praying, *tejer*.
- Christyna Johnson, MS, RDN, LDN: @encouragingdietitian (Instagram, TikTok), @encouragingRD (X)
- Your Latina Nutrition (Dalina Soto, RD, LDN): https://yourlatinanutritionist. com
- Mariposa Ancestral Practices (Michelle Mojica, LCSW): https://www. mariposaancestralpractices.com
- Womxn of Color Summit https://www.harpindermann.com/wocsummit
- National Compadres Network: https://nationalcompadresnetwork.org
- The Black Joy Project®: https://kleavercruz.com/the-black-joy-project

REFERENCES

American Psychological Association. (2010). *Model Act for State Licensure of Psychologists.* https://www.apa.org/about/policy/model-act-2010.pdf

Association of Psychology Postdoctoral and Internship Centers. (2023). *APPIC directory.* https://membership.appic.org/directory

Colon Hidalgo, D., & McElroy, I. (2021). Racial trauma perpetuated by academic medicine to those in its ranks. *Annals of the American Thoracic Society, 18*(11), 1773–1775. https://doi.org/10.1513/AnnalsATS.202105-592IP

Erickson Cornish, J. A., & Baker, J. (2023). A brief history of the Association of Psychology Postdoctoral and Internship Centers: Trends and directions for the education and training of health service psychologists. *Training and Education in Professional Psychology, 17*(2), 115–125. https://doi.org/10.1037/tep0000401

Guzman, N. (2024, November 29). You may not know the term, but Latinas know the responsibilities: Kinkeeping. Luz Media. https://luzmedia.co/kinkeeping

Jones, K., & Okun, T. (2001). White supremacy culture. In K. Jones & T. Okun, *Dismantling racism: A workbook for social change groups.* ChangeWork. https://pfc. ca/wp-content/uploads/2022/01/dismantling-racism-workbook-en.pdf

Kawaii-Bogue, B. (2020, June). *Combating anti-Blackness and White supremacy in organizations: Recommendations for anti-racist actions in mental healthcare.* Sonoma State University. https://caps.sonoma.edu/sites/caps/files/combating_anti-blackness_ and_white_supremacy_in_organizations_-_recommendations_for_anti-racist_ actions_in_mental_healthcare.pdf

Lanesskog, D., Piedra, L. M., & Maldonado, S. (2015). Beyond bilingual and bicultural: Serving Latinos in a new-growth community. *Journal of Ethnic & Cultural Diversity in Social Work, 24*(4), 300–317. https://doi.org/10.1080/15313204.2015.1027025

Le, L. (2019). Unpacking the imposter syndrome and mental health as a person of color first generation college student within institutions of higher education. *McNair Research Journal SJSU, 15*(1), 21–34. https://doi.org/10.31979/mrj.2019.1505

Lorde, A. (2017). *A burst of light: And other essays.* Dover. (Original work published 1988)

Okun, T. (2023, August). *(Divorcing) White supremacy culture: Coming home to who we really are.* https://www.whitesupremacyculture.info

Pietrantonio, K., & Llamas, J. D. (2020). Closed borders, closed hearts: Systemic oppression of Latinas in US politics: *Fronteras cerradas, corazones cerrados opresión sistémica de la gente de Latinx en la política estadounidense. Peace and Conflict: Journal of Peace Psychology, 26*(2), 110–116. https://doi.org/10.1037/pac0000459

Rosenthal, C. (1985). Kinkeeping in the familial division of labor. *Journal of Marriage and Family, 47*(4), 965–974. https://doi.org/10.2307/352340

Teran, V. G., Fuentes, M. A., Atallah, D. G., & Yang, Y. (2017). Risk and protective factors impacting burnout in bilingual Latino/a clinicians: An exploratory study. *Professional Psychology: Research and Practice, 48*(1), 22–29. https://doi.org/10.1037/pro0000126

Verdinelli, S., & Biever, J. L. (2009). Experiences of Spanish/English bilingual supervisees. *Psychotherapy: Theory, Research, & Practice, 46*(2), 158–170. https://doi.org/10.1037/a0016024

Wilcox, M., Barbaro-Kukade, L., Pietrantonio, K., Franks, D., & Davis, B. (2021). It takes money to make money: Inequity in psychology graduate student borrowing and financial stressors. *Training and Education in Professional Psychology, 15*(1), 2–17. https://doi.org/10.1037/tep0000294

9 DECIDING YOUR *CAMINO* IN BILINGUAL MENTAL HEALTH

JASMINE A. MENA AND GREVELIN ULERIO

As you travel your journey toward becoming a bilingual mental health professional, you might be unsure about whether to pursue a clinical, academic, or combined path. This chapter is designed to guide you through a self-assessment and self-reflection process to sharpen your focus and select your *camino*. This guided introspection is supported by vignettes, questions, and exercises that illuminate your interests, experiences, strengths, growing edges, and values toward the best fitting path *para ti*. In addition to highlighting the best fit for clinical and academic settings, in this chapter we explore possibilities for combining both tracks and the types of opportunities that can foster this career path. *La importancia de* formal and informal mentoring relationships, as well as organizational resources, is underscored before sending you off on the next phase of your journey.

Y AHORA, ¿QUÉ HAGO?

Si encuentras that you are vacillating between pursuing a clinical, academic, or combined bilingual mental health track, you are not alone. Regardless of where you are in your training, rest assured that there are others grappling

https://doi.org/10.1037/0000481-010
Forging Caminos: *Pathways to Becoming a Bilingual Mental Health Professional*,
M. Campos, Y. Mejia, and A. J. Consoli (Editors)

with the same almost-palpable uncertainty that comes with trying to answer the question "Now what?" Some bilingual mental health *profesionales* may start as clinicians and later transition to academic settings. Others may be firmly planted in academic positions and may end up providing direct services to fill a need in their community or a university clinic. Still others find that their bilingual skills interlace seamlessly in their clinical and academic roles. *Por ejemplo*, a professor who provides clinical supervision to students delivering bilingual services operates in both clinical and academic roles. The bottom line is this: *No hay un* single path, and your chosen path may change over the course of your career. *¡Las posibilidades son infinitas!* Assessing your personal interests, experiences, strengths, and values in bilingualism is a helpful way to facilitate the decision-making process.

A PERSONAL ASSESSMENT OF INTERESTS, LIVED EXPERIENCES, STRENGTHS AND GROWING EDGES, AND VALUES

Conducting a personal assessment is a great way to clarify your *camino*. As part of your personal assessment, it will be important to reflect on your genuine interests and lived experiences, which are rich sources of information to start your *camino*. A candid look at your strengths and growing edges and values will help you determine your next steps. Let's go!

Interests

Early experiences, such as helping family members navigate language barriers by serving as a young *intérprete*, can be the seeds of a future interest. These personal experiences, although they may start out of necessity, may grow into an interest in providing culturally and linguistically appropriate services because they show the power of language in building relationships. Alternatively, your early experiences may have helped you develop an interest in researching the role of language match in the quality and effectiveness of treatment. Either way, your interest in the importance of bilingual mental health can also grow into a desire to be appropriately recognized for having a skill that can facilitate communication and treatment (Estrada et al., 2023). Some bilingual mental health professionals are interested in both the practice and research sides of the profession. For instance, Julia[1] is deeply interested in providing psychotherapy services and the role that

---

[1]The vignettes in this chapter reflect an amalgamation of our experiences and experiences of others we have learned about over the years. The vignettes do not reflect any singular person's experience.

research plays in improving treatment efficacy. In fact, Julia has been feeling increasingly frustrated by professionals who advise her that she will have to choose between being a bilingual mental health treatment provider or a researcher. For Julia, practice is inextricably linked to research, and vice versa. Being asked to choose one feels inauthentic and forced. How might Julia feel if she were able to treat a select number of clients and use the knowledge gained to improve treatment effectiveness, write grants to fund efficacy research, and use a feedback loop to refine theory and practice?

Taking time to reflect on the ideas, practices, and communities that spark your interest and a desire to learn more is a fruitful way to decide on which bilingual mental health path suits you best. What activities do you enjoy and maybe even do well? What do you want to learn more about? What makes you feel fulfilled and satisfied with your hard work? For some, the quest to discover new knowledge through the scientific process makes a difficult research project feel effortless. For others, learning the unique narrative of each client, couple, or family, and conceptualizing the ideal approach to treatment, may be the most intellectually engaging activity. Also consider asking your friends and family when you seem happiest and most animated. They may have more insight than you realize. Yet, if you think your interests will stay the same, *piénsalo otra vez*; you might find yourself reflecting on your *camino* often, over the course of your life.

Lived Experiences

Taking stock of our lived experiences can be a great way to assess our preparedness to pursue a bilingual mental health profession. As such, identifying and classifying experiences that may intersect with our professional paths can generate clues into our readiness to *seguir adelante*. Experiences that may inform a career in bilingual mental health include a second language, positive and/or negative relationships with prominent figures in your life (e.g., parent, sibling), personal or familial psychological distress, resilience, and more. Furthermore, we may pursue a career in mental health precisely because we may have encountered the profession as a client and had a positive or negative experience that inspired us to pursue the career. Such experiences can sometimes ignite a desire to replicate a positive therapeutic relationship or to contribute to improving the profession. Regardless of what initially sparked *un deseo* to become a bilingual mental health professional, it is imperative that you seek the experiences that will equip you with the tools you will need to thrive.

Consider Iris's experiences: Iris was treated for anxiety and depression as an *adolescente*. Although she was uncomfortable with sharing her inner world with a stranger, she decided to give it a try. It helped that her therapist was culturally humble and understood that Iris's reservations, such as not saying anything that could bring negative attention to her family or culture, had some basis in her culture. Iris's experience ultimately proved beneficial, and she developed a great appreciation for the power of a positive therapeutic relationship with a therapist who is committed to cultural and linguistic competence.

This experience ignited Iris's interest in pursuing a career in bilingual mental health. Her graduate program had courses that addressed issues related to cultural diversity, and the training clinic provided services to Spanish-speaking clients, but only sporadically. Iris wondered how she might bridge the gap between the experiences she needed and what her program offered. Before transferring to a new program with a focus on bilingual mental health, she decided to talk to her professors about this developing interest and the experiences she needed. Thankfully, there were various professors and supervisors who were willing to listen to her and supportively assisted with cocrafting a plan that involved taking advanced Spanish-language courses, a summer intensive immersion experience, and a year-long externship treating Spanish-speaking clients at a community health clinic. Though not enrolled in a Latine mental health track program, Iris was able to make adjustments to support her interests.

What if Iris's professors and supervisors had not supported her interest in pursuing bilingual mental health? Though disappointing, we know this can happen. If you are in the early stages of training, you can reapply to other graduate programs and transfer. However, before doing so it might be wise to reach out to the transferring programs to inquire about transferring course credits. If you are far along in your program you could decide to complete your training there and seek additional experience after graduation. You could complete a graduate certificate in bilingual counseling and secure ongoing clinical supervision with a bilingual mental health professional (see Chapter 5, this volume). *¡Sí se puede!*

Let's take *un poco de tiempo* and think about your experiences. A great way is to pull out your updated curriculum vitae or resumé and relish in your greatness. Just kidding (only slightly)! If you do not have a curriculum vitae or resumé, list everything you have done (formal and informal) that could lend itself to the type of career you are interested in pursuing. Remember, your past experiences can give insight into what might be missing in your training, what you might have a good handle on, and new learning you would like to pursue. If you are thinking to yourself, "*Pero no sé lo que no sé,*" that is completely valid! Consider looking at your list of experiences and envision the type of role or position you would like to have. Looking at job advertisements and position descriptions on platforms like LinkedIn (https://www.linkedin.com), or PsycCareers (https://www.psyccareers.com) for positions that excite you will also help to guide your reflection on the types of experiences you would like to have.

Strengths and Growing Edges

Todes tenemos different strengths and growing edges that contribute to our uniqueness. We prefer the phrase "growing edges" over "weaknesses" because it implies that, with the right support and experiences, we can learn and grow. As such, it behooves us to identify our strengths and growing edges and use *esta información* to seek more opportunities that showcase our strengths and augment our growing edges. Unfortunately, too many evaluative processes designed to prepare us professionally overemphasize our weaknesses and underemphasize our strengths. Furthermore, some characteristics are growing edges that need to be remedied, whereas others may be perceived as weaknesses but actually reflect preferences that should be acknowledged and honored. For example, active listening is an essential skill that will support you on your clinical, academic, and combined paths. If active listening represents a personal growing edge, no matter how hard it may be, you will likely benefit from sharpening this skill. In contrast, if you need quiet time between interpersonal interactions to recharge, you may need to pick a path that will complement this personality trait. Knowing yourself and your needs is helpful for deciding on a professional path that includes the types of activities that play to your interests and strengths.

Meet Juan, an observant, reserved, and affable bilingual clinical psychology graduate student. He decided to pursue a graduate degree in clinical psychology because, having observed various family members and friends struggle with mental illness, he was interested in learning how and why psychological disorders develop. He thought a career in clinical psychology would be interesting and meaningful. However, Juan wondered if he had made the right decision because he felt emotionally drained and exhausted most days because of the heavy clinical caseload of monolingual Spanish-speaking clients. Rather than seeking social support after a long day, he desired the quiet of his apartment. He wondered what was more challenging: being heavily burdened as one of the only bilingual psychotherapists on staff or the frequent social contact. Was he on his way to burnout, or did he really prefer more opportunities for alone time in his day? What if he spent more time working on tasks that require deep concentration in solitude and not only on clinical work? Might he feel fulfilled, and maybe even less burned out, if some of his day had a mix of clinical responsibilities with designing research about clinical treatment or conducting statistical analyses? Balancing our personal styles and needs with diverse and interesting activities can be a great way to derive satisfaction and keep burnout at bay while meeting our values, interests, and needs in bilingual mental health.

Focused self-reflection may illuminate your strengths and growing edges and guide your choices in the future. To start, identify two types of experiences: some that went well and some that did not go as expected. Ask yourself these questions:

- What qualities and skills facilitated your success?
- What qualities and skills could have helped you but were (at that time) lacking?
- What else could have contributed to the outcomes?

Develop your answers with rich detail and nuance, and linger on your discoveries. With this new awareness, strive to nurture the qualities and skills that you have developed by acknowledging them often and using them intentionally. Take stock of your growing edges to determine how you could strategically seek experiences that will help you to grow in those areas; for example, one of us sought a summer training program while in graduate school to augment cultural and linguistic competence when conducting psychological assessments. Also consider external factors, such as mentoring relationships or peer collaboration, that contribute to your ability to thrive. Whatever it is, if it brings you fulfillment and motivation to keep growing, *¡consíguelo!*

Values

Values are aspirations about the type of person you want to be; you work at living up to them every day. Knowing your values is essential for making important decisions about your path in bilingual mental health and life in general. It also makes it easier to take action toward what you most treasure and to gracefully decline misaligned opportunities. Making decisions that align with your values is admittedly easier said than done because identifying your values requires deep self-reflection and awareness. Moreover, it can be hard to stay centered on our values when we are living busy, fast-paced lives filled with distorted messages about what we should be doing (or not doing), or about what represents success. Sometimes, the comparisons we inadvertently make *no tienen sentido* because we may have experiences and resources (e.g., generational wealth, a specific type of training) that differ vastly from those of others, but they leave us feeling "less than." It takes concerted effort to counteract the effects of social pressure and comparisons to find out what really matters to you and those you love. It is important to note that professional practice guidelines compel us to increase awareness of our own values (which may change over time, by the way!) as a necessary component of providing culturally appropriate services (American Psychological Association, 2017).

Consider Dani's dilemma. Dani grew up bilingual and developed a strong and positive ethnic identity and connection to other Latines. Dani envisioned themselves contributing to a community like the one in which they grew up. However, as they progressed in their education they often lamented the lack of other Latines in graduate school courses and Spanish language training opportunities. When the time came to select placements for clinical training, Dani had to make a choice: select one from the available sites or advocate for a site where they could receive training and offer services in Spanish. Maintaining their Spanish language skills over the years had not been easy, and they even felt somewhat embarrassed that their Spanish was not polished; thus, they thought it would be reasonable to accept an English-only site. How might the value Dani places on contributing to an underserved community, such as the one in which they grew up, inform their decision? One option may be for Dani to raise the issue with the training director and explore the possibility of adding new training sites to the preapproved options. Another option may be for Dani to attend one of the available sites and request Spanish-speaking clients.

¿Qué Valoro?

Imagine that you highly value justice, but you don't feel like you are having an impact; that would make for an unsatisfactory situation. Knowing your *valores* will help you to prioritize your resources—including your time and efforts—and guide your behavior. There are innumerable lists of values, including adventure, beauty, *comunidad*, courage, *confianza*, creativity, diversity, education, *familismo*, *empeño*, integrity, justice, parenting, *personalismo*, productivity, recognition, *respeto*, spirituality, *simpatía*, wisdom, and more. You could evaluate hundreds of values, *pero* to simplify your self-assessment think about the following general domains: personal, interpersonal, community, nature, spirituality, and work. For each general domain, write a few sentences to summarize your intentions in this domain (e.g., to be a compassionate, respectful, honest partner), identify the values reflected in your responses (e.g., compassion, respect, honesty), and rank the identified values on the basis of their importance to you. The top three to six values are usually the most powerful in shaping your life and will help you craft a personal mission.

MI MISIÓN

When you consider the word *misión*, what comes to mind? What or whom do you envision? In the context of your professional journey, take some time to wrestle with the question "What is my calling?" Trust that you have all the tools necessary to begin to answer this question. To do this, you will create a personal mission statement using an adapted version of Randall Hansen's Five-Step Process (Hernandez, 2024).

1. Identify four to five examples from your life or recent personal *triunfos*. This can be big or small successes from different areas of your life. Aim to identify a potential common theme or themes.

2. Elaborate on the list of values you previously created. Do not place limits on the attributes that come to mind. Next, narrow your list of values to the six that are *los más importantes*. Then, rank your values, choosing the most important to you.

3. Create a list of ways you could make a positive difference. *Idealmente*, how would you contribute best to the larger society, your family, your employer, friends, community, or other areas of your life?

4. Think about your priorities and life goals. Make a list of the *objetivos* you have for the short term (up to 3 years) and long term (beyond 3 years).

5. Using the information gained in the first four steps, start writing your personal mission statement. Try your best to keep it to one to two sentences.

Our mission statements are "To be a medium through which knowledge is distributed to improve the quality of life for others and to live mine earnestly and authentically" (Grevelin Ulerio) and "To live a life of integrity and inspire others to do the same; to have the courage to change when change preserves integrity" (Jasmine A. Mena). We recommend revisiting your *misión* every few years to ensure you are on your desired *camino*. ¿*Cuál es tu camino*?

TRADITIONAL *CAMINOS Y MÁS*

Your bilingual mental health professional *camino* may lead you to one of numerous paths. But what do they each do? Understanding the various options, including the most common activities associated with each, will help you to envision yourself in each role. As you read on, ask yourself: Are you most excited about a clinical *camino*, academic *camino*, a combination, or something else entirely?

Clinical *Camino*

Seamos honestes: The particular skill set of a bilingual mental health professional is in high demand. There are not enough qualified Spanish-speaking providers to meet the ever-growing needs of monolingual, bilingual, and bicultural communities. Latines often are unable or reluctant to seek care because of conflicting cultural values, a lack of provider cultural humility, and costs, among other reasons. Thus, if you are considering a clinical track be prepared to feel like *la última Coca-Cola del desierto* because your presence and experience will fill a large gap.

Various experiences are essential to pursuing a bilingual clinical mental health profession, including developing field-specific competency in a second language. Spanish speakers often may possess an adequate vocabulary for social interactions but need to develop mental health vocabulary and thus should pursue mental health training in both *idiomas*. In addition to language proficiency, bilingual mental health professionals need to develop cultural awareness and relevant knowledge and skills (Sue et al., 1992). Developing an awareness of one's own cultural values and biases, understanding the values and beliefs of other cultures, and developing the skills and techniques for effective intercultural interactions are key to engaging effectively with individuals of diverse backgrounds (American Psychological Association, 2017).

There are many clinical settings to consider, and learning more about them can help you decide your *camino*. For example, you may be interested in working in a hospital, a community mental health clinic, or a university counseling center. Deciding among these options may be easier if you consider the nature of the services provided as well as factors associated with the populations served, including demographic characteristics of interest (e.g., age, culture, language, socioeconomic status), approaches to treatment (e.g., individual, group, family services), and goals of treatment (e.g., addressing developmental issues, stabilizing acute psychological distress, assessment). To obtain a clearer picture of your ideal clinical setting, write down the demographic characteristics, approach, and goals of treatment that interest you most. With that in mind, consider what clinical work entails.

Activities of a Bilingual Mental Health Clinician

Clinicians are not all the same. Although some of the activities that clinicians carry out are similar from clinician to clinician, others may vary depending on the setting and role. To help you discern your *camino*, consider the following practice- and academic-oriented clinician activities.

Health Services
Bilingual clinical work encompasses directly interacting with and supporting clients who are experiencing psychological distress by conducting assessments, offering diagnoses, and delivering treatment in one or two languages. It also involves collaborating and consulting with other providers to ensure that clients receive quality care that matches their cultural and linguistic needs. Offering supervision and training to others can also be a piece of the puzzle. A clinician's full (and manageable) caseload, which includes individuals, families, and/or groups seen on a weekly basis, can vary dramatically depending on geography and setting. Note that a full-time job encompasses direct contact with clients and client-related activities (e.g., writing clinical notes, contacting other providers, attending staff meetings, translating, language brokering, preparing for sessions, adapting treatments, consultation, professional development, personal breaks).

Coordinating Care
When clinically appropriate, bilingual mental health clinicians will need to discuss the course of treatment with other providers who may or may not speak the same language as the client. For example, the clinician may reach out to a client's psychiatrist or case manager or social worker, or they may request to speak to you.

Advocacy
At times, your clinical judgment (and *intuición*) will tell you that your client needs advocacy in different life domains to help reduce distress. For example, a monolingual Spanish-speaking client may arrive to a session in a state of distress because they are having trouble understanding a notice or bill that was sent to them in English. In your role as a clinician, you can use your bilingual skills to translate these documents and help the client determine what action they would like to take. Serving as an advocate comes with the territory. Your clients may need you to advocate for them, but do not forget to advocate for yourself, too; doing so may protect your well-being. In our discussions of advocacy with bilingual clinical psychology trainees, they pointed out that if you are feeling overburdened in your role as a Spanish-speaking mental health professional, and having difficulty setting boundaries and managing guilt, you may be overcommitting. They asserted that, if you are doing more work, you should consider renegotiating the terms of the position and/or advocating for more pay.

Continuing Education
We hate to break it to you, but you will still have *tareas* as part of your professional development. After completing your degree, clinical settings will require you to obtain your license to practice. To maintain your license, you will have

to obtain the continuing education credits required by your state. Many professionals obtain these credits by attending workshops, panels, and short courses at conferences for the purpose of staying in the know about updated and relevant science and practice developments. *A la misma vez*, as a bilingual clinician, part of your continued learning will be keeping a pulse on your own language fluency and the evolution of language, including gender inclusivity. This may include speaking Spanish with your *abuelita*, keeping subtitles on your favorite *novela*, or establishing a working group with other bilingual clinicians to make sure you know how to say "posttraumatic stress disorder" in Spanish. In short, do not stop looking for novel opportunities to learn!

Academic *Camino*

Careers in academia that involve bilingual mental health can be deeply enriching. Nuances embedded in the Spanish language, such as cultural *dichos*, may be lost in translation for monolingual English-speaking researchers. Thus, having Spanish language competency improves the quality of mental health research and treatment. Furthermore, being a bilingual and bicultural researcher can shape your research questions and research designs, resulting in a more *confiable* mental health knowledge base (Roberts et al., 2020). Bilingual mental health academics and researchers are needed, and their language-based competency is valuable and enriches their professional lives (Estrada et al., 2023). *Por ejemplo*, say you are interested in researching culturally bound mental health concerns, such as an *ataque de nervios*. A monolingual English speaker might search and get the direct translation "attack of nerves" and assume that an *ataque de nervios* is equivalent to panic disorder and create their research materials with this understanding. As a bilingual academic, you may be less inclined to make this assumption, and the research you produce will be better for it.

Activities of a Bilingual Mental Health Academic

If you are interested in a bilingual mental health academic *camino*, you will have to make a few more decisions. Some questions we hope you consider are: What kind of academic setting is best for you? Will you integrate your bilingual capabilities into your research? What methods might be best suited for your bilingual participants?

Academic Settings and Roles
Academics typically work in institutions of higher education as adjunct professors, lecturers, professors of practice, and tenure-track or tenured professors. Adjunct instructors often practice, teach, and/or provide clinical supervision

to students in training on a part-time basis. Lecturers and professors of practice tend to have heavier teaching loads and may also have small clinical practices. Tenure-track and tenured professors typically have more intensive research activity compared with people in the other roles, and this may prevent many from providing direct clinical services other than through clinical supervision. Note that professors in the other roles can be, and often are, involved in various aspects of research, other scholarship, or both. Some academics may also write grant applications to fund their research activities, and others may serve as consultants on grants, in large part because of their clinical, cultural, and bilingual expertise. Which one of these settings and roles makes your heart sing?

Conceptual Considerations

Cultural awareness, knowledge, skills, and humility apply to the world of research as much as they do to clinical professionals. As a bilingual mental health professional, you could consider how your identities may inform your worldview. Your biases, if unexplored, might affect your research decisions. *Para combatir* the influence of power dynamics and researcher biases, you can collaborate with other researchers, communities, or both who are affected by the research topic.

Another consideration involves how best to measure concepts to advance research in the most inclusive and accurate manner. For example, bilingual mental health academics may consider that "Latino/a/e/x" is a pan-ethnic term that includes peoples from many diverse nations and ethnicities with myriad intersectional identities. With that in mind, do you intend to measure the experiences of diverse Latines, or would it be helpful to research the diversity within the group?

Along with intersectionality, taking the influence of context seriously is essential when interpreting findings and in guiding future research. Developing a deep respect for and understanding of the influence of context will help you challenge the tradition of psychological universality, which assumes that any participant can be replaced with any other. In contrast, as a bilingual researcher you know that one cannot simply exchange monolingual English-speaking participants with Spanish-speaking or bilingual participants and assume that the essence of the psychological truth will be unaffected. *¿Nos entiendes?* Attending to individual and systemic intersectionalities and contexts creates a more nuanced and accurate knowledge base (Torres et al., 2018).

Methodological Considerations

An academic *camino* involves practices that ensure that the specific needs of monolingual Spanish-speaking or bilingual research participants are carefully considered. For example, when it comes to recruitment, our communities might be suspicious of researchers who extract information and do not contribute meaningfully to our pressing needs, and this is understandable. As such, bilingual mental health researchers will want to first get to know the communities they enter to ensure that an alignment of priorities is forged. Other practical recruitment strategies include creating attractive and concise advertisements that potential monolingual Spanish-speaking or bilingual participants can understand. Another helpful strategy is working with culturally sensitive recruitment assistants from the community who can explain the aims of the research to potential participants and communicate your adherence to the highest standards of confidentiality so as to allay any privacy concerns. Whenever possible, allow the question of interest to determine the particular research method/design of the study. Just like you would not use a hammer for every house project, exploring a variety of approaches to generating knowledge is also fruitful. For example, consider the value that qualitative and mixed-methods research designs may bring to the topic of study. Furthermore, bilingual mental health academics may be able to increase collaboration with communities of interest by involving them in the research process; basically, *nada sobre nosotres, sin nosotres.* You can play an important role in closing the power gap between researcher and participant.

Bilingual mental health academics consider various issues related to measurement and statistics well. They consider whether measures created with non–Spanish-speaking populations are appropriate to administer to monolingual Spanish-speaking or bilingual participants. They may even conduct the research that compares the reliability and validity of a particular measure after it has been translated into a different language. The usefulness of research findings ultimately depends on the quality of the measures used to obtain those findings (Torres et al., 2018).

Finally, making meaning out of research findings will depend on how thoroughly you capture characteristics related to individual participants, social processes, and the contexts in which the participants live. At a minimum, consider inquiring about nativity, acculturation, documentation status, language preference, cultural value, generational status, and intersectional identities, as appropriate to your research. Important social processes to consider include immigration policies, discrimination, poverty, gender expression, and the impact of religion and spirituality, among others. Descriptions of the contexts may include population size and diversity, historical and policy-related events, information about the local economy, community resources, and challenges (e.g., community violence).

If you choose the academic *camino* you can expect to conduct research, mentor students in that capacity, and disseminate research through presentations at professional conferences and peer reviewed journal articles. In fact, these activities are often required for career advancement. Many academics are increasingly contributing to public knowledge by disseminating their research in more accessible formats, such as infographics, podcasts, and opinion essays, among others. Do you enjoy working with puzzles and thinking creatively to shed light on issues and solve problems that, in some cases, no one has figured out yet? If so, you may be an excellent fit for an academic *camino*.

Combined Clinical and Academic *Camino*

As you may have gleaned from our discussion of the clinical and academic *caminos*, it is possible to combine these roles. One approach is to become a clinician who practices as part of an active research team. Another approach is to maintain a clinical practice and teach on a part-time basis as an adjunct professor or lecturer. This approach usually allows you to add or remove courses from one semester to the next because such clinicians usually do not have a long-term contract. If that feels too uncertain, consider counseling centers and treatment facilities that have training programs. Clinicians contribute by teaching and providing clinical supervision to trainees who are matched for externships, practica, predoctoral internships, and postdoctoral positions.

Academics usually have less time for clinical work, but they sometimes have a small one-day-a-week practice to stay connected to clinical work and to inform their teaching. They also create treatment protocols as part of research, and sometimes they implement these protocols and train and supervise research assistant clinicians. Alternatively, you may be perfect for leadership positions, such as a director or administrator at a health service or educational institution. *Piénsalo*, a leadership position may be within your reach, and what a rewarding way this is to create positive change (see Chapter 12, this volume). With your expanding tool kit, you will likely be able to bring exceptional intercultural and interpersonal skills, oral and written communication skills, superb analytical and evaluation expertise, and an ability to treat others with empathy and compassion. We must underscore the fact that the skills you develop as a bilingual mental health professional are valuable and transferable.

Más Caminos

A veces, we forget that more traditional *caminos* are not everyone's *taza de café*. If you have gotten here and are somewhat side-eyeing or thinking to yourself, "*¿No hay algo más?*", we have got you covered. The most important thing to remember is how versatile and desirable your skills as a bilingual mental health professional will make you on the job market. *De verdad, no existen límites* with what you can do with your training. In the sections that follow, we briefly discuss *algunos caminos más* to offer a small glimpse of how to apply your skills.

Consultant

Put simply, a consultant is someone who offers a client advice and other services related to their area of expertise. In this sense, "client" means the person or organization that has brought you in or is cutting your check. As a bilingual mental health professional, you will be equipped to provide expert assessments, interventions, and consulting to improve the effectiveness of individuals and teams in various capacities. We ourselves have served as consultants. One of us, Grevelin Ulerio, has been a consultant on a grant project focused on survivors of sexual assault that had a special interest in intentionally recruiting Spanish-speaking survivors. As a member of the research team, Grevelin provided feedback on translation and cultural nuance. The idea of being considered an expert may bring up some discomfort and perhaps a bit of imposter phenomenon (it happens to all of us!). Your training as a bilingual mental health professional will provide you with the skills to understand how individuals interact with others and with systems.

Content Creator

No viene de sorpresa that in our ever-changing digital landscape there is the space and possibility to find a career in content creation. "Content creator" is a catch-all term for someone who shares material online with some level of consistency. There is a plethora of bilingual mental health professionals who use their platforms to disseminate valuable information in an effort to normalize conversations about mental health. One of our favorites is the podcast Latinx Therapy hosted by Adriana Alejandre (https://worldchannel.org/special/adriana-alejandre-decolonizing-mental-health/), a licensed marriage and family therapist who invites other mental health professionals and social media influencers to debunk myths about mental health in the Latine community. They even air Spanish segments (something you could listen to, to stay current in the language, perhaps?). Take some time to consider your niche. As you go through your training, keep the pulse of the types of clinical presentations and research you gravitate toward because this can provide potential insight into your niche. There are even folks who document their graduate training journey and share it online, such as Aeriell Armas (Instagram: @gradlifegrind). In other words, you can begin this *camino* earlier, or in tandem with others whom we have mentioned in this chapter!

There are several advantages to pursuing this kind of *camino*. First, it can offer you complete creative control over how you present your area of expertise. It is also scalable; whether you want your online content to advertise or market another project or just want to engage with your audience and create community through the use of livestreaming, it is up to you. *No todo lo que brilla es oro*. If you hope to make this *camino* lucrative, though, you must be prepared for the reality that it will not be at first. Building an audience and your brand (i.e., how you want to engage with your audience and present your message) takes time. Much of the profit from content creation comes from sponsorships, advertisement, and collaborations, which will likely begin to come around when you establish a steady audience.

Financial Considerations

A veces, el dinero manda. There is no shame in wanting financial security and taking time to reflect on what the return on your educational investments will be. It might be a good idea to review the statistics from the graduates of the programs to which you are applying, to ensure that they are mostly gainfully employed. Although we wish we could provide exact numbers, *la verdad* (like most things) is that even within *caminos* there is variability that can depend on many factors, including the passage of time. If you are interested in an academic or a combined *camino* you might find that the more senior position, the higher the baseline pay. Acquaint yourself with student loan forgiveness (https://www.studentaid.gov/manage-loans/forgiveness-cancellation), and loan repayment award programs (e.g., https://www.lrp.nih.gov) for which you may be eligible. Keep in mind that positions that qualify for loan forgiveness are often with governmental employers or nonprofit institutions. The biggest takeaway about *dinero*, regardless of which *camino* you are inclined toward, is that it is okay to think it over, discuss it with a mentor, or be confused about it. We want to reiterate that your skills are marketable, which means you will have bargaining power!

MAXIMIZING MENTORSHIP RELATIONSHIPS IN DECIDING YOUR *CAMINO*

You are part of an extensive social network that may hold the information you need to help you determine your next step in your career. In fact, your network is inherently a form of social capital (Yosso, 2020). If you need to build a network, look at Chapter 6 (this volume) for some helpful *consejos*. Peruse the list of professional organizations at the end of this chapter, and reach out to the ones that align with your goals. Most require a fee to join and give you access to listservs, events, and trainings. For example, the National Latinx Psychological Association (https://www.nlpa.ws/) offers all these benefits and has a mentoring program you can opt into if you are looking to get connected directly to someone in the field. Although reaching out may feel like a risk because you are advocating for yourself, *inténtalo*, because it may bear fruit. It is not only who you know, but also who they know, that may help advance your career. Perhaps a former high school teacher has a colleague who works in the school district in which you would like to become a psychologist. *¡Une nunca sabe!* Strive to stay in touch with the people with whom you cross paths, and share your *camino* with them.

Formal and Informal Mentoring Relationships

The key difference between formal and informal mentors is that formal mentor relationships tend to be short term in nature and structured around a particular expertise. A formal mentor is often someone who has volunteered to advise and consult another person or several people, such as an academic advisor. Formal mentors agree to guide you by sharing their expertise. Over time, a formal mentoring relationship can sometimes change into a natural one. A natural mentoring relationship is an organically formed relationship with a nonparental adult who has more experience than you do and who provides support and guidance (Zimmerman et al., 2005). Put plainly, a natural mentor is someone who provides emotional and instrumental support and potentially serves as a role model, as seen in the relationship of the authors of this chapter. As an undergraduate student, Grevelin was mentored by Jasmine, who was her professor, but did their relationship end on graduation day? Not at all! Who might be some natural mentors in your life? How did you meet them, and how do you each maintain the relationship? Natural mentors often see you through more life stages than formal mentors, which is beneficial to your success. Natural mentors can help in recentering, grounding, and humbling you when needed. Both formal and informal mentors can help you decide on your bilingual mental health *camino*. Having a variety of people who can support you can provide the stabilizing foundation necessary for you to decide your *camino*.

Maximizing Mentoring Relationships to Decide Your *Camino*

Maximizing your mentoring relationship will require effort and intention on your part. If you have a mentor in mind, we strongly encourage you to discuss your career prospects with them. Arrive to that meeting with your responses to the self-reflection prompts from this chapter, and see what your potential mentor has to say. If your mentor does not have the resources you need, they likely know someone who does.

Consider looking at your mentor as a launching pad of sorts. Part of using your mentoring relationships wisely involves following through on their suggestions. Talking with folks who are on a *camino* in which you are interested could help you determine whether it is the right one for you.

Consider Marleny's interaction with her mentor. Marleny is a bilingual doctoral student in clinical psychology. She began graduate school during the COVID-19 pandemic and is less inclined to pursue the more traditional *caminos*. After doing her own self-assessment, Marleny solidified her passion for advocacy for university students of marginalized identities. Marleny bashfully shared this with her academic advisor, anticipating that she would be advised against pursuing this less traditional path. Instead, Marleny's advisor suggested that perhaps she might enjoy a more administrative role, such as a university dean of students, and noted that her bilingual and bicultural skills and experiences would be an asset. Marleny's advisor knew someone within their network who was a dean of students and set up an email introduction. Marleny followed up and conducted an informal interview with her advisor's colleague to obtain a better understanding of the job. When seeking mentorship-making career decisions, keep in mind that you have the final say. Mentors can provide *consejos* and guide you toward potentially helpful resources, but they cannot, and should not, make decisions about your *camino* for you. Stand firm.

SUMMARY AND CONCLUSIONS

The fact that you have gotten this far in the book should offer insight into how much you value being a bilingual mental health professional. This profession has its twists and turns, but it also offers rich rewards. Knowing that your commitment to linguistic and cultural competence could change a person's life in treatment, lead to the highest quality research, or both, will, we hope, propel you forward on your *camino*.

Although in this chapter we described career pathways separately, we must emphasize that most professional careers are not linear. In fact, you may be committed to one trajectory today and find yourself somewhere you did not expect tomorrow. That is not only okay but also a potentially exciting part of your journey! Unfortunately, there is no magic wand or one-size-fits-all checklist we can provide that will guarantee that you are on the correct path. The truth is that there is no single right path, only the right path *for you at this time*. Remembering to offer yourself leniency and compassion if and when that path changes will ease your discomfort. You will also benefit from sharing your challenges and successes with those in your social network, including formal and informal mentors; this will remind you that you are not alone. Finally, allow your *camino* to evolve and be guided by your interests, experiences, strengths, growing edges, and values because, when challenges inevitably arise, you will take comfort in knowing that you are following what matters most to you.

TAKEAWAYS

- Conduct a periodic personal assessment, and engage in deep reflection, because these are valuable steps in your development, and your answers will steer you on your path.

- If you do not already have access to an established training experience that meets your bilingual needs, create it! For example, create a consultation group with other bilingual professionals who work with Spanish-speaking clients. Or perhaps set up an informal working group to simply practice Spanish. The possibilities are endless!

- When in doubt, *¡busca ayuda!* Your mentors and loved ones have funds of knowledge both about you and the world that can help you to get to and through your *camino*.

REFLEXIONES

- How do your interests, experiences, and strengths align with bilingual mental health?
- How might learning experiences and training address your growing edges?
- What do your *valores* and your *misión* tell you about your ability to find fulfillment in a bilingual mental health profession?
- Can you envision yourself more easily in a clinical, academic, or combined *camino*?
- Who are your formal and informal mentors? Where might you find mentors, peers, and future collaborators?

RESOURCES

Recommended Reading

American Psychiatric Association. (2023). *DSM-5-TR manual diagnóstico y estadístico de los trastornos mentales: Texto revisado*. Editorial Médica Panamericana.

Gutierrez, V., Rafiee, C., Bartelma, E. K., & Guerra, V. (2010). *An English–Spanish manual for mental health professionals*. Createspace.

Swazo, R. (2013). *The bilingual counselor's guide to Spanish: Basic vocabulary and interventions for the non-Spanish speaker*. Routledge. https://doi.org/10.4324/9780203136386

Associations

- The National Latinx Psychological Association (https://www.nlpa.ws): This group aims to promote and advance the psychological well-being of Latine communities. It offers a variety of resources for bilingual mental health professionals, including networking opportunities, job postings, and continuing education courses.

- Hispanic Neuropsychological Society (https://hnps.org): The Hispanic Neuropsychological Society aims to promote the competent practice of neuropsychology with Spanish-speaking populations. It offers a variety of resources for bilingual mental health professionals, including conferences, training programs, and research opportunities.

- Latinx Therapy (https://latinxtherapy.com): This is a bilingual podcast and online directory of bilingual therapists whose mission is to destigmatize mental health struggles in Latine communities. Clients can search for bilingual therapists. It also provides resources for students and professionals.

- American Psychological Association Division 53, the Society of Clinical Child and Adolescent Psychology (https://sccap53.org), Bilingual Psychologists Special Interest Group (https://tinyurl.com/mvkdpk35): This group is composed of bilingual providers and training programs; its members are interested in compiling resources, and they support the development of practice guidelines. They advocate for student training and client services and help connect trainees with mentors.

REFERENCES

American Psychological Association. (2017). *Multicultural guidelines: An ecological approach to context, identity, and intersectionality, 2017*. https://www.apa.org/about/policy/multicultural-guidelines.pdf

Estrada, F., Angèle, B., & Martinez, F. (2023). *Ya era tiempo* (It's about time): Latinas/os training to be counselors share the meaning of obtaining recognition for their Spanish proficiency. *Journal of Hispanic Higher Education, 22*(1), 3–17. https://doi.org/10.1177/15381927211005071

Hernandez, G. (2024, April 2). *The five-step plan for creating personal mission statements*. LiveCareer. https://www.livecareer.com/resources/careers/planning/creating-personal-mission-statements

Roberts, S. O., Bareket-Shavit, C., Dollins, F. A., Goldie, P. D., & Mortenson, E. (2020). Racial inequality in psychological research: Trends of the past and recommendations for the future. *Perspectives on Psychological Science, 15*(6), 1295–1309. https://doi.org/10.1177/1745691620927709

Sue, D. W., Arredondo, P., & McDavis, R. J. (1992). Multicultural counseling competencies and standards: A call to the profession. *Journal of Multicultural Counseling and Development, 20*(2), 64–88. https://doi.org/10.1002/j.2161-1912.1992.tb00563.x

Torres, L., Mata-Greve, F., Bird, C., & Herrera Hernandez, E. (2018). Intersectionality research within Latinx mental health: Conceptual and methodological considerations. *Journal of Latina/o Psychology, 6*(4), 304–317. https://doi.org/10.1037/lat0000122

Yosso, T. J. (2020). Whose culture has capital? A critical race theory discussion of community cultural wealth. In L. Parker & D. Gillborn (Eds.), *Critical race theory in education* (pp. 114–136). Routledge. https://doi.org/10.4324/9781003005995-8

Zimmerman, M. A., Bingenheimer, J. B., & Behrendt, D. E. (2005). Natural mentoring. In D. L. DuBois & M. J. Karcher (Eds.), *Handbook of youth mentoring* (pp. 143–157). Sage. https://doi.org/10.4135/9781412976664.n10

10 EL CAMINO CLÍNICO

Cultivating Your Clinical and Cultural Identity

KIMBERLY ALBA AND JORGE CIENFUEGOS SZALAY

Bienvenides y felicidades. After much thought and exploration, you have decided to extend your *camino* as a bilingual and bicultural clinician and healer. To begin, it is crucial we contextualize the content in this chapter. We position ourselves as White Latine bilingual and bicultural clinicians who draw from our own experiences, privileges, struggles, and connections to our communities to address how we have navigated our development as clinicians. For us, our bilingual clinical identity is inextricably intertwined with our Latine culture, and thus we developed and wrote this chapter with this framework in mind, with a specific focus on bilingual Latine clinicians. Given the lack of representation of Latine individuals in our field, we also center this chapter with the intention of addressing this disparity. Similarly, we recognize the inherent privileges of our positionality and thus actively use our resources to amplify racially marginalized Latine voices and underrepresented narratives.

We also hope our insights resonate with a more extensive audience, including bilingual individuals who may not identify as bicultural or Latine. If you are one of these readers, we extend a warm welcome and celebrate that you,

https://doi.org/10.1037/0000481-011
Forging Caminos: *Pathways to Becoming a Bilingual Mental Health Professional*,
M. Campos, Y. Mejia, and A. J. Consoli (Editors)

too, play a vital role in the dismantling of colonial practices and in advancing bilingual mental health practices. We encourage you to engage with this content with awareness of your social location and a willingness to consider how the insights shared throughout relate with your own experiences, regardless of cultural and ethnic identity. We hope this chapter serves as a valuable resource for anyone interested in exploring the intersection of language, culture, and clinical practice.

To embark on this *camino*, we define the terms *clinician* and *healer*. Language and definitions ground us in our values, serving as vehicles for social change (Kendi, 2019). The term *clinician* refers to those who participate in the direct clinical care of mental health disorders, offering diagnostic impressions, treatment planning, and psychotherapy services (Citizen Advocates, 2021). According to the American Psychological Association (2022), the practice of clinical psychology includes the comprehensive treatment of mental health issues for diverse groups, in addition to consultation, training, education, supervision and research. Although these definitions identify the different responsibilities of a clinician, we also believe that clinicians accompany societies in healing and change. In our intentions to decolonize mental health, we recognize that the mental health field originated from the healing practices of communities of color. Core traditions and rituals have been stolen, diluted, and packaged into Western mental health theories and concepts, limiting psychology's effectiveness with communities of color, including Latine folx.

We encourage you to consider a blending of the terms *clinician* and *healer* because we intend to center your growing clinical identity in Latine, Indigenous, and African cultural healing traditions that have existed for millennia despite attempts to erase and silence core practices. We believe a healer is someone who accompanies a person and/or communities in a trajectory of *sanación* by bearing witness to storytelling and guiding the use of practices (many innate to the individual and their community) that soothe the mind, body, soul, and transgenerational wounds. We also believe healers engage in advocacy, empowering the voices of others and connecting with other healers in their efforts to effect change. We acknowledge that we are providing a general description of the term and that many of you may hold layered roles as healers, some identifying as *curanderxs, brujxs*, or different roles in your religious and spiritual practices. Give yourself a moment to reflect on the language and definitions you will use to describe your role as a clinician and healer using our recentering cues: sets of questions that will guide you in evolving and reclaiming your Latine clinical and cultural identity throughout this chapter.

Recentering Cue

- What are your social locations, and how do you introduce yourself when accompanying others in bilingual and bicultural spaces?
- Which healer identities, terms, and layers resonate with you?

A DONDE EL CORAZÓN SE INCLINA, EL PIE CAMINA: ARRIVING AT YOUR CLINICAL IDENTITY

As you consider the language and principles you will choose, let's explore your arrival to your *camino clínico*. You likely considered various paths within our field. You imagined yourself in those roles, your contributions to and impact on each. If your decision to grow your clinician and healer identity was anything like ours, you were mostly led by your *corazón. A donde el corazón se inclina, el pie camina*. Your heart is open to accompanying people in their pain, joy, and recovery. Your heart yearns to collaborate with a community of healers while also guiding the next generation. Your heart values a *camino* of self-discovery and self-healing, which are integral features of becoming and being a wholesome clinician. Your heart also wishes to liberate your communities through advocacy, transgenerational healing, and education. Your heart is a source of *intuición*—an intuition that is spiritually rooted in the beliefs and desires of your *ancestres* and that has been grown by elders, families, and communities. In choosing this *camino* with consideration and mostly your heart, you have made a collective decision that will have an everlasting mutual impact on your *comunidad*—one that can be both revitalizing and heavy to carry, a duality we discuss throughout this chapter.

By recognizing the spiritual and cultural forces guiding your evolution as a clinician, you are reclaiming protective elements of our roots as Latine people. Latine folx have historically embraced spirituality as a means of guidance, strength, and resilience (Santiago-Rivera et al., 2002). As they navigate Western medicine and White spaces, many Latine clinicians are constantly met with cultural conflicts, forcing them to quiet and even abandon spiritual guidance. As Latine mental health students and professionals, we face unique pressures of adopting opposing values to survive doctoral programs and keep positions, resulting in heightened levels of burnout and degree incompletion (Castellanos et al., 2006).

Recentering Cue

- When did you begin to recognize your healer identities?
- How were your healer identities embraced/celebrated and/or quieted in your community?
- How have spirituality and intuition served as protective guides for you?

EVOLUCIONANDO: GROWING A BILINGUAL AND BICULTURAL CLINICAL IDENTITY

Your cultural and clinical identities are inextricably linked. Cultural identities exist in connection to other identities, including, but not limited to, race, ability, immigration status, ethnicity, financial standing, educational experience, sexuality, gender, and religion. We discuss core values and clinical goals from our lived experiences and current day literature while encouraging you to consider your unique interpretation depending on your intersecting identities. We also discuss the borderland spaces you share with those in your *comunidad*. Latine bilingual and bicultural clinicians have a unique role in understanding borderland spaces in *acompañamiento*. This process requires ongoing reflection and support as clinicians learn to hold space for layered and emotionally potent experiences, heal themselves, and guide the healing of others.

Biculturalism

Latine folx in the United States are constantly responding to living on "the margins of two worlds" (Castellanos et al., 2006, p. 138) and navigating two cultural knowledge systems, also known as *biculturalism*. Being a bicultural person requires ongoing negotiation of competing value systems given that White-centered spaces differ in their focus on individualism, the acquisition of power, and perspective-challenging. Cultural conflicts become more pronounced during key developmental periods when Latine folx are faced with the tasks of evolving their Latine (and other) identity; core values; and growing in unfamiliar, White spaces. This is especially true as you enter the mental health field as a clinician. Despite the millions of Latine folx who live in the Untied States and the mental health field's significant roots in the traditions of people of color, there is underrepresentation of Latine and Spanish-speaking mental health professionals. In addition, although there is a growing body of literature on decolonizing mental health and the provision of Latine, bilingual, and bicultural practice, being exposed to it during your clinical training and professional development remains a rarity. Entering the field with a clear understanding of your identity statuses, cultural and clinical values, the challenges you will face, and networks for support and continued learning will help you carry the weight of reclaiming your Latine identity.

Recentering Cue

- Consider your intersecting identities. Reflect on your areas of privilege and subjugation.
- How do your identities, bicultural or otherwise, influence your core values?
- How have you successfully or unsuccessfully negotiated cultural conflicts in the past?

Conexiones y Colectivismo

We believe biculturalism is a superpower that serves as a cultural meta-perspective that heightens your ability to connect and make an impact on your communities (Rivera, 2023). *Conexiones* in Latine culture are founded in *personalismo*. As you begin your clinical and healing work with others, especially with the Latine community, *personalismo* will play an integral role in building therapeutic alliances. While participating in the initial phases of *acompañamiento*, you will notice a natural inclination to connect to your community using elements of humor and warmth. You may notice a curiosity about small moments of their lived experiences, asking questions that may be perceived by others as too personal. Members of your community may also begin to initiate these moments, asking you about your weekend or the *cafecito* you had that morning. You both take the time to get to know one another and form a trusting relationship (*confianza*), which will fuel their recovery. For bilingual clinicians, we encourage you to explore and cultivate how your bilingualism fosters meaningful strategies for *conexión*.

Cultural conflicts may arise because Western medicine and psychology emphasize clinician–patient boundaries, time constraints, and productivity. Throughout your training there will be a focus on the use of boundaries that uphold power structures in the therapeutic alliance instead of neutralizing them to form accompanying relationships with communities. The Western value on productivity is revealed in clinical objectives that primarily monitor symptom reduction. Taking the time to build *confianza* may be undervalued. Because of this same principle of *personalismo* and *simpatía*, Latine folx will not voice their dissatisfaction with culturally insensitive boundaries and recovery trajectories, resulting in stagnant healing and discontinuation of care. As a bicultural clinician, ignoring your rootedness in *conexiones* will leave you feeling disingenuous, and isolated from your *comunidad*, contributing to higher levels of burnout. It is important to note that boundaries have their function, and it is even more crucial that you critically think about your boundaries and if they are interfering with culturally sustaining care. *La cultura cura*—in other words, "our culture heals"—and when we adopt Western medicine approaches without considering their impact we miss an opportunity to heal with our *comunidad*.

Related to *conexiones* is the value of *colectivismo*, a prioritization of the well-being of the *comunidad*. Our interpretation of this value is not to abandon the individual's sense of self and self-care but to consider the power of togetherness in an oppressive society. Latine folx's emphasis on family and community is an adaptive value that has helped them overcome and heal from colonialism, civil wars, immigration, racism, and complex trauma histories. *Colectivismo* and *familismo* will reveal themselves at all stages of your clinical work.

As mentioned, your decision to become a clinician is a collective one. Because you have this personal value and the experience of existing in community, when embarking in clinical spaces these values will shape the way you understand the person in front of you. You will see their challenges and strengths in the context of their generational lineage, family, and communities. You will be more likely to include discussions about family members in sessions and encourage their participation. In practicing within these borderland spaces you will experience a felt sense of ethnic and cultural connection that reduces burnout (Delgado-Romero et al., 2018). At the same time, you will see an overlap in negative familial experiences, creating a risk for compassion fatigue. This is true for work in all clinical interactions; in psychology it is referred to as *countertransference*. Navigating Latine clinician–patient borderland spaces holds different weight because challenges are deeply rooted in colonial trauma and systemic racism. For example, as a Latine immigrant or second-generation Latine folx you may uniquely understand the hardships of an immigrant family whose members are being separated by deportation and robbed of their value of togetherness.

Latine clinicians' value of collectivism extends beyond clinical relationships to those with colleagues, staff, mentors, and teams. A cultural clash arises because of Western values in individualism. This may translate to a minimal understanding of family inclusion in clinical work or a lack of familial and community programming and communal spaces. Among clinicians, although teamwork is promoted there are unspoken values of individualism, competitiveness, and power acquisition that facilitate promotions and career advancements. Because Latine clinicians value collective growth and navigate their work spaces with this in mind, they are less likely to be in positions of leadership. It is important to renegotiate values of collectivism and resort to consultation and *mentoría* to facilitate your growth while using avenues that are true to your *identidad*.

Recentering Cue

- How do you embody *conexiones, colectivismo, familismo,* and *personalismo*?
- Do your clinical boundaries support or interfere with your connection to others?
- How may your experiences of *colectivismo* translate to your clinical work? What challenges may you face?

Mi(s) Lengua(s)

We now arrive at a pivotal aspect of our bicultural identity: *el lenguaje.* Many of us will exhibit a wide spectrum of proficiency in both Spanish and

English, ranging from native fluency to varying degrees of bilingualism. It is important to recognize that these varying levels of language proficiency can influence our bicultural identity and shape our sense of self, our cultural connections, and the ways in which we engage with our respective *comunidades*. A large majority of us may also use *Spanglish*, a hybrid language or form of code-switching whereby Spanish and English may be mixed in a variety of ways (Martínez, 2010).

Spanglish can be traced back to historical interactions between English- and Spanish-speaking communities across the globe, which often were rooted in colonization and migration. The mixing of these languages was and continues to be a result of power dynamics, acculturative processes, and the attempted imposition of one language over another. In a sense, Spanglish then also represents a linguistic resistance against the dominance of a single colonial language by embracing elements of both languages. It is a reminder of the complicated—and at times violent—history that has shaped our communities and our bilingual identities. It may have emerged because of colonialism yet it also represents resilience and the ability to adapt, a celebration of cultural tenacity. By reclaiming and reshaping language, Spanglish empowers us to navigate and express our identities in ways that transcend colonial boundaries and promote cultural inclusivity.

As bilingual clinicians, using Spanglish holds great importance, insomuch that the very use of it recognizes and celebrates one's bicultural identity. By incorporating Spanglish into our work, we bilingual psychologists can create a safe and inclusive space for the with whom we communities we work who also navigate multiple languages and cultures and find themselves in other borderland spaces. It allows for a more authentic and relatable therapeutic relationship because it validates and acknowledges the unique linguistic and cultural context of bilingual individuals. The use of Spanglish also reinforces the idea that language is not a barrier but a bridge, allowing us to connect more deeply with our clients and communities, which in turn allows us to gain a richer understanding of their experiences. Embracing Spanglish as part of our professional identity allows us to tap into the nuances, humor, and cultural references that may be lost in a strictly monolingual approach, ultimately enhancing the therapeutic rapport and promoting a more humane, safe experience.

We feel it is also important to highlight the challenges that may come with attempting to integrate Spanglish into our professional identities as bilingual clinicians. We have likely encountered external pressures, such as the urge to solely conform to English or Spanish. This is especially true for those of us who have been trained clinically in White-centered spaces that enforce English-only or Spanish derived from the *Real Academia Española* (https://www.rae.es/). As we navigate graduate and professional worlds, there may be expectations or norms that favor adherence to English, which can create a sense of internal conflict and uncertainty and often lead to forced code-switching.

The desire to conform to a monolingual approach may lead to doubts about the validity or professionalism of using Spanglish. However, it is essential for bilingual clinicians to recognize that their bilingualism is an asset and that Spanglish can be a valuable tool for effective communication and therapeutic connection. Efforts to discourage us from using Spanglish can be seen as a manifestation of a colonial perspective that seeks to erase or devalue aspects of our bilingual identities. Language is not only a tool for communication; it encompasses a complex web of cultural, historical, and personal meanings. By not integrating Spanglish into our professional identity there is also a risk of perpetuating the monolingual and monocultural norms that have marginalized both us and our communities.

We also acknowledge that overcoming the urges to conform requires confidence in one's linguistic abilities and an understanding of the cultural and contextual need of using Spanglish in therapy. This may be particularly difficult for those of us who are attempting to reclaim Spanish as an act of defiance of oppression, or for those who have never trained or been supervised by bilingual or Spanish-speaking clinicians yet have been in positions where they have delivered therapeutic services in Spanish. Some of us may also experience feelings of insecurity or incompetence when delivering service in Spanish because we may perceive our professional identity as being perceived as more competent in English. For example, psychological nomenclature may be more accessible in English for those of us who completed our training in primarily English-speaking training sites. These factors underscore the importance of seeking bilingual-specific supervision and consultation to continuously empower Latine (Spanish-speaking) clinicians in navigating their professional bilingual and bicultural identities with more ease and confidence.

Finally, we find it important to recognize the experiences of Latine clinicians who strongly identify with and take pride in their Latine culture and identify as monolingual English speakers. We consider it essential to approach this discussion with sensitivity and wish to avoid inadvertently suggesting that one's level of bilingualism determines their authenticity as a Latine individual. Language is undoubtedly significant, but it is just one aspect of a multifaceted bicultural identity. There are numerous other meaningful ways for us to connect with ourselves and our communities, including shared cultural values, traditions, and community involvement. Although we have used Spanglish as the main example throughout this section, we honor the rich variety of languages spoken throughout Latin America. We recognize that Latine clinicians with knowledge of other languages may encounter additional barriers.

Recentering Cue

- In what ways do you find strength and pride in your bilingual identity?
- How do you navigate your bilingual identity in monolingual spaces?
- How do you navigate spaces where you are made to feel that one language is preferred over the other?

Liberación

You will likely arrive at your *camino clínico* with the hope of being a part of your community's liberation from the emotional, social, physical, spiritual, economic, and political effects of colonialism. Latine activism rose from a long-standing yet multifaceted history of imperialism and oppression. Psychotherapists in Latin America helped spread Liberation Psychology (Burton & Guzzo, 2020; Moane, 2003) during a period of oppressive regimes and dictatorships. At the same time, many *liberadorxs* of the time also expressed anti-Black, anti-Indigenous, and anti-immigrant views that are important to label and dismantle as we embark on our own liberation work. Our mission to extend our *acompañamiento* beyond the therapy room is rooted in a liberation lineage, and we must be intentional in working to liberate all the members of our *comunidades*, especially those historically marginalized within and by our *comunidades*.

Valuing liberation presents itself in various ways each with a common thread, unique to the Latine clinician. Latine healers find themselves facilitating *testimonios* that detail people's lived experiences with injustices and their sequelae: pain, suffering, and generational wounds. In bearing witness to *testimonios*, Latine clinicians also identify and uphold the person's and the community's innate strength, resourcefulness, and use of spiritual guides. The sharing of *testimonios* creates an overflow of borderland spaces for the Latine clinician and community as they explore collective trauma and suffering, and clinicians are gifted with a chance for redemption where they recognize their strengths and heal their own trauma (Rivera, 2023).

Liberation also takes the form of advocacy, translating to Latine clinicians empowering others to speak their truth to the world. Latine clinicians, together with those they accompany in care, also use their privilege as professionals and mental health experts to express the needs of their community and demand social change. In your clinical work, *liberación* may be carving out time outside of your individual psychotherapy sessions to advocate against disparities within, for example, schools, workplaces, health care, judicial systems, and immigration processes. You may extend yourself because of the limited number of Latine bicultural and bilingual clinicians and resources: *¿Si yo no lo hago, entonces quién?* A Latine clinician may reflect on the collective decision to expand their *camino clínico*, feeling the weight of making a collective impact in a world that upholds values and systems of imperialism and marginalization. If we do not seek the duality in liberation, which includes rest, we will grow in fatigue, damaging our well-being—another version of oppression. *Recuerda, quien mucho abarca, poco aprieta.* This does not mean we cannot follow our hearts and all their intentions; it means that we cannot do it all at once, without rest and alone time. In the next section, we further explore how to promote self and collective liberation across White-centered spaces.

Recentering Cue

- What does *liberación* mean to you?
- How do you participate in advocacy now?
- How do you rest, recover, and recharge from your liberation efforts?

TÚ Y YO SANÁNDONOS: COLLECTIVE HEALING IN WHITE-CENTERED SPACES

As mentioned throughout this chapter, embarking on a career in the mental health field as bilingual and Latine individuals brings about unique opportunities and challenges shaped by our minoritized identities. Although our journey to develop our professional identities predominantly unfolds within English-dominant, White-centered spaces—leading to a complex interplay of cultural and systemic dynamics—we are also uniquely positioned to work closely with our communities. Through engaging, addressing, and healing the pain caused by systems of oppression and colonization, our lived experiences provide us with invaluable insights into how said systems have affected both the collective and individual well-being of our people. This work is both an honor and a responsibility as we stand alongside our communities in the pursuit of liberation and justice. It is also important to highlight how this work may exacerbate our own negative and traumatic experiences (Rivera, 2023). When working with our communities, topics such as poverty, persecution, violence, discrimination, and migration are likely to appear, indirectly placing us in positions where we ourselves may be (re)traumatized. Although we are made to be acutely aware of our own vulnerability, we can use these shared experiences as a trauma-informed frame to guide our work (Saakvitne, 2002).

Our journey toward healing our communities also is deeply interconnected with how we heal ourselves. Offering our communities an experience that differs from our own, for example, can contribute to our own personal growth and healing as Latine individuals in White-centered spaces (Rivera, 2023). By witnessing the resilience and growth of those we accompany we may find solace and hope in knowing that our efforts have positively influenced someone who has experienced similar challenges and traumatic experiences. Through this connection, we find mutual empowerment and embark on a transformative journey of healing, both individually and collectively. As we continue to strive for the well-being of our community, we find our own wounds being tended to, our own resilience strengthened, and our own sense of purpose affirmed.

We must also recognize that despite sharing cultural and ethnic backgrounds, our experiences may differ significantly from those of others. This understanding underscores the importance of incorporating an intersectional lens into our therapeutic work (Crenshaw, 2013). By doing so, we enter the therapeutic space with an awareness that our unique identities interact with systems of oppression, giving rise to distinct perspectives and realities. This lens enables us to actively acknowledge and honor the diverse identities within ourselves and our communities, allowing us to offer more nuanced and inclusive therapeutic support. We recognize the complex interplay among race, ethnicity, gender, sexual orientation, socioeconomic status, among other variables. By valuing and centering these experiences, we create a space for healing that respects and empowers the unique journey of the individuals with whom we work. Incorporating an intersectional lens into our work not only serves to address the diverse needs of our clients but also aids us in navigating the complexities of the mental health field as bilingual and Latine clinicians and healers. Using this lens allows us to critically examine the power dynamics and systemic biases that shape our professional contexts, and it forces us to critically examine how our own positions of privilege interact with these systems. Through this lens, we can advocate for change, challenge the dominant narratives, and promote equity and justice. By doing so, we work toward the creation of a more affirming and responsive environment that honors and uplifts the voices and experiences of our communities.

We deem it important to highlight barriers that exist beyond our immediate control yet nonetheless significantly affect our work as Latine clinicians in White spaces. These barriers have profound implications for our ability to develop as professionals, influence how we provide effective care, and dampen our ability to contribute to the well-being of our communities.

They may also hinder our advocacy efforts and contribute to burnout rates. By acknowledging these external barriers, we aim to raise awareness and advocate for continued systemic changes that promote equity and inclusivity for our communities. The barriers we discuss in the following section are not intended to be an exhaustive list (and have been mentioned briefly throughout this chapter) but rather are intended to highlight some of the external significant challenges that we, as Latine clinicians, encounter in our work.

Underrepresentation

Like many other fields in the United States, psychology has been dominated by White professionals. Currently, only 7% of psychologists in the United States identify as Latine (American Psychological Association, 2022), and only 5.5% identify as Spanish speaking (Smith, 2018). The lack of substantial representation of Latine mental health professionals may leave many of us uncertain about how to navigate academic and professional circles within the field. Moreover, it may perpetuate systemic barriers for other aspiring Latine mental health professionals because the limited presence of mentors can result in reduced influence on policies and curriculum development, perpetuate systemic biases, reinforce existing power imbalances, and hinder recruitment and retention because of a lack of equitable environments for Latine therapists. For this and many other reasons, we have centered this chapter on bilingual and bicultural experiences. We hope more Latine and bilingual individuals join the mental health field in order to expand the growth and healing of our communities.

Cultural and Linguistic Barriers

Latine mental health professionals operating in White spaces encounter cultural barriers with regard to norms, values, and communication styles, which contribute to feelings of isolation. For example, many of our Latine cultures emphasize warmth and interconnectedness and take a collectivist approach to community, in contrast to Western cultures, which often value an individualistic approach. These differences may lead to misunderstandings, misinterpretations, and difficulties in establishing a supportive environment for professional growth. Moreover, they place the onus on the minoritized individual to find ways to bridge these cultural gaps and promote understanding. This can contribute to feelings of isolation and burnout. A dearth of culturally relevant resources for Latine clinicians compounds these feelings of isolation.

Racism

A significant challenge Latine mental health professionals encounter is being on the receiving end of racism, bias, and stereotyping. We may face preconceived notions about our expertise, be subjected to racial and ethnic aggressions, and grapple with hostile work environments. Moreover, Latines are often treated as a monolithic group, obscuring the incredible diversity of races, ethnicities, nationalities, cultures, and experiences all of us bring to the workplace. This monolithic perspective overlooks the disparities and intersectional experiences within the Latine community and can further reinforce inequalities. It is also necessary to shed light on the embedded racist ideas and structures that perpetuate the marginalization of Afro-Latine and Indigenous Latine folx within our community.

As White Latine healers specifically, we must face the ways in which we (and our lineage) avoid our White privilege and ignore the racialized realities of Afro-Latine and Indigenous Latine individuals, specifically, in our workspaces (Adames et al., 2020). It is our ongoing responsibility to hold a mirror up to ourselves and our *ancestres*, as we exist in racist systems, and label our racial privilege and Whiteness. We must also explore and address how we have benefited from racism and how our White privilege has influenced our clinical trajectories in the fields of mental health and academia. If you are a White Latine clinician, consider the following: How does your Whiteness influence the opportunities presented to you so far (e.g., acceptance into doctoral program, workplace environment, burnout levels)? How do you continue to exclude Afro-Latine and Indigenous voices when discussing the Latine experience and collective liberation? Notice your reactions to these reflective points. To engage in collective healing, we must first (and continuously) acknowledge the racial injuries within our community, actively participate in repair, advocate for societal justice, and amplify the nuanced experiences of racially oppressed Latine folx. By using a lens of intersectionality and positionality, we can work toward dismantling internalized, interpersonal, institutional, and structural racism for all Latine folx.

Recentering Cue

- How has working with your community made you reflect on your own experiences as a bicultural individual? For those of you who may not identify as bicultural, what are ways your bilingual identity has allowed you to connect to other communities outside of your own?

- For those of you who are White Latine, in what ways are you holding up racist practices? How are you actively working to dismantle racism within yourself and the Latine community?

- How do you incorporate, or envision incorporating, an intersectional lens into your work?

¡ESX SOY YO! RECLAIMING AND CELEBRATING BILINGUALISM AND BICULTURALISM

As we continue to grow as professionals, the impact of working in White-centered spaces does not go unnoticed by our minds and spirits. At times, we may find ourselves lost, or disconnected from the reasons why we started a *camino clínico*. As Latine clinicians, we bring a lived experience and first-hand knowledge of the diverse cultural backgrounds, traditions, and values that shape the Latine community. This understanding allows us to connect with our Latine clients on a deep level, recognizing the unique challenges they may face and providing culturally attuned care. By centering (and recentering) our Latine identity, we can draw on our own experiences of navigating the complexities of biculturalism, bilingualism, discrimination, and immigration and enable ourselves to foster a sense of solidarity and trust with the communities with which we work. This shared cultural identity can create a safe space where clients feel understood, validated, and empowered to explore their own identities and seek support from someone who genuinely relates to their experiences. By recentering our identity as Latine healers, we ultimately can not only leverage our strengths to provide impactful and effective therapeutic interventions but also embrace and reconnect with our communities, culture, and the core values that drove us to heal in the first place.

Seeking support and connecting with other Latine and bilingual clinicians can further provide a sense of community and validation when we feel lost or disconnected. This aids us by cultivating a sense of belonging and camaraderie that can counter the feelings of isolation that may arise in White-centered spaces. Sharing common experiences, challenges, and successes with others who understand the nuances of being a Latine healer creates a unique bond and fosters a supportive network to lean on: *Dime con quién andas, y te diré quién eres*. A way this can be achieved is through joining professional organizations or clinical consultation groups that are specifically tailored to the experiences of Latine clinicians. These dedicated spaces offer opportunities for professional development, knowledge exchange, and skill enhancement in a culturally relevant context. They also provide protected opportunities for dialogue, collaboration, and learning as well as access to resources, research, and best practices that are specifically applicable to working with Latine communities, helping us reconnect to our values. Integrating ourselves into these spaces allows us to celebrate and embrace our cultural heritage, maintaining a strong connection to our roots while contributing to our professional development. Moreover, the shared understanding and mutual support in these groups empower us to navigate the complexities of our work with greater confidence, resilience, and strength.

Recentering Cue

- List the ways in which you recenter yourself and your community.

- For readers who do not identify as Latine, consider the ways that you recenter with your cultural backgrounds. How can you join Latine communities in recentering their cultural identities, and what areas of growth may you need to address to do so in a culturally sustaining and sensitive way?

HASTA LUEGO: A COMMITMENT TO RECLAIMING OUR BILINGUAL IDENTITY

We have reached the end of our chapter and a pivotal moment for self-reflection and commitment to continuously reclaiming and grounding yourself in your Latine *identidad* and *comunidad*. Recentering your identity as a Latine clinician requires a commitment to cultural rootedness and sustainment, self-reflection, and ongoing learning from those in our community. By embracing our bicultural identity and using it as a foundation for therapeutic work, we Latine healers can provide a more holistic and culturally responsive approach that honors and values the diverse experiences we and our communities bring into the therapeutic, healing space. This process requires an active engagement with our own biases, areas of privilege and subjugation, an openness to continued learning from our community, and a willingness to change our practice to meet the ever-changing needs of those we accompany in care. We strive to empower ourselves and our *comunidad* by celebrating our bicultural identities. A continuous reclaiming of who we are will fuel our *camino clínico* and path toward collective liberation. In solidarity with oppressed communities everywhere, *hasta luego*.

TAKEAWAYS

- Your decision to evolve your bilingual and bicultural identity is rooted in your culture, family lineage, and ancestry. In reclaiming your roots, you will grow in congruence with your values and intentions as a bilingual and bicultural healer and clinician.

- Latine communities share values, many which have protected them from the wounds of colonialism and oppression. Understanding your unique experience of these values will help you integrate them into your accompaniment of communities, especially as you explore the nuances of navigating borderland spaces and negotiating cultural conflicts in White-centered spaces.

- Integrating our bilingualism into our professional identities may be challenging, but it is paramount for our growth as Latine healers. By doing this, we honor our ancestors and foster a safe therapeutic environment by deepening understanding, enhancing rapport, and validating the unique linguistic and cultural context of our communities.

- As we work closely with our communities, we can address the impact of oppression and colonization, drawing from our own lived experiences. The healing of our communities is thus interconnected with our own healing as Latine individuals in White-centered spaces. By incorporating an intersectional lens into our work, we also hold space for Latine individuals whose experiences differ from ours.

- Embracing our bicultural identity and making continuous efforts to recenter ourselves in this identity allows us to connect deeply with our communities. It also enhances therapeutic approaches that honor and value diverse experiences, allowing us to actively engage with biases and adapt our work to meet evolving needs.

REFLEXIONES

- Narrate why you decided to take your *camino clínico*. List three intentions as you embark on this journey.

- Reflect on your experience with Latine values related to *espiritualismo, biculturalismo, bilingüismo, colectivismo, personalismo,* and *liberación.* How will these values, and others, shape your accompaniment of communities in care?

- Think about your connection to your languages. What other ways do you believe your bilingual identity enhances your clinical work?

- What does it mean to you to engage in healing as a healer yourself, and how does this self-healing journey influence your ability to support and empower your clients?

- How do you envision your career trajectory in terms of providing culturally sustaining supervision for Latine mentees, and what steps do you plan to take to ensure that you can effectively support and nurture their professional growth as emerging clinicians?

RESOURCES

Recommended Reading

Buqué, M. (2023). *Break the cycle: A guide to healing intergenerational trauma*. Dutton.

Kokaliari, E., Catanzarite, G., & Berzoff, J. (2013). It is called a mother tongue for a reason: A qualitative study of therapists' perspectives on bilingual psychotherapy— Treatment implications. *Smith College Studies in Social Work*, *83*(1), 97–118. https://doi.org/10.1080/00377317.2013.747396

Medina, L., & Gonzales, M. R. (2019). *Voices from the ancestors: Xicanx and Latinx spiritual expressions and healing practices*. University of Arizona Press.

Moreno, R. (2023). *Get rooted: Reclaim your soul, serenity, and sisterhood through the healing medicine of the grandmothers*. Hachette.

Zapata, K. (2020, February 27). Decolonizing mental health: The importance of an oppression-focused mental health system. *Calgary Journal*. https://calgaryjournal.ca/2020/02/27/decolonizing-mental-health-the-importance-of-an-oppression-focused-mental-health-system

ONLINE RESOURCES

Websites

- Dr. Mariel Buqué: https://www.drmarielbuque.com
- Latinx Therapy: https://latinxtherapy.com
- Latinx Therapists Action Network: https://ltan.org
- Therapy for Latinx: https://www.therapyforlatinx.com
- National Latinx Psychological Association: https://www.nlpa.ws

YouTube Channels

- The First Gen Psychologist: https://www.youtube.com/@thefirstgenpsychologist/streams
- Institute of Chicano/a Psychology: https://www.youtube.com/@xicanpsych
- Latinx Therapists Action Network: https://www.youtube.com/@latinxtherapistsactionnetw1627
- National Alliance on Mental Illness, "*Compartiendo Esperanza*: Mental Wellness in the Latinx/e Community": https://www.namiwa.org/compartiendoesperanza

Video

- Browning Counseling, "Working With Latinx Clients": https://www.youtube.com/watch?v=kufMHe9ttYs

Podcasts

- Anzaldúing It: https://soundcloud.com/anzalduingit
- La Cura: https://www.mijentesupportcommittee.com/la-cura-podcast
- Latinx Therapy: https://latinxtherapy.com/podcast
- Latinx and Queer: https://podcasts.apple.com/us/podcast/latinx-queer/id1627233321
- The Latinx Mental Health Podcast: https://podcasts.apple.com/us/podcast/the-latinx-mental-health-podcast/id1453357829

REFERENCES

Adames, H. Y., Chavez-Dueñas, N. Y., Jernigan, M. M., & Sanchez, D. (2020). *We must do better: A toolkit for non-Black Latinxs who choose to address their anti-Blackness.* IC-RACE. https://icrace.org/wp-content/uploads/2020/06/final-antiblackness-.pdf

American Psychological Association. (2022). *Demographic tool: Demographics of the U.S. psychology workforce* [Interactive data tool]. https://www.apa.org/workforce/data-tools/demographics

Burton, M., & Guzzo, R. (2020). Liberation psychology: Origins and development. In L. Comas-Díaz & E. Torres Rivera (Eds.), *Liberation psychology: Theory, method, practice, and social justice* (pp. 17–40). American Psychological Association. https://doi.org/10.1037/0000198-002

Castellanos, J., Gloria, A. M., & Kamimura, M. (2006). *The Latina/o pathway to the PhD: Abriendo caminos.* Stylus.

Citizen Advocates. (2021, July 21). *How to become a mental health counselor, clinician or therapist.* http://tinyurl.com/5n6s4sju

Crenshaw, K. (2013). Demarginalizing the intersection of race and sex: A Black feminist critique of antidiscrimination doctrine, feminist theory and antiracist politics. In K. Maschke (Ed.), *Feminist legal theories* (pp. 23–51). Routledge.

Delgado-Romero, E. A., De Los Santos, J., Raman, V. S., Merrifield, J. N., Vazquez, M. S., Monroig, M. M., Cárdenas Bautista, E., & Durán, M. Y. (2018). Caught in the middle: Spanish-speaking bilingual mental health counselors as language brokers. *Journal of Mental Health Counseling, 40*(4), 341–352. https://doi.org/10.17744/mehc.40.4.06

Kendi, I. X. (2019). *How to be an antiracist.* One World.

Martínez, R. A. (2010). Spanglish as literacy tool: Toward an understanding of the potential role of Spanish–English code-switching in the development of academic literacy. *Research in the Teaching of English, 45*(2), 124–149. https://doi.org/10.58680/rte201012743

Moane, G. (2003). Bridging the personal and the political: Practices for a liberation psychology. *American Journal of Community Psychology, 31*(1–2), 91–101. https://doi.org/10.1023/A:1023026704576

Rivera, E. P. (2023). *Working with other immigrants brings the parts that I lost back to me: The experiences of Latin American immigrant therapists working with Latin American immigrant populations* (Publication No. 656) [Doctoral dissertation, University of San Francisco]. University of San Francisco Scholarship Repository. https://repository.usfca.edu/diss/656

Saakvitne, K. W. (2002). Shared trauma: The therapist's increased vulnerability. *Psychoanalytic Dialogues, 12*(3), 443–449. https://doi.org/10.1080/10481881209348678

Santiago-Rivera, A. L., Arredondo, P., & Gallardo Cooper, M. (2002). *Counseling Latinos and* la familia: *A practical guide.* Sage. https://doi.org/10.4135/9781452204635

Smith, B. L. (2018, June 1). Spanish-speaking psychologists in demand. *Monitor on Psychology, 49*(6), 68. https://www.apa.org/monitor/2018/06/spanish-speaking

11

EL CAMINO ACADÉMICO

Bilingual Professional Identity in Academia

VANESA MORA RINGLE AND RAQUEL SOSA

Being a bilingual academic in psychology is incredibly fulfilling, but you can feel undervalued at times. The academic *camino* splits into narrower *caminos*, and some of these allow more use of your bilingual abilities, such as when you conduct research that focuses on issues of language. For the most part, if you want to make use of bilingual abilities you will certainly be able to do so within the academy. Working in academia comes with a unique set of perks and challenges, and being a bilingual academic can be a strength that one can leverage, *si une quiere*. In this chapter, we delve into the structural landscape of academic settings and the unique experiences and challenges faced by bilingual academics. Being a bilingual academic opens doors to diverse cultural perspectives and academic opportunities, including advocating for and promoting a more linguistically equitable society. We explore the multifaceted aspects of navigating academia in two languages, from research and teaching to administration and personal identity.

It is possible that you are reading this from your undergraduate *camino* in psychology or other related fields, or maybe you are currently pursuing your graduate degree. Wherever you are, you have likely interacted with a professor, perhaps even one who became a key educator and/or mentor or guide in

https://doi.org/10.1037/0000481-012
Forging Caminos: *Pathways to Becoming a Bilingual Mental Health Professional*,
M. Campos, Y. Mejia, and A. J. Consoli (Editors)

your academic journey. Professors can be influential people in our lives, and in academic settings they can use their influence for a lot of good, *¡especialmente si hablan dos idiomas!* Along the *camino académico del cual te queremos contar*, imagine professors as wise, tall trees with strong roots (because it takes many years of education and training to become a professor) who help provide comforting shade to (sometimes weary) travelers on this path. Or perhaps envision professors as gardeners who nurture students' growth and help them flourish intellectually. Whatever the analogy, professors are one of the first and core representatives of the field to budding psychologists such as yourself. They are also one of the first living examples we see that show us how our career can look.

Imagine you are a bilingual professor guiding future professionals: *Eres alguien que realiza investigaciones, las cuales, muchas veces, tienen impacto en la comunidad; alguien que enseña, y también trabaja duro para convertir a las universidades en lugares más seguros para las personas bilingües.* If this kind of work sounds appealing to you, we recommend you read the rest of this chapter closely and persist on this *camino. ¡Necesitamos más profes bilingües!*

LAS OPCIONES SON DIFERENTES, ASÍ QUE DEPENDE DE TI

Primero, queremos destacar que although this chapter mostly focuses on working in academia as a bilingual professor we can still find ways of manifesting our bilingual values at every point in our academic journeys. We certainly do not have to wait until we are professors! We can embody our bilingual values in academia in many different ways. For example, as an undergraduate you can look for opportunities in research laboratories or other spaces where you can make use of your Spanish-speaking ability, especially if by doing do you can give back to your communities. You can also do the same if you have completed your bachelor's degree and are looking for post-bachelor's research jobs. It can be easy to disregard your bilingual abilities in academia because of systemic and structural language inequity issues. We want to encourage you to adopt bilingual pride, which we review in the section *"Mi Corazón Late en Dos Idiomas*: Being Your Whole Bilingual Self in Academia," regardless of where you are on your academic journey!

The general path of an academic goes something like this: First, obtain a bachelor's degree; then, attain a doctoral degree (most likely a PhD); and finally, become a professor at a university. But that general, three-step path *¡excluye mucho!* Academics, or professors, have common responsibilities and varied levels of influence within institutions of higher education. These responsibilities and related tasks include research; teaching; service; administration; professional development; and, sometimes, public engagement. We think it is generally helpful to review the background on the structure of academia and higher education, including the concept of tenure, which is unique to academia.

Institutions of higher education can be categorized in different ways, and it is important to know and distinguish among them because they have different implications for the work you do as a bilingual academic. One important categorization is based on the level of research activity at the institution; another is whether the institution awards doctoral degrees or only undergraduate degrees. Institutions that award only undergraduate degrees, including associate's-level degrees, such as community colleges, are referred to as Primarily Undergraduate Institutions. Note that institutions that grant doctoral degrees are typically associated with increased research activity.

The Carnegie Classification of Institutions of Higher Education (n.d.-a) groups institutions according to how integral research is to a given university. R1 institutions are universities in the United States that demonstrate a *very high research spending and doctorate production*. R1 universities are characterized by their robust commitment to research, which is reflected in their funding (at least $50 million for research and development) and a significant number of doctoral degrees awarded across various majors (at least 70 research doctorates). R2 institutions are universities in the United States with *high spending and doctorate production*; these universities spend at least $5 million annually on research and development and award at least 20 research doctorates. Carnegie created a new category for the 2025 classifications, titled "Research Colleges and Universities," which are universities that spend more than $2.5 million annually on research (Carnegie Classification of Institutions of Higher Education, n.d.-b); this category could include liberal arts colleges and regional institutions that are primarily teaching focused but integrate meaningful research. To find out whether a university corresponds with one of these categories, visit the Carnegie Classification site (https://carnegieclassifications.acenet.edu/) and search for the university. Carnegie states that they update classifications every 3 years, so be sure to look at the most updated one.

Tenure, which grants a professor permanent employment at their university and protects them from being fired without cause (Academic Positions, 2024), is one more distinct feature of the academic sphere and is offered only through tenure-track faculty positions. In essence, tenure provides professors with both job security and academic freedom. Accordingly, some see it as one of the biggest perks of being a professor. Tenure, along with other benefits, make tenure-track professor positions quite appealing and coveted. For more information, and a step-by-step guide on applying for tenure-track faculty positions, please read *The Professor Is In* (Kelsky, 2015). *Repasemos* details about what it means to be an academic within these various higher education environments, with more information and emphasis on a research-focused track, which is our own (i.e., the authors') current academic path. Keep these notes about the general structure of academia in the back of your mind as you read and reflect on what setting may make the most sense for you as a bilingual academic.

Postdoctoral Fellowships and Other Academic Positions

One thing to consider before applying for a tenure-track professor position is whether a postdoctoral fellowship might be right for you. Postdoctoral positions can include teaching, research, and some clinical responsibilities. Note that a completely clinical postdoctoral fellowship with very limited or no research responsibilities may not position you well for obtaining professor positions upon completion.

You may also want to consider other, non–tenure-track academic positions, such as visiting assistant professor, teaching assistant professor, and/or adjunct instructor. If your primary passion is teaching and supervising students, you may particularly enjoy teaching in assistant professor and adjunct instructor positions. Most people in these positions spend their time teaching and in service (e.g., supervising students), and you can actually be an adjunct instructor as a doctoral student. However, please note that these positions do not typically come with an opportunity for tenure.

The Academic *Camino* and the Tenure-Track Process

Faculty and administrators who work in academia typically are identified by a specific rank or position title. For example, some titles of positions that may be temporary include adjunct faculty/instructor or lecturer. The three levels of professors are assistant, associate, and full professor. Ranks also describe the degree of promotion you earned, with full professor being the highest rank among the three, and associate professor, the lowest, with a rank of full professor indicating that one has attained tenure. A tenure-track professor is a faculty member on a career path that leads to tenure. This position involves a probationary period, typically 5–7 years, during which the professor must demonstrate excellence in teaching, research, and service.

The tenure-track process includes being evaluated annually as an assistant professor for retention. At the end of the first 6 years in the position (or earlier, if faculty believe the person is ready), the departmental tenure committee, typically known as the Retention, Tenure, and Promotion Committee or Personnel Review Committee, reviews the professor's work and then makes a recommendation to the person who conducts the next level of review, usually the head or chair of the department. A favorable recommendation for tenure is likely to include promotion to associate professor. If tenure is not awarded, the person will have to find employment elsewhere (at some institutions, a terminal year is given). The departmental tenure committee typically evaluates a professor's work in three areas: (a) research, (b) teaching, and (c) service to the university (depending on the institution, this could involve service to the community and to the profession). Each of these areas includes a number of activities. For example, research may include obtaining funding in the form of grants, and teaching may include mentoring students.

In order for the committee to review a professor's work in these areas, the candidate puts together a tenure dossier, which typically includes a curriculum vitae, a list of publications, a comprehensive teaching portfolio (which could include class evaluations by students and peer observations), a tenure statement, a list of awards/grants, and details about university service (Academic Positions, 2024). The department or college also will seek external evaluations of the candidate's dossier from impartial scholars in the field who have no conflict of interest with the candidate (e.g., are not the candidate's former advisor, have not published with the candidate). These evaluative letters may include an assessment of the candidate's impact on the field and whether the writer believes the candidate should be awarded tenure.

For bilingual academics, the dossier might include publications in Spanish and university service positions that align with their bilingual identity, such as being part of developing bilingual mental health concentrations in their department. You may find throughout this process that your evaluators may not value your work in Spanish as much as your work in English, and you may have to provide evidence of its impact, or justify it. If your institution does not see the value of your bilingual work, you may want to think about other universities that would value it.

The review committee (which may consist of full professors, although that is not always the case) reads the entire dossier and writes a letter that includes a recommendation. Some tenure committees may weigh parts of the tenure dossier higher than others depending on the classification of the school and the rank (e.g., R1 institutions may place more emphasis on research publications than on university service at the assistant professor level when one is seeking tenure and promotion to associate professor). In addition to the committee review, there are many other decision makers in the process. These could be the department head, the chair, the dean of the college, the dean of faculty affairs, and then the provost (typically referred to as the chief academic officer) and the university president or chancellor, who will make the final tenure decision. A professor who is awarded tenure usually is promoted to associate professor. Five to 7 years after being promoted to associate professor, one can apply for promotion to the full professor rank (Academic Positions, 2024). For more information on the tenure track process for Chicana and Latina faculty, please see Pérez (2021).

¿CUÁLES SON LAS RESPONSABILIDADES DE UN ACADÉMICO?

The university's Carnegie classification may dictate the size of a professor's teaching load. For example, a Primarily Undergraduate Institution may entail a heavier teaching load, such as a 3-3, or teaching three classes in the fall semester and three classes in the spring semester. This can require a lot of preparation work, especially if the professor has not taught the course in the recent past. Bilingual academics can use existing networks or build networks to work in *comunidad* with other professors through listservs, such as the one provided by the National Latinx Psychological Association (https://www.nlpa.ws), and ask professors who have taught a similar course for their syllabi and class materials. This would help decrease the preparation time associated with finding reading materials or coming up with a syllabus from scratch.

An R1 university may have less of an emphasis on teaching, with teaching loads as low as 1-1 (i.e., teaching one class in the fall semester and one class in the spring semester). The teaching load ultimately is dependent on the university, and although the teaching load may be less at an R1 or R2 institution, research and service expectations will also factor into hours spent on the job. Thus, it is important to reflect on what you like to do more of, teaching or research. *Si te gustan las investigaciones*, consider applying for R1 and R2 faculty positions. As stated earlier, tenure-track positions come with expectations, so if the expectations for tenure have a heavy research component you will also want to identify what kind of support that position is going to offer you to help you meet those expectations. For example, do they have a support system in place for grant applications, start-up funds, computer/software resources, course buyouts (i.e., a release from teaching a course for a particular semester or academic year to dedicate more time to research, administrative duties, or other projects)? For bilingual academics who are looking to use their bilingual skills in their research, look for universities that have a Latinx mental health concentration in their program, existing bilingual faculty/leadership, or a high bilingual or Latinx student/community population.

Professors also advise students. In graduate school, a professor may accompany and guide advisees in their journey more closely compared with a professor who supervises undergraduates. Bilingual academics may consider using Spanish in the name of their research group/collaborative/laboratory or their teaching materials, speaking Spanish with their bilingual advisees, and encouraging their advisees to also speak Spanish in academic places. Faculty also may engage in service at their university by being a part of research or program committees; serving as an advisor to a university club; or participating in shared governance (i.e., whereby faculty and administrators work together to make decisions that affect the university), such as serving on the academic senate.

You may also consider taking a leadership role in academia and getting involved in academic administration. These positions include a higher number of administrative responsibilities and may hold more institutional power than other faculty positions. Administrators' primary responsibilities, instead of research, teaching, and service, like tenure-track or tenured faculty, involve managing and overseeing institutional operations, which typically also include the development of a strategic plan. A department chair may focus on orienting and answering questions for students and faculty, managing the department budget and teaching schedule, working on ensuring accreditation, or supervising staff and leading department meetings. Academic deans have administrative responsibilities at the broader college level. They may focus on upholding and enforcing expectations for the faculty and facilitating the growth of and development in their college. Provosts oversee budget allocations, develop and implement academic programs, and plan for faculty recruitment and retention, among other responsibilities. Persons in these positions may have a lot more say in the hiring and recruitment of bilingual faculty, which may be attractive to academics who want to transform their department. For example, a department chair may be in charge of leading faculty searches and could advocate for bilingualism to be a part of the desired qualifications in the faculty search description; they may also have a larger say in actually offering the faculty position to bilingual candidates and in negotiating for higher pay for them.

EN LAS BUENAS Y EN LAS MALAS

There are certainly pros and cons to being an academic, and we want to be transparent about some of the drawbacks and benefits you may experience if you choose this route. The tenure-track process can be extensive; however, depending on your career goals and personal priorities navigating it may be worth the many challenges. First, a tenured position allows for job security. In fact, one of the reasons tenure was created was to foster academic freedom by allowing faculty to engage in any research focus, choose what to teach in the classroom, and present and publish research findings. Faculty's research can have quite an impact. Faculty can leverage their expertise and research to address social justice issues; shape policy; and provide professional expertise to the media, on legal matters, and to state and federal institutions (American Psychological Association [APA] Task Force on Inequities in Academic Tenure and Promotion, 2023). In addition, faculty work with students, and providing this sort of mentorship can feel quite rewarding. For example, you may have advisees that you meet with on a frequent basis; in these mentoring relationships you can pass along your wisdom and help them grow throughout their academic journey. In addition, students have their own wisdom and lived experience, so the growth can be reciprocal. Furthermore, being a professor brings significant social capital in the form of professional networks, institutional resources, credibility, and community influence. Academics also usually have a 9- to 10-month work schedule, so they may have more flexible summers where they may be able to visit *familia*. However, this does not mean that academics have summers off: Professors are likely to continue to conduct research and engage in writing during the summer. Some professors may decide to teach during the summer, especially as an adjunct or assistant professor, to generate more income. Furthermore, during the school year you may also have more flexibility than traditional 9-to-5 jobs. For example, a faculty member may be able to attend a doctor's appointment during the day or take their family member to the doctor, volunteer at their child's school classroom, provide home care for an ailing partner or relative, or be at the picket line when others are on strike.

There are also some negative experiences in academia. At universities with high research activity (R1s and R2s) there might be a publish-or-perish environment that entails a pressure for faculty to publish constantly lest they not obtain tenure and/or promotion. This may not align with your values and commitment to service. For example, professors may want to focus on community-based actions and collaborate with communities in their research endeavors, which may take longer to complete. Some professors value qualitative research, which often helps illustrate the full narrative of bilingual communities; however, their colleagues may have biases against qualitative research and believe it is not as rigorous or valid as quantitative research (APA, 2021). Other professors may want to concentrate on presenting their research findings in media outlets, where it might actually reach key community members, rather than in journals, whose audience is mostly academics or other researchers. We recommend you pay attention and try to discern whether this type of pressure exists at your potential place of employment.

Depending on the specific field you want to go into, faculty positions—specifically, tenure-track faculty positions—may be scarce and competitive. In addition, these positions may not always be readily available in your geographic location, and thus you may have to consider moving in order to land a tenure-track position, something that may be in opposition to your values (e.g., being far away from family). Aside from limited options and competitiveness, compensation at the assistant professor level (depending on your university) may not be appealing, especially for recent graduates who have accrued debt throughout their educational journey, or first-generation students who are seeking financial freedom and stability. In addition, although faculty have advanced education and develop years of expertise, salaries do not necessarily eventually compensate them properly, at any rank, because of the countless hours of unpaid labor (e.g., hours spent for licensure, leadership, and service) they have put in. These are all factors to consider when you are applying for faculty positions. *Pero como con todo en la vida, si este es tu camino, ¡no pierdas la esperanza! Hay comunidades académicas que están encontrando diversas maneras de sobrellevar estos desafíos y tú también puedes encontrar una posición que coincide con lo que necesitas, quieres y mereces.*

Just like being a student in graduate school, in academia there is a hidden curriculum (i.e., unwritten norms, practices, and expectations for academic advancement) that just intensifies social inequities for marginalized faculty. For example, new faculty may not know how to gain resources for their research because of a lack of transparency surrounding how to land those resources at their university. As another example, an assistant professor may not know about the inner workings of how to obtain a new tenure-track position at another university or how to navigate the transition at their current university (Kelsky, 2021). Bilingual faculty may not know the funding opportunities available to them to conduct bilingual research, or they may be looking for local resources to help improve their students' clinical skills (e.g., local practicum sites where bilingual students can do therapy in Spanish). Universities should aim for more transparency regarding their tenure process; if not this leaves the onus on the faculty to figure it out. This is where mentoring is really helpful, and it is important to connect with faculty who you got to know through your academic journey. If you do not have close connections with other faculty there are also programs that help faculty succeed. For example, the American Association of Hispanics in Higher Education Faculty Fellowship Program (https://www.aahhe.org/

faculty-fellows-program) helps Latinx faculty have successful careers in academia and guides assistant professors in obtaining tenure. This group also offers the Graduate Student Fellowship program (https://www.aahhe.org/graduate-fellows-program), which is geared toward students who are preparing for faculty positions. These programs can assist in filling in the gaps and help you understand the hidden curriculum.

Systemic Issues in Academia

Although the rates of graduate students of color is increasing, promotion, tenure, and retention of faculty of color are still unjustifiably low. For instance, despite the fact that approximately 40% of the U.S. population consists of people of color (U.S. Census Bureau, 2020), only 24.6% of faculty identify as faculty of color, and most of them are assistant professors (National Center for Education Statistics, 2024). Among Latinx professors, only 5.53% are assistant professors, 5.15% are associate professors, and 4.12% are full professors (National Center for Education Statistics, 2024). There are many systemic issues in academia that affect faculty of color and bilingual academics. Faculty of color who are bilingual are often completing invisible labor, that is, unrecognized or uncompensated work that supports students and institutions, such as translating, mentoring, or serving on diversity committees, and they may experience a mismatch of values between the academic culture and their cultural values (Settles et al., 2019). Often, faculty of color and bilingual faculty are few in number in their department, which could lead to cultural and linguistic isolation at an individual level and possibly result in extra emotional labor (Pettit, 2019). For example, faculty of color and bilingual faculty may be tokenized in the form of routinely being assigned diversity work at the university level and be automatically seen as a role model and emotional support for graduate students of color (APA Task Force on Inequities in Academic Tenure and Promotion, 2023). This can create an extra emotional burden that other faculty do not experience. In addition, faculty who engage in this work often are not acknowledged for it during their tenure and promotion reviews (Babcock et al., 2017).

Academia rewards individual accomplishments, rapid and frequent publishing in journals with high impact factors, and citation counts (Dougherty & Horne, 2022). This may not always align with the values of bilingual faculty or faculty of color, who may want to focus on research that is meaningful to their community and spend more time in community-based participatory projects that require more effort (Few-Demo et al., 2016). Overall, faculty of color face discrimination that is manifested through microaggressions, conflicts between the institution's values and their cultural values, social isolation, and mentorship difficulties (Griffin, 2020). These difficulties are also amplified for gender-diverse faculty of color (APA Task Force on Inequities in Academic Tenure and Promotion, 2023).

Awareness of these systemic issues is important before starting your career in academia because these experiences do not contribute to a rewarding work environment and can lead faculty of color to leave academia. Scholars have talked about their journeys with respect to leaving academia and finding meaningful outlets elsewhere to continue doing the work they are passionate about. As an example, listen to Episode 11 of the *Get Me Outta Here Please!* podcast hosted by Drs. Hilary Anand and Grace Chen (2022). As a bilingual faculty member of color, it is important to know what your values are and to recognize the parts of academia with which you align and the parts with which you do not. It is important to be surrounded by colleagues who understand and support you and a university that acknowledges, recognizes, and compensates you for your work. *Más que nada es importante sentir auto confianza y reconocer que la academia es solo una parte pequeña de nuestra identidad y experiencia como seres humanos.*

¡SI! QUIERO SER AN ACADEMIC: *LA IDENTIDAD Y EL TRABAJO* OF AN ACADEMIC PROFESSIONAL

Tal vez, despite the varied challenges in being an academic as a bilingual person of color you, like some of us, still want to pursue *este camino. ¡Qué bueno y qué alivio!* As you read earlier in this chapter, there are very few of us here, so if academic scholarship is what you like, we need you! *Y queremos apoyarte en este camino* with the information and reflections we share here. As you will read in the rest of this chapter, there are various things we can do as academics that increase language equity and bilingual inclusivity in the academy. As a professor, you certainly are in a position of more power, and you can leverage this in various ways to increase access and benefits for other bilingual people of color.

Our identity is multifaceted and multidimensional, comprising various influences and factors. Depending on our professional contexts, there may be aspects of our identities, such as the languages we speak, that become more or less salient or relevant, often because of the cultural values inherent to a particular setting. In academia there are opportunities for multilingual work, but because of systemic and structural racism they are not automatically built in, so to speak, so we have to seek them out. In other words, languages other than English are valued less, or are valued almost solely within the confines of a languages department. As such, if you are considering *este camino* you may want to reflect on how important it is to you to be able to fulfill the language aspects of your identity within a professional context. There are certainly ways of incorporating this cultural asset and value, but these opportunities are not common, and your academic path may include more exploration and trial and error. Those of us navigating this path are continuously working on figuring out how to bring this aspect of our identity and values into our work.

The dominant cultural and linguistic values and practices in society at large also govern academia. This includes language and, as in other professional settings, the English language reigns supreme in academia. One consequence of this is a systematic and structural undervaluing of languages other than English, especially Spanish, in institutions of higher education. Thus, as in K–12 education, everyone at U.S. colleges and universities is expected to be proficient and communicate predominantly in English. Thus, as an academic, professor or otherwise, your multilingual abilities may take a backseat, but they certainly do not have to, and we hope they will not!

Despite these inherent structural language inequities in academia, or perhaps to combat them, there are several reasons we hope to encourage more bilingual academics. First and foremost, the need and concomitant demand *ison gigantes!* This is because the number of people in the United States who prefer to speak languages other than English, especially Spanish, is growing. Thus, academic settings in the United States are going to have to adapt and evolve to meet this change. And guess who can help with this? Bilingual academics! There is an increasing amount of academic work that requires bilingual skills. For example, in terms of research, there is much work that needs to be done in Spanish, including the training of students; conducting the research; analyzing data collected in Spanish; and partnering with communities, such as in community-based participatory action research. Establishing academic–community partnerships in which patients/clients are served, apart from any research pursuits, also will require bilingual abilities. And that is just to name a few things! So, if the bilingual aspect of your identity is important to you, please know that *te necesitamos en la academia.*

ORGULLO BILINGÜE

¿Entonces, what does it mean to bring your full bilingual self into academic work? In the broadest possible sense, there are essentially two ways that are not mutually exclusive, and in combination may prove to be quite fulfilling.

One way involves integrating issues of language or multilingualism into your research, teaching, service, and administration work in academia. The other way is less concrete or pragmatic and consists of a way of being, or having an overall approach of openness and pride about your multilingualism and multiculturalism.

Conducting Research That Aligns With Your Bilingual and Multicultural Values

As previously discussed, most academic positions consist of varying degrees of research work, thus, pursuing research that centers issues of language and culturally responsive care is an excellent way to do meaningful work as a bilingual academic. In fact, issues of language and language equity are relatively underresearched in the fields of psychology and mental health care (see the "Resources" section at the end of this chapter). Scientific journals are also increasingly publishing abstracts in both English and Spanish (e.g., the *Journal of Latinx Psychology*), so this may be another way to pursue and promote language equity through research in the academy. The publication of research in both English and Spanish is especially important because it increases access to scientific information for members of the public who prefer to speak and read in Spanish.

If you feel unsure where to start in your pursuit of language-related research questions, we recommend looking through research articles to get a sense of who is doing this work. Finding other researchers with similar backgrounds (bilingual, Latine), interests, and experiences is a key way to establish relationships that will help you grow in your empirical pursuits (and further your social support system, which is very much needed in academia). We can assure you that your Latine colleagues are more than eager to collaborate and love hearing from others who are interested in this type of research. You might also consider cross-field collaborations with *gente* in other fields, such as linguists, cognitive psychologists, educational psychologists, and neurolinguists. Folx in these fields sometimes specialize in conducting empirical work that examine issues of language from innovative and intersecting angles.

Teaching That Aligns With Your Bilingual and Multicultural Values

Being a bilingual professor also opens doors for exciting teaching opportunities. You could pursue teaching courses in Spanish, especially in topics directly related to your research or clinical areas of expertise. Note that because there may be fewer models of teaching courses related to issues of mental health in Spanish in the United States, some extra preparatory work may be necessary to design such courses for higher education settings. In addition, bilingual professors can each language-related courses in various academic departments and at various levels, such as in the areas of international studies, global affairs, ethnic studies, cultural studies, and foreign language. Bilingual professors can also pursue teaching opportunities in professional schools and programs, such as law schools, medical schools, and social work programs, where they can offer courses related to their field of expertise while incorporating bilingual and multicultural perspectives.

Bilingual Issues in Academic Service and Administration

As we have described, academics have other responsibilities besides teaching, and these can also lend themselves to addressing or incorporating bilingualism and language equity into academia. These include graduate student supervision/mentorship; various administrative activities; leadership roles; and involvement in other scholarship activities, such as fellowships and visiting scholar programs. Professors are the gatekeepers of graduate education in a significant way. Whether at an R1 or R2 institution, professors often are responsible for reviewing graduate school applications and making recommendations about who gets in. *Por eso*, having bilingual folx of color in these positions can make a big difference in who gets a spot at the academic table. This can also include helping shape a department culture that values and prioritizes issues of diversity and equity in the graduate admission process and in overall education, including language equity and fostering an inclusive and supportive environment for multilingual/multicultural academics in training.

Graduate admissions are just the beginning of professors' important supervision work. Professors serve as supervisors and mentors and are an essential and significant support to students throughout their journeys, especially during the arduous *camino* of graduate education. As some of you have probably experienced, professors support a student's master's thesis; dissertation; independent research projects, and many other academic pursuits, such as conference presentations and fellowship applications. This often includes reading many drafts, providing feedback on drafts and other materials, writing recommendation letters, and providing overall guidance, among many other things. As such, professors play a pivotal role not only in the recruitment but also the retention of graduate students of color in graduate education. It is important to have professors who are multilingual, with whom students of color share a background and to whom they can relate, who engage in mutual encouragement and ultimately optimize each other's support system in the academy. You may also be involved in clinical supervision and, in this role, you will likely have opportunities for training and supervising bilingual trainees and supporting them as they serve Spanish-speaking clients.

As a bilingual academic in a leadership position, you can engage in system-level advocacy and change by influencing institutional policy. As an academic, you can hold positions of leadership, such as program director, chair, or dean, which grant more power to help shape department- and/or college-level policy and practices. Shaping policies at universities is important because they can prioritize (or not) issues of equity and diversity, including cultivating an environment and infrastructure that supports bilingual folx in the academy. In health services and allied psychology programs this can make a big difference in terms of creating and fostering a structural support system for bilingual graduate trainees who are trying to provide services in both English and Spanish or another language when their clinical education is exclusively in English. As an academic leader, you can help address system-level equity-related questions and needs, such as addressing questions like "How can we increase access to resources that Spanish-speaking clinical trainees need when serving Spanish-speaking clients?" and "What additional resources do Spanish-speaking clinical trainees need, and how can we increase departmental awareness of these needs?" Note that because Latines currently make up a very small percentage of professors, you will find even fewer of them in leadership positions, but there are some, and we hope their numbers will continue to grow. *¡Quizás el liderazgo académico pueda ser una de tu metas y aspiración!*

Other academic work might include the pursuit of various activities such as pursuing competitive scholarly fellowships and writing and publishing in various outlets for purposes other than research. One delightful and adventurous way for professors to make use of their Spanish-speaking and academic abilities is by conducting scholarly work (research and teaching, among other things) in a Spanish-speaking country. Ideally, you might find an opportunity in a Latin American country to which you have a connection! There are national and institution-based fellowships; you have probably heard of one of the most prestigious ones: the Fulbright Scholar Program for faculty and postdoctoral fellows (https://fulbrightscholars.org). Check the program's website see if your university offers support for completing these applications; you can also try reaching out to past recipients. *Más aun*, if you have a desire to use your Spanish language writing abilities in the United States (this can feel very rewarding, especially if Spanish is your first language), there are opportunities to do that as an academic that may also count toward your tenure. This may take the form of contributing to the development and publication of clinical manuals in Spanish or writing book chapters in Spanish (or Spanglish!).

"MI CORAZÓN LATE EN DOS IDIOMAS": BEING YOUR WHOLE BILINGUAL SELF IN ACADEMIA

Now that we have covered various activities in which you can engage that align with your values as a bilingual academic, we switch to considering a way of being as a bilingual professional. This approach to being a bilingual academic is more elusive, *¡pero es muy importante!* And really, it is something that we hope to convey and encourage, directly and indirectly, for every bilingual professional *camino* discussed in this book. We are referring to being proud of your bilingualism, seeing it as the magnificent cultural asset that it is, and finding ways of living that out professionally.

Many of us have experience with *assimilation*, or the adopting of a dominant culture over one's heritage culture. In many ways, U.S. society demands that minoritized people of color assimilate to the dominant culture to succeed. Unfortunately, this is to the detriment of our individual well-being, the well-being of our *comunidades*, and our cultural heritage and assets. Assimilation to the dominant culture within academia is tempting and easy to fall into, and in its most extreme form it erases a big part of our multicultural identity. We have such amazing backgrounds and experiences, and we should not have to hide or restrain *nuestra cultura* to belong in academia. Adopting and living out this posture of cultural pride is one of the best ways we can think of to combat the strong pull of assimilation in academia. Language is a big and important part of our identity, especially our ethnic identity. As such, if we want to be fully ourselves, and accomplish fulfilling work, it helps to be proud and make use of our Spanish language abilities, even in academia.

As we keep in mind the great diversity within bilingual English–Spanish speakers, and the intersectionality of identities, we want to recognize that many bilingual Spanish-speaking academics may not have experience with assimilation and that the dominant White culture in the United States is, in fact, their culture, or is aligned with their values and worldviews. We want to encourage those readers to reflect on their social location and access to power and privilege; leverage these to amplify efforts to dismantle the various forms of oppression in academia; and promote equity, especially language equity in the academy.

PLATIQUEMOS DE ALGUNOS TEMAS PRÁCTICOS Y (QUIZÁS) TUS PRÓXIMOS PASOS

We want to wrap up our discussion of what it is like to be on the bilingual academic *camino* by considering some potential steps you can take down this path to thrive and have a fulfilling career as a bilingual person of color. First, it is helpful to seek information and understand the programs and departments within universities that interest you. We cannot simply make assumptions about a program's or department's values and support on the basis of its location or other such factors. In general, it might help to consider the background (research and otherwise) of the faculty in these departments. Who are the graduate students? Are their backgrounds similar to yours? What values are noted on the department's website? How does the department embody those values? What values are listed in the program manuals? Do you get an overall sense that the institution is welcoming to and inclusive of people of color?

Of course, there are many other factors that inform and affect the decision-making process when considering and applying for jobs in academia (e.g., location, family). You may want or need to prioritize those other factors over a program's values, and that is completely okay. It will still be very helpful to take that next step of applying, or perhaps accepting an offer, with a general sense of the department's values and climate, so you can adjust your expectations accordingly. *Desafortunadamente*, there are few programs that truly value multiculturalism and even fewer that provide structural support for bilingual academics. However, this should not deter you from going after these academic jobs! Remember that there are already a few of us navigating this path, so it is our hope that, little by little, we will effect some change toward valuing and supporting language equity and bilingual faculty. It is also definitely possible to still do meaningful and fulfilling work within departments (the majority of them) that do not yet fully embrace language diversity and equity.

Applying to Academic Jobs

When applying for postdoctoral or faculty positions, reflect on whether you want to share the bilingual/multicultural aspects of your identity during this step *en el camino*. If you do want to share, how will you do this? Most of these jobs require a cover letter, a research statement, a teaching statement, and a diversity statement as part of the application process. Consider how you might convey this aspect of your identity through those statements. This is also connected to decisions about having an overall bilingual theme and how that is reflected on your website and other social media accounts (if you have them). During interviews, how might you convey aspects of your bilingual background and experiences? Maybe it will be during your job talk (i.e., your presentation during the job interview process)? Maybe during individual interviews? Maybe it does not make sense to bring it up at all?

Deliberating and Negotiating Job Offer(s)

Now, let's assume you get an academic job offer. This, too, is an important step on the path of a bilingual academic. How will you negotiate for compensation (monetary or otherwise) that accounts for your bilingualism? This is all the more important if the position comes with responsibilities to do work in both English and Spanish. Either way, it is critical that you include your bilingual abilities as a point for negotiating a higher salary and other resources. The likelihood that your Spanish language abilities will be used at one point or another is very high. If you conduct research with Spanish-speaking populations, you are likely to have a long list of extra steps you have to take, and resources you need, and negotiating for those resources will be separate from negotiating your salary. Your dialogues about the experiences of a bilingual academic in a predominantly English-speaking setting will depend of how attuned to this issue the person you are negotiating with (dean and/or chair) is. Prepare to speak to all of the extra work inherent in your bilingual contributions, especially if the department has not yet provided other structural supports for doing work in both English and Spanish. In terms of general negotiation tips, there is an episode on Adam Grant's (2020) *Worklife with Adam Grant* podcast that discusses this at length that may be helpful.

PARA CONCLUIR

In some ways, academia is like other professional *caminos*, but it also has a significant hidden curriculum. We hope this chapter has shed some light on what is hidden, especially for people who have historically been excluded from this space. For the most part, if you want to make use of your bilingual abilities you will certainly be able to within the academy. We can embody our bilingual values at any point on our academic paths and do not have to wait until we become professors. As an undergraduate, you can look for opportunities in research laboratories or other spaces where you can make use of your Spanish-speaking powers, especially they entail opportunities to give back to our communities. Being a bilingual academic in psychology is incredibly fulfilling, so we encourage you to take pride in your bilingual abilities!

TAKEAWAYS

- Gaining insight into how academia works will be helpful as you determine whether this is the professional *camino* for you.

- Pay attention to the professional activities that feel fulfilling to you. If they are related to research and teaching, the academic path may be right for you.

- Take pride in your bilingual and multicultural background, even in academia! If you do not feel that sense of pride, consider why that might not be the case and what is getting in the way.

REFLEXIONES

- Who are the people that I can reach out to for mentoring with respect to faculty positions?
- Do I like conducting research? Do I like research being a big component of my professional responsibilities?
- Do I like teaching? Do I like teaching being at the center of my professional responsibilities?
- Do I enjoy mentoring/supervising graduate students in research and other scholarly pursuits?
- How do I feel about advocating for issues of language equity in academia?
- Am I prepared to negotiate for fair compensation that takes into account my bilingual abilities?
- How am I embracing a posture and way of being of cultural pride in academia?

RESOURCES

Recommended Reading

- Mojica Rodriguez, P. D. (2021). *For brown girls with sharp edges and tender hearts: A love letter to women of color*. Seal Press.

Online Resources

- American Association of Hispanics in Higher Education, Inc., Faculty Fellowship Program: https://www.aahhe.org/faculty-fellows-program
- American Association of Hispanics in Higher Education, Inc., Graduate Student Fellowship Program: https://www.aahhe.org/graduate-fellows-program
- Carnegie Classification of Institutions of Higher Education: https://carnegieclassifications.acenet.edu
- National Center for Faculty Development & Diversity: https://www.ncfdd.org
- The Professor Is In: https://theprofessorisin.com/

REFERENCES

Academic Positions. (2024, April 3). *What is tenure track?* https://academicpositions.com/career-advice/what-is-tenure

American Psychological Association. (2021, October). *Role of psychology and the American Psychological Association in dismantling systemic racism against people of color in the United States.* https://www.apa.org/about/policy/resolution-dismantling-racism.pdf

American Psychological Association Task Force on Inequities in Academic Tenure and Promotion. (2023, August). *APA Task Force Report on promotion, tenure and retention of faculty of color in psychology.* American Psychological Association. https://www.apa.org/pubs/reports/inequities-academic-tenure-promotion.pdf

Anand, H., & Chen, G. (Hosts). (2022, February 14). Leaving academia and defining one's own professional journey (Episode 11) [Audio podcast episode]. In *Get me outta here please!* Psych Grad Corner. https://psychgradcorner.libsyn.com/ep-11-leaving-academia

Babcock, L., Recalde, M. P., Vesterlund, L., & Weingart, L. (2017). Gender differences in accepting and receiving requests for tasks with low promotability. *The American Economic Review, 107*(3), 714–747. https://doi.org/10.1257/aer.20141734

Carnegie Classification of Institutions of Higher Education. (n.d.-a). *Carnegie Classification of Institutions of Higher Education®.* https://carnegieclassifications.acenet.edu

Carnegie Classification of Institutions of Higher Education. (n.d.-b). *2025 Research designations.* https://carnegieclassifications.acenet.edu/carnegie-classification/research-designations

Dougherty, M. R., & Horne, Z. (2022). Citation counts and journal impact factors do not capture some indicators of research quality in the behavioural and brain sciences. *Royal Society Open Science, 9*(8), 220334. https://doi.org/10.1098/rsos.220334

Few-Demo, A. L., Piercy, F. P., & Stremmel, A. J. (2016). Balancing the passion for activism with the demands of tenure: One professional's story from three perspectives. In P. A. Matthew (Ed.), *Written/unwritten: Diversity and the hidden truths of tenure* (pp. 201–221). University of North Carolina Press. https://doi.org/10.5149/northcarolina/9781469627717.003.0012

Grant, A. (Host). (2020, March 23). The science of the deal (Season 3, Episode 3) [Audio podcast episode]. In *Worklife with Adam Grant.* TED Audio Collective. https://podcasts.apple.com/us/podcast/the-science-of-the-deal/id1346314086?i=1000469312967

Griffin, K. A. (2020). Institutional barriers, strategies, and benefits to increasing the representation of women and men of color in the professoriate. In L. W. Perna (Ed.), *Higher education: Handbook of theory and research* (Vol. 35, pp. 1–73). Springer. https://doi.org/10.1007/978-3-030-11743-6_4-1

Kelsky, K. (2015). *The professor is in: The essential guide to turning your Ph.D. into a job.* Three Rivers Press.

Kelsky, K. (2021, May 14). *How to hop from one tenure track job to another.* The Professor Is In. https://theprofessorisin.com/2021/05/14/how-to-hop-from-one-tenure-track-job-to-another

National Center for Education Statistics. (2024). *Characteristics of postsecondary faculty.* https://nces.ed.gov/programs/coe/indicator/csc

Pérez, P. A. (2021). *The tenure-track process for Chicana and Latina faculty.* Routledge.

Pettit, E. (2019, October 22). When faculty of color feel isolated, consortia expand their networks. *The Chronicle of Higher Education*. https://www.chronicle.com/article/when-faculty-of-color-feel-isolated-consortia-expand-their-networks

Settles, I. H., Buchanan, N. T., & Dotson, K. (2019). Scrutinized but not recognized: (In)visibility and hypervisibility experiences of faculty of color. *Journal of Vocational Behavior, 113,* 62–74. https://doi.org/10.1016/j.jvb.2018.06.003

U.S. Census Bureau. (2020). *2020 census: Demographic data map viewer.* https://www.census.gov/library/visualizations/2021/geo/demographicmapviewer.html

12 ¡YA PUES!

Intentional, Comprehensive Bilingual Mental Health Training Now

MACIEL CAMPOS, YESSENIA MEJIA, AND
ANDRÉS J. CONSOLI

Haciendo y deshaciendo se va aprendiendo.

Integrating the *caminos* that have brought us to this point is crucial for envisioning the future of bilingual (English–Spanish) mental health training and professional development. We hope a mini "rest stop" at the metaphorical *mirador* will give us the opportunity to appreciate all we have accomplished thus far and inspire enthusiasm for exploring the road ahead in Latinx and bilingual mental health in the United States.

As we arrive at the final stop on the *caminos* of this book, we detail anticipated needs within the field, in the context of long-existing and emerging determinants of health. We reckon with inequitable representation in leadership to inspire readers with aspirations of *liderazgo* in this field to serve as stewards of equity and justice and rebuke White supremacy. We offer guided reflections that address the relevance of advocacy and engagement, in particular with respect to leadership roles. We discuss foreseeable barriers in advocacy and do so in a radically genuine manner to prepare you

https://doi.org/10.1037/0000481-013
Forging Caminos: *Pathways to Becoming a Bilingual Mental Health Professional,*
M. Campos, Y. Mejia, and A. J. Consoli (Editors)

for the *caminos* ahead. We share tips and recommendations for managing such barriers, engaging upper management structures and complex systems in problem solving for language equity and prioritizing self-care. Mental health education, training, research, service delivery, and advocacy must embrace and affirm bilingual abilities if the field wants to remain vibrant and relevant in an increasingly diverse U.S. society.

Lifelong learning, commitment to professional growth, and intentionality are key to *transformar el presente y cocrear el futuro* of bilingual mental health training. The authors of the preceding chapters, our expert *guías*, have forged intentional *caminos* and paved the way to this apex in championing bilingual professional training and development in the mental health field. Each *camino* has been curated to spark and sustain your inspired commitment to becoming a bilingual mental health professional and shape your *metas* in this specialized field. The *sabiduría* abundantly and generously shared thus far is our *legado generacional*, equipping us for centering and maximizing our bilingual talents and skills at each *paso* of building a career as a bilingual mental health scientist–practitioner. Our *guías* started us all with descriptions of the ins and outs of preparing for your professional and academic goals in bilingual mental health during and after your undergraduate education. They explored opportunities for fostering your bilingualism and understanding your academic and professional options. They shared *consejos* for applying to graduate school, choosing a compatible program, and showcasing your bilingualism in preparation to successfully transition into graduate education. Their shared *testimonios* intended to inform expectations for burgeoning bilingual and bicultural Latinxs to thrive and unapologetically take up space in graduate school settings.

In demanding intentional and comprehensive bilingual mental health training, our *guías* have provided dedicated intentionality for competencies, ethics, supervision, and mentorship that prioritize bilingualism as a specialized skill set. *Al fin*, as you grow into the final stages of your academic training and start your early career, *exploramos* navigating the internship and postdoctoral process for bilingual and Latinx applicants and pursuing lifelong learning in equity and bilingual professional identity formation. The voice of *liberación* resonates throughout the book *y retumba* in direct calls for centering *afrolatinidad e indigeneidad* within bilingual mental health training and development, challenging long-standing and -upheld oppressive practices and mestizaje racial ideologies (see Chapter 4, this volume). *Sin duda*, all *caminos* lead to demanding deliberate and comprehensive bilingual mental health training *ahora*. *Confía* that you are equipped to harness your personal *sabiduría* and experiences, and those of your *guías*, to claim your role in envisioning and launching bilingual mental health training, leadership, and advocacy.

FUTURE NEEDS AND CONSIDERATIONS

The *paisaje* that awaits is one with peaks of resilience and valleys of pressing concerns for bilingual professional training and development. The advancements in the Spanish language, changing Latinx population needs, and evolving treatment approaches warrant urgent commitment and dedication to comprehensive bilingual mental health training and professional development. Psychology has yet to systematically address the historically unmet diverse needs in the training of bilingual mental health professionals. As we make strides in endeavors to address such needs, it behooves us to consider further anticipated needs highlighted by current events, such as the ones mentioned later in this chapter. Continuing your unlearning to better understand these anticipated needs will be imperative for your leadership and advocacy in bilingual mental health.

The Evolution of *Latinidad* and Spanish

Growing interrogations and rejections of *latinidad* as a construct have apexed in "Latinidad is canceled" (Flores, 2021) movements, exposing a disconnect between the Latinx/e/o/a label and the multiple identities it purports to include. As stewards of equity and justice, the work of bilingual scientists–practitioners with Latine and bilingual Spanish-speaking *comunidades* will need to be anchored in inclusivity and a radical reckoning with intra-oppression. *No se puede tapar el sol con un dedo,* and so it is the responsibility of bilingual scientists–practitioners to be informed about these critical dialogues. We encourage you to complement key how-to's from this volume with ongoing unlearning and relearning as you achieve positions of leadership and engage in service, research, teaching, and advocacy. Fortunately, there are plentiful avenues, such as workshops, seminars, and conferences, that promote your unlearning of ideologies anchored in colonialism and White supremacy, foster your self-awareness, and acquaint you with seminal literature and progressive experts in this field. Explore and challenge preconceived notions and biases you might have about the relevance of antiracism work within bilingual mental health. For example, you might notice thoughts such as "Racism is a *gringo* issue," or some of you might find yourselves denying privileges associated with your proximity to Whiteness.

The advancement of bilingual mental health hinges on such radical intro-spection and creating space for Black, Indigenous, and Spanish-speaking colleagues and communities.

Scholars and activists alike have ushered in increased attention and ten-sions directed at efforts toward inclusivity within the Spanish language, which is traditionally a gendered one. Although we honor the various pros and cons identified by groups that have different perspectives, we orient ourselves to the primary goal of inclusivity. Consider that rejections of lan-guage fluidity and evolution may in part be founded in White supremacy and colonialism that decry alternative possibilities as threats to hegemony. If you are experiencing gender-inclusive language as challenging, awkward, or clumsy, we encourage you to practice self-awareness of your privilege and maintain the goal of inclusion. Other concerns that continue to be high-lighted within Spanish include the propagation of *machismo*, homophobia, and transphobia. Words matter, and *dichos* like *"Calladita te ves más bonita"* are the building blocks for intrinsically sexist policies and practices.

We recommend encouraging people to self-identify without imposing labels. Actively include Spanish-speaking people of historically (and inten-tionally) excluded identities in determining how they wish to be part of *latinidad*, if at all. There is great promise for growth and insight when we consider how people connect meaningfully with their chosen identities. Further understanding the evolution of *latinidad* as a construct, the Spanish language, and intersectionality is salient for the future of bilingual mental health training and development; it must not be ignored.

La Pandemia: COVID-19

Spanish-speaking Latinx communities in the United States continue to be disparately plagued by individual and global traumas. The beginning of the 2020s featured the COVID-19 global pandemic, which has dispro-portionately affected racially and ethnically minoritized and economically disenfranchised *comunidades* (Lee et al., 2023; Mental Health America, n.d.). This has resulted in disparities in death rates, long-term disability, unemployment, and homelessness for many Latinxs in the United States (Krogstad et al., 2020; Mental Health America, n.d.; Morales, 2020). As much of the world resorted to remote options for schooling, work, and socialization, many Latinxs experienced reduced opportunities because of systemic issues, in particular what has been commonly referred to as "the great digital divide," which is characterized by markedly limited access to technology among minoritized groups (Hodges & Calvo, 2023). Continued differential access to technology has further exacerbated preexisting challenges in academic performance and well-being for Latinx youth in the United States (Dorn et al., 2020; Fernandez, 2020). Stay-at-home orders intended to promote safety and well-being predisposed multigenerational households often found in our *comunidades* to faster COVID-19 transmission, greater proximity to substance misuse, and increased exposure to domestic violence (Czeisler et al., 2021). The resulting trauma, grief, isolation, and anxiety have proven to be a disastrous recipe for a nationwide mental health crisis.

"Give Me Your Tired, Your Hungry, Your Poor"?

Global destabilization resulting from climate change, political persecution, war, poverty, and the economic exploitation of natural resources continues to generate the displacement of marginalized communities and fuel forced and voluntary immigration among many, including folx from Latin America. Defor-estation of the Amazon rainforest, the rise of autocracies, and radically active and intentional anti-Blackness and anti-Indigeneity throughout Latin America are few among the life-and-death matters that are driving migration and immigration patterns with urgency. For many excluded from access to financial and legal means to immigrate, *la Bestia, yolas, la jornada,* become a perilous yet desperate and necessitated means that point in one direction: *el Norte.*

The duplicitous role of destabilizer and refuge is a historical one for the United States. Explicitly xenophobic changes in immigration policies targeting Latinxs have been supplemented with reductionist verbal brandings, such as "the triangle" to refer to the independent nations of El Salvador, Guatemala, and Honduras; repeated references to drug and weapon cartels; and threats of invasions of gangs, such as the MS-13 gang (which, ironically, is rooted in the United States). The resulting humanitarian crisis at the Mexico–United States border has been reflected in widely disseminated images of children detained in cages. Families with undocumented or mixed statuses have experienced intensified fear and dread as the raids by the U.S. Immigration and Customs Enforcement increased in frequency. Widely broadcasted images of White border patrol agents on horses assaulting Black Haitian refugees with whips, eerily reminiscent of slavery in the United States, served as reminders of the intersectionality of race and immigration, which permeates all national boundaries, including those across Latin American countries. Hopelessness, grief, and depression affect many undocumented youth who struggle to understand their future in the United States as propositions such as the Deferred Action for Childhood Arrivals (known as DACA) continue to lack resolution.

"El Sueño Americano"

Many Latinxs often find employment opportunities in front-line sectors that include agriculture, hospitality, factories, construction, and child care. Baseline vulnerabilities in these occupations include long hours, low wages, and higher risks of injury, as seen in the Baltimore Francis Scott Key Bridge tragedy in early 2024, in which six construction workers, all immigrants from Honduras, El Salvador, Guatemala, and Mexico, were killed (Kurtz, 2024). Added impacts from the COVID-19 pandemic, unregulated markets, and climate change jeopardize wages, opportunities, and, ultimately, quality of life. The underpayment of Latina workers has continued this decade, highlighting how much longer it takes Latinas to earn what White men do in the United States (Equal Pay Today, n.d.). These factors are reflective of a caste-oriented employment system that makes Latines vulnerable to increased psychosocial stress. The gentrification of traditionally African American and Latinx communities in major U.S. cities has additionally contributed to increased rents; priced-out resources, such as at chain supermarkets and other stores; and the eventual displacement and erasure of our *comunidades*. Gun violence and ongoing challenges in reaching agreements on new gun legislation have touched the lives of countless people living in the United States. Mass shootings, such as the one at the Pulse nightclub in Orlando, Florida in 2016, which specifically targeted the lesbian, gay, bisexual, transgender, intersex, queer/questioning, asexual+ community, and at the Robb Elementary School in Uvalde, Texas in 2022, are recent gun violence events that have particularly affected our *comunidades*. The marginalization of many Latinxs increases their vulnerability to gun-related and other forms of violence, and does not receive the same national attention as when Latinx individuals are alleged as perpetrators of gang-related violence, for example.

This brief synopsis highlights an anticipated explosive increase in needs for the Latinx Spanish-speaking community. It is now *tu turno* to harness your knowledge and advocate for and lead in bilingual mental health. You are entrusted with tapping into the innovation that is at the heart of this work, to become acquainted with these needs and changes, champion equity and inclusion, dismantle coloniality, and advance bilingual mental health training that is responsive to our *comunidades*. This chapter invites you to accept the torch and create *los nuevos caminos* toward intentional and comprehensive bilingual mental health research, service, and advocacy.

HOW TO BE AN INTENTIONAL LEADER IN BILINGUAL MENTAL HEALTH

Intentional leadership in bilingual mental health is built on community, collaboration, dedication, innovation, and *compromiso*. On this *camino*, we recommend understanding the wide range of possibilities for leadership, including opportunities to envision and create them if they do not exist. In Chapter 9, you learned how to identify and center your values, strengths, growth edges, and expertise. Consider referring back to it, to identify leadership roles that complement your strengths and values, or to review how to use awareness of your growth edges to prepare for leadership positions. As an intentional leader, you will understand how the salient themes pertinent to bilingual mental health as reviewed here inform your leadership in this field. Although leadership can indeed be fulfilling, exciting, and promising, *no todo es color de rosa*; you will therefore also need *conocimiento* of the anticipated barriers in advocacy for bilingual mental health, along with problem-solving skills.

Para el gusto se hicieron los colores: There are many titles and roles in leadership that might be available to you on the basis of your interests, preferences, and skill set. The key will be understanding how your professional goals and goals within bilingual mental health overlap and learning what existing opportunities can be a match. If you have your eye on a particular position, learn more about the skills, traits, and experience most favored in this leadership opportunity. Refer back to Chapters 6 and 9 to leverage supervision and mentorship spaces in which you can understand the responsibilities inherent to this particular role and how to hone your skills in preparation to work toward such a role. Leadership positions usually rely on skills such as innovation, communication, collaboration, coordination, multitasking, and effective problem solving. *Anímate* to think about how these skills are inherent to bilingual mental health and how you possess and implement them in your everyday work and life. It is our experience that the bilingual brain, particularly when required to translate, interpret, and broker between two languages, is well familiarized with innovative problem solving, multitasking, and collaborative communication. You have been in training for leadership and can pivot toward such a role to intentionally advance bilingual mental health.

Un vistazo: Fernanda has her eye on the open training director position for the clinical predoctoral internship program at her mental health clinic. Her interests and goals include training, supervision, and program development. From supervision meetings and mentorship relationships, Fernanda understands that this leadership position requires coordination with varied graduate programs, developing and evaluating the training program, timely completion of necessary documentation and paperwork, and assessing trainee competencies. On the basis of her training and early career experiences, as well as supervision feedback and evaluations, Fernanda is confident in her impeccable organizational skills, enjoyment of collaboration and relationship building, and creative program development.

Like you, Fernanda has committed herself to intentional bilingual training in mental health services and has a sound understanding of the pertinent and relevant learning themes. She has ingenious ideas to further much-needed bilingual mental health services and is highly motivated to contribute to the field. With no formal practices or policies for bilingual mental health training within the program, Fernanda identifies an opportunity to showcase her leadership skills in a way that reflects her commitment to her values and interests. Fernanda reaches out to her trusted mentor, Alejandro, and they both brainstorm possible *pasos* for shaping her *camino* in leadership. As a result, Fernanda *toma el volante* and works on standardizing a Spanish–English interview format for assessing the bilingual skills of self-identified bilingual applicants to the training program. She soon becomes the trusted expert in bilingual mental health at her program, forging her path toward a formal leadership position, such as training director. Fernanda makes her aspirations clear to colleagues both inside and outside of her employment system and meticulously identifies training programs that are compatible with her interests and professional goals. Fernanda is positioning herself to soon be a training director who develops bilingual training. We check back with Fernanda's *camino* later in this chapter. For now, here are some questions for you to consider: What are the qualities a leader should possess? What are your leadership aspirations? In what ways do you already embody a leadership role?

Here is a list of possible leadership roles and opportunities that we encourage you to consider: clinical director; director of clinical training; director of a program; chair of a department; director of a division; lead researcher or principal investigator; dean of a college; director of Inclusion, Diversity, Equity, and Accessibility (IDEA); president of a university; chief of psychology at a hospital; supervisor; chair of a special interest group; member or chair of an executive board or organization; secretary, member-at-large, or president of a professional organization; leader of a work group; leader of a presidential initiative; consultant; mentor; advisor; systems manager.

"Si Quieres Moños Bonitos, Aguanta Jalones": Liberation and Fallacies in Leadership

Unsurprisingly, mental health systems, including academia and health care, operate under and uphold systemic and structural oppression that is embedded in White supremacy and anti-Blackness. These mental health systems value and emphasize individuality, compliance, productivity, and power (Okun, 2021). They do so via embedded mechanisms, such as rigid hierarchies, unilateral decision making, rigid strategic plans, and "expert" mindsets.

Your leadership will not be immune to this; therefore, proceed with intentionality, and contribute to shifts that benefit bilingual mental health training. Leadership includes the navigation of competing demands that at times may not align. The advocacy and leadership needed in bilingual mental health training must be anchored in social justice, equity, and liberation. *El amor no quita conocimiento,* and we would be lying to you if we told you that you will encounter no resistance on a transformative, socially just leadership journey. Should you be up for this *camino,* please know that many resources are available for leaders in mental health to engage in *liderazgo* approaches and styles that center antiracism, decolonization, and liberation and leverage the privilege, power, and access inherent in leadership positions that are geared toward aims of social justice and equity (Miville et al., 2017).

"Remember Who You Are" —Mufasa, *The Lion King*

We can all probably think of at least one example of someone who seemed to forget who they were, or lost their way as they moved through leadership positions. These positions at times bring greater proximity to administration and less proximity to what many consider groundwork. We strongly encourage you, as a bilingual reader, to prioritize and consider ways to maintain your *conexiones* to bilingual mental health and the vision and values that drove you to leadership. Many leaders who prioritize this connection will say that the best way to do so is to carry on doing the work by continuing to deliver patient care or directly interact with research participants, for example. Stay up to date with salient issues that affect bilingual mental health professionals, and maintain frequent contact with this *comunidad.*

Leadership positions bring access to power, privilege, and shareholders; this is your *oportunidad* to amplify and bring attention to issues of equity that pertain to bilingual mental health. Explore ways to center values such as collectivism, collaboration, and direct communication, and unlearn White-dominant narratives around "professionalism" that are meant to penalize marginalized people, such as urgency, tone policing, overvaluing pedigrees, and nontransparent communications (Training Resources for the Environmental Community, 2023). As in other parts of your *camino,* we encourage you to engage in social location, power, and privilege analyses. Be honest with yourself about ways in which you continue to perpetuate oppressive approaches.

Un vistazo: ¿Te acuerdas de Fernanda? Well, she has gained recognition among her colleagues after her efforts to standardize bilingual interviews with bilingual applicants. As a result, she now oversees a series of innovative endeavors geared toward dedicated bilingual mental health training in her setting. She continues to build her portfolio and curriculum vitae to work toward the internship director position. On the basis of her own *experiencias* and those shared by her bilingual colleagues and supervisees, Fernanda determines that the next area that merits her attention is increased support and differential compensation for bilingual mental health providers. To this end, she engages in needs assessments with her colleagues, gathering data about current and projected needs and the use of bilingual services. Fernanda completes literature reviews on bilingual mental health and advocacy and engages her colleagues in supportive spaces that center collaborative problem solving. She continues groundwork, directly supporting the bilingual community she accompanies. Fernanda stays up to date with pertinent issues related to bilingual mental health and affected communities. She has earned *el respeto y la confianza* of her bilingual colleagues and the bilingual community; she is a leader. Having increasing access to leaders with decision-making power, Fernanda sees the opportunity for advocacy. Fear looms as she feels her body tense, her heart race, and her stomach *un nudo*. Rocking the boat is foreign in a lifetime of *simpatía y armonía*. Connecting to her values, maintaining community, and engaging in her own self-care practices, Fernanda decides to rip off the proverbial bandage and begin her advocacy for differential supports and compensation for her bilingual colleagues.

Mauricio, a bilingual manager, also frequents leadership spaces where decisions are made. And although Fernanda recognizes Mauricio as a bilingual colleague, her *intuición* helps facilitate a keen awareness of the ways she and Mauricio differ in their values and ideology. During a discussion of differential supports for bilingual professionals, Mauricio reminds Fernanda that their work is *para la comunidad* and that compensation, for example, does not compare to the profound need of those they serve. In an effort to validate Fernanda's plight, he offers his personal *sabiduría*, suggesting that Fernanda look into other opportunities, such as private sector work, on the side, to complement her income. Mauricio expresses deep appreciation of and admiration and respect for Fernanda's contributions to bilingual mental health training and services at their setting, which have emphasized the need for them. He reminds her that *unicornios* like them have to continue augmenting and delivering bilingual services; otherwise, what will the community do without them? No pain, no gain: *Si quieres moños bonitos, aguantas jalones.* Fernanda wavers briefly, questioning her own audacity to advocate for differential compensation when her *comunidad* is in need. Her personal work in social justice, liberation, and antiracism reroute her to her *camino* of intentional leadership that intuitively aims to protect against *jalones*.

Now that we know more about Fernanda's *camino*, let's check in: What parts of the leadership role feel more comfortable to you or aligned with you? Have you encountered some Mauricios along the way? If so, how have you handled these interactions? How do you feel about rocking the boat? Does that feel safe to you in your current environment?

"Te Conozco Bacalao, Aunque Vengas Disfraza'o"

Leaders are well-versed visionaries. They pursue a mission with conviction, and others look up to and trust them for guidance and mentorship. Leadership does not necessarily entail formal titles or positions. When you lead without a formal title, it might offer you more flexibility, role diversity, and opportunity to pursue your passions and interests; however, your access to power and privilege may be limited. Some people find that informal positions of leadership untether them from upholding the unjust and inequitable system policies and practices that are intrinsically embedded in formal leadership positions. In the example of Fernanda, she is able to achieve and is perceived as a leader among her colleagues and the community she accompanies. The limitations of her reach are also evident because she does not have decision-making capacities that more formal positions, such as directorships, bring. Mauricio, on the other hand, in his formal title as manager, has a greater capacity for decision-making power and privilege to engage in advocacy. Nonetheless, we see how Mauricio upholds oppressive practices under the guise of prioritizing *"la comunidad."* His behaviors and *"consejos"* for Fernanda are stark reminders of Zora Neale Hurston's (1996, cited in Noxolo, 2009) wise words that "all skinfolk ain't kinfolk" (p. 56). Herein lie the dangers of leadership under pan-ethnic monolithic *latinidad* constructs that ignore diversity of experiences and fail to recognize pressing issues of antiracism, equity, and liberation within Latinx communities.

Throughout this book we have contended with the notion that people who have joined this *camino* may have radically different experiences with bilingualism, Spanish, English, and *latinidad*, shaped by their positionality. Some benefit from the status quo and might hesitate to use the privileges they have. *Te invitamos* to explore and challenge biases about bilingualism. Reflect on the dialectical nature of bilingual experiences in the United States: joy and pain, privilege and oppression. For example, it is not uncommon for Spanish-language learners to credit their initial bilingual interests to Latinx caretakers or nannies from childhood, without recognition of these caretakers' personal sacrifices in acquiring this gain. On this journey, we must avoid co-opting and extracting actions that characterize colonial paradigms. Table 12.1 contains a list of common forms of extraction and ways to reorient them to a coconspirator approach.

TABLE 12.1. Common Forms of Extraction and Ways to Reorient to Coconspirator Approaches

Extraction	Coconspirator approach
Making decisions about hiring bilingual staff without any further investment in bilingualism	Defer these decisions to bilingual staff
Making decisions about bilingual mental health without involving bilingual mental health professionals	Ask, involve, respect, and trust bilingual mental health professionals
Performative praising of bilingual mental health professionals for their contributions	Promote bilingual mental health professionals
"Wishing" bilingual mental health professionals could be paid more	Put your money where your mouth is; conspire with bilingual mental health professionals
Using Spanish to get "in"	Champion the prioritization of recruitment and retention of bilingual staff who are people of color

DOS IDIOMAS, UN CAMINO . . . Y UN SALARIO

It reads like a telenovela, only it is a harsh reality: For decades now, bilingual mental health professionals have been referencing the notion of "twice the work" for one salary. Like us, you, too, might remember the Spanish-speaking adults in your life encouraging you to hold on to your *español* because *"Nunca te faltará trabajo"* and *"Te pagan más."* Well, they were half-right. So, what is at stake here? Promotion rates to advanced titles and positions of leadership are lower for Latines, including Afro-Latines, Black, and Indigenous folx and bilingual Spanish speakers (Colvin, 2021). Similar trends occur even in settings that primarily accompany Latine and Spanish-speaking populations. If you find this hard to believe, look up the executive committee or C-suite of your agency and/or institution. Experiences of burnout, low confidence, resentment, and being overworked are widely documented in literature addressing bilingual mental health services. In addition, many Latine, Black, and Indigenous folx are often first-generation higher education students with historical exclusion from financial and social capital. In these cases, the *camino* to higher education and presumed social mobility is riddled with increased student loan debt; longer and less reliable work commutes from more affordable communities; and pressures to maintain scholarships, stipends, or other forms of financial assistance (Kawaii-Bogue, 2020). All these themes are intertwined, so differential compensation; support;

and equitable hiring, promotion, and retention practices are the foundation of intentional bilingual mental health.

"You Are My Other Me" (In Lak'ech: *"Tu Eres Mi Otro Yo"*)

Bilingual leaders *como nosotres* need to be intentional in our advocacy for bilingual mental health and assert, once and for all, that bilingualism is not a soft skill. Professional bilingualism, especially when paired with cultural contextualization of shared lived experiences, biculturalism, and immersion, is a complex set of many diverse skills worthy of support, recognition, attention, and dedication. There should be *no más* extraction of our work, time, energy, and abilities to uphold colonial practices that exploit our skill sets. The *lucha* for bilingual mental health is not just for you as a leader, or for your colleagues as bilingual scientists–practitioners, as some would have you think. Your *lucha* is not selfish—do not be led astray by the Mauricios of institutions. Your advocacy is needed because it is in the intentional bilingual leadership, in the equity and justice for bilingual professionals, that these professionals can provide dedicated, ethical, equitable, and liberated *acompañamiento*. We are interconnected and, when anchored in community and justice, your *prosperidad* is my *prosperidad*. Remember, some of you are leaders in your own right, whether that may be as a first-born/eldest child, a generational cycle breaker, a community role model, a first-generation college student, or a first-generation bilingual speaker navigating systems *entre dos mundos*. Whichever it may be, you were born for this role, with everything and everyone that came before leading you to this here-and-now.

Allies, Accomplices, and Coconspirators, Oh My!

How you choose to advocate and enact change as a bilingual leader will depend on many factors, including, but not limited to, your values, work setting, personality style, or your zodiac sign, if we ask Walter Mercado (Scorpio, Libra, and Pisces representation here!). In the paragraphs that follow, we offer a range of tips and considerations to inform your advocacy efforts. Do keep in mind the greater context of White- and English-centered systems and culture in which your advocacy must likely happen. We cannot stress enough our recommendation to continue the work of acquainting yourself with White supremacy culture in systems, leading from an antiracist stance, and maintaining self-awareness within your own leadership (see Chapter 4). Throughout such work you will likely come across the terms "ally," "accomplice," and "coconspirator." In your leadership *camino* you will likely use all three styles of advocacy, depending on your bandwidth and what is at stake, among many other factors. If you are not familiar with these terms, the main differences identified in social justice circles include the level of activity and risk: Accomplice and coconspirator roles are generally thought to be more active with respect to advocacy efforts when compared with an ally role because they usually undertake tasks that leverage their privilege and involve risk (Hughes-Hassell et al., 2019).

As you assume these advocacy roles, we share here a variety of tools to use on your leadership *camino*. Examples of pressing themes for bilingual professionals include proper recognition, differential compensation, recruitment, retention, promotion, intentional support, relevant training, culturally and linguistically attuned approaches, ethics, competencies, supervision, and mentorship. If you find yourself in a setting where there is a contingent of professionals who are bilingual and/or Latinx, consider using surveys and focus groups to inform a needs assessment that helps you understand their experiences with and attitudes toward the bilingual themes you are advocating for and to create relevant support spaces for bilingual professionals. White- and English-centered systems value data and evidence; part of your work as a leader in bilingual mental health will involve compiling the data, research, and literature (ahem, *este libro*) in a way that duly recognizes, honors, and celebrates bilingual mental health training and development; is anchored in the principles of social justice; and is aligned with the system. Please keep in mind that although "data" may be highly valued in White- and English-centered systems, you can define the data as qualitative, for example, to be consistent with your values as a bilingual mental health leader (see Chapter 7).

Next, identify who your allies, accomplices, and co-conspirators might be, as well as the gatekeepers and shareholders with decision-making capacities. As leaders in bilingual mental health, it is our duty and responsibility to make other leaders aware of the pressing needs within bilingual mental health as well as how to monitor progress and adherence to the changes agreed upon and their implementation. Educate your leadership counterparts on the necessity of culturally and linguistically attuned implementation of practices in your setting and the ethical parameters and competencies in which these are anchored. Stay connected with other bilingual and Latinx mental health professionals working toward similar advocacy efforts so as to inform your own efforts, collect data, and build community. This is especially true if you are the only or one of few bilingual professionals in your setting. Your advocacy efforts will likely depend on your capacity, availability, values, and personal style.

"I Have Come to Accept That the Life of a Front Runner Is a Hard One" —Pelé

In the capitalist–industrial complex there are many reasons why it may be challenging to bring to fruition your efforts for intentional bilingual mental health training. These barriers might include unwilling colleagues and leadership, a lack of support, a lack of funds or a workforce, and competing demands. Activists have taught us that a common anticipation in advocacy is that of loss. Losses will range from professional to social to personal, affecting promotions, performance expectations, and evaluations, as well as your own well-being. We share this to prepare, not deter you. Many of us are no strangers to bumpy *caminos* and are familiar with systems' tendencies to resist change and maintain the status quo. Rationalization, denial, invalidation, and gaslighting are among the many possible responses to your advocacy. At times, opposers will even use antiracist and IDEA underpinnings against your advocacy, conflating equity with equality or citing reverse racism, for example. They might describe bilingualism as a soft skill, claim your use of Spanish is voluntary, cite culturally attuned healing practices as not reimbursable, and use human resources policies to sidestep bilingual mental health advocacy. In many institutions, true investment in bilingual mental health is perceived as not profitable and therefore not worthy. Gatekeepers can be swift, and their responses may seem logical and sensible (remember Mauricio). But *tú te pusiste las pilas* and are bringing your fiercest *jogo bonito* of *sabiduría y experiencia* to these dialogues.

Just as many factors inform your advocacy style, similar factors will inform how you respond to these anticipated barriers. We encourage you to give yourself grace and always socially locate yourself within your professional setting when you reach such crossroads. Each response will have pros and cons for different people and different stages of professional and personal development.

Leveraging Systems, Resistance, and the In Between

We refer to leveraging systems as offering you the seat at the proverbial table with the goal of inserting yourself into important discussions that pertain to bilingual mental health. This approach includes identifying buy-ins for systems and gatekeepers while at times making trade-offs or exchanges of resources. Identify what motivates your system or setting. For example, differential compensation can improve hiring rates of bilingual professionals, a buy-in for systems. A larger bilingual workforce requires more commitment from leaders like you to supervise and mentor, which is a trade-off. When leveraging systems, you are usually operating within the socially approved parameters of your workplace culture and their standards for "professional-ism." These tend to promote conformity and consistency with the status quo in the workplace and are avoidant of discomfort. Examples include following a chain of command in communications, providing data, and assuming the front-line work while rendering final decision-making capacity to broader leadership in a hierarchical system. To maximize your success in leveraging systems, identify a champion who shares your motivation to advance bilingual mental health and has privilege in decision making; prepare proposals with data; and connect your arguments to enterprise-wide performance goals, mission, vision, and values.

Surges in IDEA and antiracism in different companies are opportunities to craft proposals in accordance with these social justice initiatives. Keep in mind, however, that many organizations *van para donde sople el viento* and are quick to dismantle IDEA initiatives if there is enough backlash, as has been seen in many academic institutions in the mid-2020s. On this note, remember that accountability is key. Have a plan for holding yourself and shareholders accountable and following up. As you develop your plan, manage your expectations. *Mafalda*, the cartoon character created by Argentine Joaquín Salvador Lavado Tejón, who is known as Quino, and her pet turtle, *Burocracia*, remind us of the slow-moving nature of systems. Be prepared for waits and concessions, and identify your thresholds ahead of time.

We recommend that you write a pros and cons list, considering the importance, duration, and impact of each. General pros for leveraging include raising awareness about issues that are pertinent to bilingual mental health, learning more about the subject (e.g., data, needs), educating others, becoming familiarized with systems and key shareholders, implementing change within system limits, *cosechando* relationships, and working toward professional goals. Cons might include engaging with bureaucracy, making concessions, valuing inconsistent behavior, experiencing extraction, making more sacrifices than other shareholders, and being recruited into performative politics.

"Les Falta Sazón, Batería y Reggaetón" –Bad Bunny

¿Qué sientes when you see the word "resistance"? Although it often carries neg-ative connotations, it is a key advocacy tool in the context of an oppressive status quo that marginalizes bilingual mental health. Resistance is widely documented throughout history's activism and civil rights movements and can become an option when benefits outweigh the costs of leveraging

systems or when most options for leveraging systems have been exhausted to little or no avail. Before you proceed with this option, we recommend you have conversations with trusted supervisors and mentors to discuss the status of your advocacy thus far because the risks that you are about to undertake can be big. Losses in social capital might precede the gains (Smith, 2018). Resistance will work best when you are located in a supportive environment with fellow co-conspirators.

When you identify a plan of action that outlines issues, demands, desired outcomes, and understanding of past advocacy efforts, be honest with yourself in centering your values and understanding what you are willing to endure before anticipating repercussions. Let's check in again: *Cómo te sientes* reading about the very real possibility of risks and losses when leading and advocating? Are you scared? Is your heart racing? It is completely normal if at this point you are revisiting the section about leveraging systems and deciding that resistance is not for you. Pause and take a few deep breaths. Close your eyes and think of Dolores Huerta, Victoria Santa Cruz, their sacrifices and risks, and envision a liberated and intentional future for bilingual mental health. Remember this is a marathon, not a sprint. Big-scale resistance in the form of walkouts, strikes, or protests are more impactful yet also might feel riskier. Such actions take a lot of preparation and organization. If you are not ready to engage in this level of resistance, you can also consider other acts, such as vocalizing concerns in meetings, or starting and delivering petitions, for example. You can also imbue day-to-day actions with resistance by affirming your identity and the advocacy you represent. For example, we love writing in Spanish without translations (look it up!), welcoming people in Spanish, quoting *dichos* or lyrics of songs in Spanish, including the *acentos* in our names, or rocking hoop earrings with a red lip.

Pros of resistance might include greater alignment with your values, authenticity, and engaging in social responsibility. Cons might include disciplinary action; demotions; and loss of promotions, networks, and employment. Everyone has different experiences and thresholds; we encourage you to understand how these risks and gains might affect you in the context of what is important to you. As with most things in life, you can also try to combine leveraging systems and resisting, or you can alternate between both approaches.

Know when to stop. Leaving a particular struggle does not mean failure and is, at times, necessary to advance your cause and to preserve your well-being. Leaving also offers opportunities for growth and re-envisioning in ways that are more aligned with ourselves. Become well acquainted with your personal and professional limits. Examine your commitment to efforts in leadership and advocacy. Identify barriers that are interfering with your commitment, explore solutions, and keep inventory of your progress. Advocacy and leadership can be exhausting and overwhelming. Most leaders and advocates are attracted to the big picture, which can lead us to miss smaller wins or progress, contributing to more stress. If you see that the transgressions of your limits and progress outweigh your commitment, this may be a strong indicator that it is time to withdraw from a particular effort. Leaving can be temporary, and there is nothing wrong with taking a pause to catch your breath. We recommend that leadership and advocacy in bilingual mental health be rotated among coconspirators with the goal of allowing for rest and self-care.

Leadership is not a monolith role or title; you can embody leadership in bilingual mental health in many spaces. Some may see having a seat at the *mesa* as overrated and view the *mesa* as not made for them. Yet, the *mesa* exists, and many will have the skill set and bandwidth to take a seat there at different stages in their lives. Others will create a separate, inclusive, and reenvisioned *sala*. Both are needed. Values consistent with reenvisioning usually include justice, equity, alignment, egalitarianism, community, liberation, creativity and creation, balance, and spirituality. Leadership and advocacy require restoration and self-awareness. Accordingly, we recommend therapy as an important tool in furthering your self-exploration in this process and caring for yourself.

Thoughtfully and intentionally consider the importance of coalition building and development. Bilingual mental health in the United States, be it training, research, service, funding, advocacy, or leadership, is not a matter pertinent to Latines exclusively. It is a topic dear and relevant to all Ethnic Acknowledging Psychological Associations (Consoli & Myers, 2022) in the United States, so joining forces with them all is paramount because *la unión hace la fuerza*. Familiarize yourself with the work of groups and task forces such as the Coalition of National Racial Ethnic Psychological Associations, the American Psychological Association's Commission on Ethnic Minority Recruitment, Retention and Training in Psychology, and the like. Moreover, consider that building is a life-long endeavor and that destroying is quick. In other words, commit yourself to the long game and honor the work done, starting with, for example, the often-overlooked 1993 publication by APA's Office of Ethnic Minority Affairs titled *Guidelines for Providers of Psychological Services to Ethnic, Linguistic, and Culturally Diverse Populations*, which was published in APA's flagship journal, the *American Psychologist*. As Santayana (1905) stated, "Those who cannot remember the past are condemned to repeat it" (p. 284).

LOS CAMINOS DE LA VIDA . . .

We have arrived at the *fin* of this *camino*, but there are many more ahead. With diverse identities that have shaped a range of lived experiences, all the contributors to this book share one commonality: their demonstrated commitment to intentional bilingual mental health training and development. We are confident that their *sabiduría, experiencia, consejos*, and *amor* permeate every intentional page of this book. *Apreciamos el mutuo acompañamiento* on this *camino* to becoming a bilingual mental health scientist–practitioner and, most important, the *camino* home to our most authentic selves. *Nos despedimos* with the *confianza* that you are ready to not only embark on the *caminos* discussed here but also to build new, promising ones. Head high, *voz firme, y pa'lante*.

TAKEAWAYS

- Stay informed about changing needs and relevant themes within bilingual mental health that are affecting bilingual and Latinx communities. Remember to diversify your resources.

- Leadership transcends formal titles. Consider all possibilities to lead, and follow what is consistent with your mission and values.

- Advocacy is central to leadership in bilingual mental health. Identify allies, accomplices, and coconspirators, and keep an eye out for the "ol' okey doke"/*el bacalao disfraza'o*.

- Self-awareness is key. It is important to engage in social location and power analyses and to know what risks you are willing to take.

REFLEXIONES

- What other needs and shifts do you anticipate within bilingual and Latinx mental health?
- In what ways have you already assumed leadership in bilingual mental health? What are your aspirations for leadership?
- What is your preferred style of advocacy? What personal successes and barriers do you anticipate for yourself?
- Who are your *gente*? How do you support and back each other?

¡CONSEJOS!

- Give yourself grace.
- *Cuídate.*
- *Y* remember the motto, *estar bien para servir bien.*

RESOURCES

Recommended Reading

American Psychological Association Task Force on Race and Ethnicity Guidelines in Psychology. (2019, August). *APA guidelines on race and ethnicity in psychology.* American Psychological Association. https://www.apa.org/about/policy/guidelines-race-ethnicity.pdf

de Carvalho-Filho, M. A., Tio, R. E., & Steinert, Y. (2020). Twelve tips for implementing a community of practice for faculty development. *Medical Teacher, 42*(2), 143–149. https://doi.org/10.1080/0142159X.2018.1552782

Powell, W., Agosti, J., Bethel, T. H., Chase, S., Clarke, M., Jones, L. F., Lau Johnson, W. F., Noroña, C. R., Stolbach, B. C., & Thompson, E. (2022). *Being anti-racist is central to trauma-informed care: Principles of an anti-racist, trauma-informed organization.* National Center for Child Traumatic Stress. https://tinyurl.com/3w7yxmdj

Online Resources

- Gender in Language Project: https://www.genderinlanguage.com

REFERENCES

American Psychological Association, Office of Ethnic Minority Affairs. (1993). Guidelines for providers of psychological services to ethnic, linguistic, and culturally diverse populations. *American Psychologist, 48*(1), 45–48. https://doi.org/10.1037/0003-066X.48.1.45

Colvin, C. (2021, June 30). *Women, BIPOC face roadblocks to C-suite, Gartner reports.* HR Drive. https://www.hrdive.com/news/women-bipoc-promotion-c-suite/602584

Consoli, A. J., & Myers, L. J. (2022). Alternate cultural paradigms in psychology: Long overdue recognition and further articulations. *Journal of Humanistic Psychology, 62*(4), 471–487. https://doi.org/10.1177/00221678211048114

Czeisler, M. É., Lane, R. I., Wiley, J. F., Czeisler, C. A., Howard, M. E., & Rajaratnam, S. M. W. (2021). Follow-up survey of US adult reports of mental health, substance use, and suicidal ideation during the COVID-19 pandemic, September 2020 [Research letter]. *JAMA Network Open, 4*(2), e2037665. https://doi.org/10.1001/jamanetworkopen.2020.37665

Dorn, E., Hancock, B., Sarakatsannis, J., & Viruleg, E. (2020, December 8). *COVID-19 and learning loss—Disparities grow and students need help*. McKinsey & Company. https://www.mckinsey.com/industries/public-sector/our-insights/covid-19-and-learning-loss-disparities-grow-and-students-need-help#

Equal Pay Today. (n.d.). *Latina equal pay day*. https://www.equalpaytoday.org/latina-equal-pay

Fernandez, A. (2020, July 7). *Latinx: The expendables of the COVID-19 crisis*. Latinos for Education. https://www.latinosforeducation.org/2020/07/07/latinx-expendables-covid19-crisis

Flores, T. (2021). Latinidad is cancelled: Confronting an anti-Black construct. *Latin America & Latinx Visual Culture, 3*(3), 58–79. https://doi.org/10.1525/lavc.2021.3.3.58

Hodges, J. C., & Calvo, R. (2023). Teleservices use among Latinx immigrant families during the Covid-19 pandemic. *Children and Youth Services Review, 145*, 106778. https://doi.org/10.1016/j.childyouth.2022.106778

Hughes-Hassell, S., Rawson, C. H., & Hirsh, K. (2019). Allies and antiracism. In S. Hughes-Hassell, C. H. Rawson, & K. Hirsh (Eds.), *Project READY: Reimagining equity and access for diverse youth* [Online curriculum]. https://ready.web.unc.edu/section-1-foundations/module-14

Kawaii-Bogue, B. (2020, June). *Combating anti-Blackness and White supremacy in organizations: Recommendations for anti-racist actions in mental health care*. Sonoma State University. https://caps.sonoma.edu/sites/caps/files/combating_anti-blackness_and_white_supremacy_in_organizations_-_recommendations_for_anti-racist_actions_in_mental_healthcare.pdf

Krogstad, J. M., Gonzalez-Barrera, A., & Noe-Bustamante, L. (2020, April 3). *U.S. Latinos among hardest hit by pay cuts, job losses due to coronavirus*. Pew Research Center. https://www.pewresearch.org/fact-tank/2020/04/03/u-s-latinos-among-hardest-hit-by-pay-cuts-job-losses-due-to-coronavirus/

Kurtz, J. (2024, March 28). The Baltimore bridge collapse is an immigration story. *New Jersey Monitor*. https://newjerseymonitor.com/2024/03/28/the-baltimore-bridge-collapse-is-an-immigration-story

Lee, D., Kett, P. M., Mohammed, S. A., Frogner, B. K., & Sabin, J. (2023). Inequitable care delivery toward COVID-19 positive people of color and people with disabilities. *PLOS Global Public Health, 3*(4), e0001499. https://doi.org/10.1371/journal.pgph.0001499

Mental Health America. (n.d.). *BIPOC communities and COVID-19*. Retrieved May 27, 2024, from https://www.mhanational.org/bipoc-communities-and-covid-19#_edn12

Miville, M. L., Arredondo, P., Consoli, A. J., Santiago-Rivera, A., Delgado-Romero, E., Fuentes, M., Domenech Rodriguez, M., Field, L., & Cervantes, J. (2017). *Liderazgo*: Culturally grounded leadership and the National Latina/o Psychological Association. *The Counseling Psychologist, 45*(6), 830–856. https://doi.org/10.1177/0011000016668413

Morales, E. (2020, May 18). *Understanding why Latinos are so hard hit by COVID-19*. CNN. https://www.cnn.com/2020/05/18/opinions/latinos-covid-19-impact-morales

Noxolo, P. (2009). "My paper, my paper": Reflections on the embodied production of postcolonial geographical responsibility in academic writing. *Geoforum, 40*(1), 55–65. https://doi.10.1016/j.geoforum.2008.06.008

Okun, T. (2021). *(Divorcing) White supremacy culture: Coming home to who we really are*. https://www.whitesupremacyculture.info

Santayana, G. (1905). *The life of reason: Reason in common sense*. Scribner's.

Smith, M. D. (2018, September 28). *A vision of social justice for mental health care* [Keynote address]. Rebellious Psychiatry 2018 Conference, Yale University, New Haven, CT, United States. https://www.youtube.com/watch?v=0oUxa2RUy4k

Training Resources for the Environmental Community. (2023). White supremacy culture and professionalism. https://www.trec.org/wp-content/uploads/2023/04/WSC-and-Professionalism-v423.pdf

Index

marginalization of, 211
race-neutral representation of, 71
Alejandre, Adriana, 191
Alliance for Latino Behavioral Health
Workforce, 102
Allies, 253–254
American Association of Hispanics in
Higher Education, 143
Faculty Fellowship Program, 227–228
Graduate Student Fellowship program,
228
American Council on the Teaching of
Foreign Languages (ACTFL), 72–74
American Dream, 245–246
American Psychological Association (APA),
100
accreditation by, 41, 42
APIC recognized by, 157
Bilingual Psychologists Special Interest
Group, 161
Center for Workforce Studies, 159
financial assistance from, 58
internship development by, 158
on italicizing Spanish words, 142
mentoring programs of, 125
on practice of clinical psychology, 200
Society of Latinx Womxn in Psychology,
143
Analyzing data, 141, 148
Ancestral cultural wealth and wisdom,
140–143, 161
Anti-Blackness, 9
labeling and dismantling, 207
in mental health systems, 248–249
supervisors'/mentors' modeling of, 111
Anti-immigrant views, labeling and
dismantling, 207
Anti-Indigeneity
labeling and dismantling, 207
supervisors'/mentors' modeling of, 111
Antiracism, 256
APA. *See* American Psychological
Association
APIC (Association of Psychology Internship
Centers), 157
APPIC. *See* Association of Psychology
Postdoctoral and Internship Centers
Applying for jobs, 235
Armas, Aeriell, 191
Assimilation, 234
Assistant professors, 222, 227, 228
Associate professors, 222, 228

Association of Psychology Internship
Centers (APIC), 157
Association of Psychology Postdoctoral
and Internship Centers (APPIC),
157–160, 170, 172
Association of State and provincial
Psychology Boards, 158
Authenticity, 63
in academic career, 230–231, 234
in clinical work, 206
in internship interviews, 164
Award opportunities, 144
Aztlán, 143

B

Barriers
anticipated, responding to, 255
for Latine clinicians in White spaces,
209–211
Belonging, sense of. *See also*
Community(-ies)
through connecting with Latine and
bilingual clinicians, 212
through cultural and linguistic
validation, 30–34
Bias, 211
Biculturalism, 202–208
bilingualism and bicultural identity,
204–207
in clinical work, reclaiming and
celebrating, 212–213
connections and collectivism in,
203–204
and liberation, 207–208
in research, 187
Bilingual assessments, 165
Bilingual audit, of graduate programs, 89
Bilingual identity, 9, 202–208
Bilingualism, 11–22
in academic careers, 219–220, 230–231,
234
asserted as professional skill, 253
and bicultural identity, 204–207
in clinical work, reclaiming and
celebrating, 212–213
current standards of bilingual training,
18–21
Latinidad as social construct, 17–18
Latinx population in United States, 12–13
owning your association with, 136–137
rethinking, 62–63

About the Editors

Maciel Campos (she, her, *ella*), PsyD, is a bilingual (English–Spanish) clinical psychologist licensed in the state of New York, United States, and program director for the Child & Adolescent Outpatient Psychiatry Center at Kings County Hospital, part of NYC Health + Hospitals. She was born and raised in Brooklyn, New York, to immigrant parents from the Dominican Republic and El Salvador. She is a first-generation United States–born *hija* and first-generation higher education graduate.

A proud graduate of New York City public schools across Brooklyn and Queens, Dr. Campos obtained her bachelor's degree from what is now Macaulay Honors College at Hunter College, City University of New York. She completed her doctorate in psychology at Adler University in Chicago and did her predoctoral clinical internship at the New York–Presbyterian Morgan Stanley Children's Hospital, part of the Columbia University Irving Medical Center. Dr. Campos has dedicated her career to treating families affected by chronic medical illnesses, treating individuals across the life span and accompanying bilingual Spanish- and English-speaking communities of color in culturally humble and linguistically attuned care. Dr. Campos is also trained in dialectical behavior therapy (DBT) and has dedicated the greater part of her experience as a DBT therapist applying cultural and linguistic considerations to interventions. As a senior clinical psychologist, Dr. Campos was also the program director of the Home-Based Crisis Intervention program at Morgan Stanley Children's Hospital. Previously a voluntary assistant professor of clinical psychology in the Division of Child & Adolescent Psychiatry at Columbia University Irving Medical Center, Dr. Campos has held supervisory and teaching roles in psychology and psychiatry training programs, emphasizing evidence-based treatments, cultural humility, and bilingual training. In this capacity, she codeveloped supportive training programming and supervision for bilingual trainees and early-career professionals.

Dr. Campos was honored with the inaugural Margaret Morgan Lawrence Memorial Award for Community Child and Adolescent Mental Health Care in the Division of Child & Adolescent Psychiatry at Columbia University Irving Medical Center for her dedication to community mental health care. She continues these pursuits in her current role as program director of the Child & Adolescent Outpatient Psychiatry Department at Kings County Hospital and voluntary clinical assistant professor at SUNY Downstate Health Sciences University. In addition to giving presentations and conducting workshops focused on bilingual training and DBT with Latinx families, Dr. Campos's interests include staff wellness and burnout prevention. In 2018, Dr. Campos had the honor of joining a multidisciplinary team that provided post–Hurricane Maria mental health aid relief efforts in San Juan, Puerto Rico.

Yessenia Mejia (she, her, *ella*), PsyD, is a bilingual–bicultural (English–Spanish) clinical psychologist, first-generation eldest daughter of immigrant parents, and proud *Neoyorquina*. Dr. Mejia graduated from the school–clinical doctoral program at Ferkauf Graduate School of Psychology, Yeshiva University, and completed her predoctoral and postdoctoral training at New York–Presbyterian/Columbia University Irving Medical Center, working predominately with Latinx children and families in Washington Heights.

Dr. Mejia currently holds a clinical assistant professor appointment at the Department of Child & Adolescent Psychiatry, Grossman School of Medicine, New York University (NYU), and she accompanies the Latinx community of Sunset Park, Brooklyn, through her staff position at the Family Health Centers of NYU Langone. Dr. Mejia's work is grounded in understanding cultural considerations of evidence-based practices and the importance of cultural and linguistic competency when providing care to Latinx communities. As a bilingual and bicultural clinician, Dr. Mejia's interests include integrating anti-oppressive practice and social justice frameworks in psychotherapy, developing opportunities for early-career bilingual bicultural psychologists, and addressing mental health disparities that affect marginalized communities.

Dr. Mejia also serves as a cochair of the National Latinx Psychological Association's Bilingual Issues in Latinx Mental Health Special Interest Group, which aims to provide support to bilingual psychologists throughout the nation in the form of consultation groups, didactics, the exchanging of resources, and the creation of support spaces for mental health providers.

Andrés J. Consoli (he, him, *él*), PhD, is a bilingual (English–Spanish) professor in the Department of Counseling, Clinical & School Psychology, and a faculty affiliate at the Department of Chicana and Chicano Studies, the Department of Spanish and Portuguese, and the Latin American & Iberian Studies Program, at the University of California, Santa Barbara (UCSB). He was born and raised in Buenos Aires, Argentina, where he received a *licenciatura* degree in clinical psychology at the Universidad de Belgrano (1985). Dr. Consoli earned a master's (1991) and doctorate in counseling psychology at UCSB (1994) and received postdoctoral training in behavioral medicine in the Department of Psychiatry and Behavioral Sciences at the Stanford University School of Medicine (1994–1996). Prior to joining UCSB, Dr. Consoli was a professor and associate chair of the Department of Counseling, College of Health & Social Sciences, at San Francisco State University (1996–2013). He is a member of Fundación Aiglé, Argentina, a visiting professor at the Universidad del Valle in Guatemala, and is a licensed psychologist in California.

Dr. Consoli served as vice president for international affairs of the American Psychological Association (APA) Division 17: Society of Counseling Psychology (SCP; 2020–2023); president of the National Latinx Psychological Association (NLPA; 2014); member-at-large of APA's Division 52: Society for Global Psychology (2011–2013); president of the *Sociedad Interamericana de Psicología* (SIP; 2007–2009); and president of the Western Association for Counselor Education and Supervision (2001). He also served as senior member of the Board for the Coalition of National Racial and Ethnic Psychological Associations' Leadership Development Institute, representing NLPA (2022–2025), and on the Council of National Psychological Associations for the Advancement of Ethnic Minority Interests (2014–2016), chairing the council in 2016.

In 2015, Dr. Consoli received the Interamerican Psychologist Award for distinguished contributions to the advancement of psychology in the Americas, granted by SIP. In 2020, he received the Excellent Contribution Award for remarkable contributions to international research, program development, and teaching/mentoring by the SCP's International Counseling Psychologists section. Dr. Consoli is a fellow of both APA and of the Society for the Exploration of Psychotherapy Integration.

Dr. Consoli's professional and research interests involve transnational collaborations, multicultural supervision, psychotherapy integration and training, systematic treatment selection, ethics and values in psychotherapy, access and utilization of mental health services within a social justice framework, and the development of a bilingual (English–Spanish) academic and mental health workforce. With more than 100 publications to his name, he is the lead editor of the multinational book *Comprehensive Textbook of Psychotherapy: Theory and Practice* and a coauthor of the binational book *CBT Strategies for Anxious and Depressed Children and Adolescents: A Clinician's Toolkit.*